# COVID-19 AND SPEECH-LANGUAGE PATHOLOGY

This collection is the first of its kind to examine the impact of the COVID-19 pandemic on the caseloads and clinical practice of speech-language pathologists.

The volume synthesises existing data on the wide-ranging effects of COVID-19 on the communication, swallowing, and language skills of individuals with COVID infection. Featuring perspectives of scholars and practitioners from around the globe, the book examines the ways in which clinicians have had to modify their working practices to prioritise patient and clinician safety, including the significant increase in the use of telepractice during the pandemic. The volume also reflects on changes in training and education which have seen educators in the field redesign their clinical practicum in order to best prepare students for professional practice in an age of COVID-19 and beyond, as the field continues to grapple with the long-term effects of the pandemic.

Offering a holistic treatment of the impact of COVID-19 on the work of speech-language pathologists, this book will be of interest to students, researchers, and clinicians working in the discipline.

**Louise Cummings** is Professor in the Department of English and Communication at The Hong Kong Polytechnic University. Her research interests in speech-language pathology are pragmatic disorders, language impairment in COVID-19, and communication in neurodegenerative disorders. In 2020, she published the volume *Language in Dementia* with Cambridge University Press.

# Routledge Research in Speech-Language Pathology

Series editor: Louise Cummings

*Routledge Research in Speech-Language Pathology* looks beyond traditional areas of study within the discipline to showcase topics historically underserved in research on communication disorders, highlighting fresh perspectives on issues of key importance in speech-language pathology. The series offers comprehensive treatments of communication disorders and the work of speech-language pathology with an eye toward pushing the field forward, critically examining challenges in addressing disparities in speech-language pathology and exploring the latest developments in related disciplines with implications for the future of research on communication disorders. Volumes in this series will be of particular interest to students, scholars, and clinicians in speech-language pathology, speech and language therapy, and clinical linguistics, as well as related fields such as special education, psychology, neurology, psychiatry, social work, and nursing.

**Language Case Files in Neurological Disorders**
*Louise Cummings*

**COVID-19 and Speech-Language Pathology**
*Louise Cummings*

For more information about this series, please visit: www.routledge.com/ Routledge-Research-on-Speech-Language-Pathology/book-series/RRSLP

# COVID-19 AND SPEECH-LANGUAGE PATHOLOGY

*Edited by Louise Cummings*

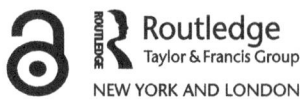

Routledge
Taylor & Francis Group

NEW YORK AND LONDON

Cover image: Getty Images

First published 2023
by Routledge
605 Third Avenue, New York, NY 10158

and by Routledge
4 Park Square, Milton Park, Abingdon, Oxon, OX14 4RN

*Routledge is an imprint of the Taylor & Francis Group, an informa business*

ISBN: 978-1-03219-0-075 (hbk)
ISBN: 978-1-03219-0-068 (pbk)
ISBN: 978-1-00325-7-318 (ebk)

DOI: 10.4324/9781003257318

Typeset in Bembo
by Apex CoVantage, LLC

# CONTENTS

# CONTRIBUTORS

**Stephen M. Camarata** received a doctorate from Purdue University and completed a postdoctoral fellowship at the University of Arizona. His expertise includes speech and language intervention in children with autism spectrum disorder, Down syndrome, hearing loss, and specific language impairment. He is the past chair of the NIH study section on Developmental Disabilities and Child Psychopathology, the current chair of the NIH study section on Communication Disorders Research, and an editor-in-chief for the *Journal of Speech-Language-Hearing Research*. He has published over 100 papers and two books related to development, *Late Talking Children: A Symptom or a Stage* and *The Intuitive Parent*.

**Ashley E. Cameron** holds a bachelor of psychology from the Queensland University of Technology and a master of speech-pathology studies from the University of Queensland. She completed her PhD at the University of Queensland, where she investigated approaches to enhance the participation of individuals with acquired communication difficulties. Dr Cameron has worked as a speech-language pathologist for Queensland Health since graduation. She is also the lead of the Allied Health – Translating Research into Practice initiative programme, which supports the Queensland Health workforce in translating knowledge within healthcare settings.

**Vivian Nga-Ying Chai** obtained a bachelor's degree in translation from the Chinese University of Hong Kong and a master's degree in speech therapy from The Hong Kong Polytechnic University. She has a wide-ranging interest in rehabilitating communication disorders in children and adults in Hong Kong. During the pandemic, she completed her master's thesis on investigating the psychosocial implications of the COVID-19 lockdown on individuals with aphasia and their caretakers in Hong Kong. She currently works as a qualified speech therapist in an early education and training centre (with a primary caseload of preschool children) at the Hong Kong Christian Service.

**Sara A. Charney** is a speech-language pathologist who specialises in voice, swallowing, and upper airway disorders at Mayo Clinic in Arizona. She received her master's degree in communication sciences and disorders from Vanderbilt University and her BS in cognitive science degree from Occidental College. She completed her clinical fellowship at the NW Clinic of Voice and Swallowing at Oregon Health Science University. Her research interests include voice and swallowing disorders, including those secondary to head and neck cancer, as well as inducible laryngeal obstruction. She has recently developed an interest in the potential long-term impact of COVID-19 on the field of speech-language pathology.

**Alexander Chern** is a resident physician in otolaryngology – head and neck surgery at NewYork-Presbyterian Hospital (Columbia and Weill Cornell campuses). He received his MD from Vanderbilt University School of Medicine and his BS in molecular biophysics and biochemistry from Yale University. His research interests include music perception and cognition, cochlear implantation, and the effects of hearing loss on the brain. Since the start of the COVID-19 pandemic, Dr Chern has been investigating otolaryngologic manifestations of the disease, as well as the wider implications of the pandemic on the field of otolaryngology – head and neck surgery.

**Louise Cummings** is Professor in the Department of English and Communication and Associate Dean for Research in the Faculty of Humanities at The Hong Kong Polytechnic University. She teaches and conducts research in pragmatics, clinical linguistics, and health communication. She is the author and editor of 18 books, including most recently *Language Case Files in Neurological Disorders* (Routledge, 2021); *Fallacies in Medicine and Health* (Palgrave Macmillan, 2020); *Language in Dementia* (Cambridge University Press, 2020); and the *Handbook of Pragmatic Language Disorders* (Springer, 2021). She is editor of the book series *Routledge Research in Speech-Language Pathology* and online series *Cambridge Elements in Health Communication*.

**Emerald J. Doll**, MS, CCC-SLP, is the supervisor of the Adult Voice Clinic and a practicing speech-language pathologist at University of Wisconsin (UW) Hospital and Clinics. She specialises in voice and upper airway disorders with an emphasis on vocal performers, including singers and actors, and patients with heavy vocal demands and needs. She received her bachelor of music and master of science in speech-language pathology from the University of Wisconsin – Madison.

**Anthony Pak-Hin Kong** is Associate Professor in Human Communication, Development, and Information Sciences at the University of Hong Kong. His research interests include aphasia, discourse analyses, and neurogenic communication disorders in multilingual speakers. His research has received continuous funding from the National Institutes of Health, the Hong Kong government, and multiple (inter)national universities and private foundations. Apart from serving as a consultant to provide research, clinical, and/or professional consultations to many (inter)national agencies, such as Aphasia United, Project BRIDGE (Building Research Initiatives by Developing Group Effort, USA), the Hong Kong Hospital Authority, and the Hong Kong Society for Rehabilitation, Professor Kong is currently Section Editor (Inaugural Linguistics Section) of *PLOS-ONE* and Editorial Board Member of *Perspectives of the ASHA Special Interest Groups*.

**Dustin Kai-Yan Lau** is Associate Professor in the Department of Chinese and Bilingual Studies, Faculty of Humanities at The Hong Kong Polytechnic University. He has worked as a speech therapist and clinical instructor in a variety of settings, which equipped him with frontline experience in assessing and treating clients with different communication disorders. His research interests lie mainly in psycholinguistics and neurolinguistics. He is also interested in developing clinical assessments and evidence-based treatments for different communication disorders in Chinese.

**Anna Miles**, PhD, is a practising speech-language therapist with over 25 years of experience working in the acute and community setting. She is a researcher, lecturer, and clinician in the area of voice and swallowing disorders at the University of Auckland. Dr Miles runs a hospital-based student teaching clinic as well as an outpatient voice and swallowing rehabilitation clinic. She is the New Zealand Speech-Language Therapists' Association Clinical Expert in Adult Dysphagia and COVID-19 and chaired the Dysphagia Research Society's COVID-19 Taskforce from 2020 to 2021. Dr Miles has approximately100 peer reviewed publications and around 1,000 citations. The Swallowing Research Laboratory in the Centre of Brain Research at the University of Auckland, led by Dr Miles, strives to improve the lives of people with swallowing difficulties through improved assessment, treatment, and medical education.

**Ranjini Mohan**, PhD, CCC-SLP is an Assistant Professor in the Department of Communication Disorders at Texas State University, USA. Dr Mohan earned her PhD in cognitive neuroscience and gerontology at Purdue University. Her research explores the behavioural and electrophysiological bases of cognitive-linguistic processes in typically aging adults and those with neurogenic disorders. During the COVID-19 pandemic, Dr Mohan has been studying the effects of the disease on swallowing and its implications for speech-language pathology services. She has extensive clinical experience performing diagnostic and evidence-based treatment for adults in acute, subacute, and outpatient settings both in the US and in India.

**Bijoyaa Mohapatra**, PhD, CCC-SLP, is an Assistant Professor in the Department of Communication Sciences and Disorders at Louisiana State University, USA. Earlier, she received her PhD from the University of Georgia, USA. Her research interests include psychophysiological measurement of cognitive, communicative, and affective behaviour and complementary-alternative treatment practices in the rehabilitation of adults with acquired brain injury. Dr Mohapatra is currently engaged in research topics exploring the speech–language pathologist's role in COVID-19 management and remote delivery of rehabilitation services to improve quality of life in persons with aphasia. She also holds the Certificate of Clinical Competence from the American Speech-Language-Hearing Association.

**Janet Ho-yee Ng** is the Speech Therapy Unit director and a senior clinical associate in the Department of Chinese and Bilingual Studies of The Hong Kong Polytechnic University. In addition to teaching communication disorders and professional ethics, she oversees the curricular content and assessments of clinical education in the postgraduate speech therapy programme. She chaired the Hong Kong Association of Speech Therapists from 2005 to 2010. She has been appointed the founding chairperson of the Professional Council of the Hong Kong Institute of Speech Therapists, leading the management of the Register of Speech Therapists accredited by the Department of Health in Hong Kong.

**Megan Overby** is an Associate Professor in the Department of Speech-Language Pathology at Duquesne University, where she teaches courses in telepractice and a variety of paediatric-based communication disorders. After founding the department's telepractice service model, Professor Overby now researches the pedagogy of telepractice and assists the department in the clinical application of telepractice to paediatric and adult clients. Her publications include journal articles titled "Qualitative perspectives of effective telepractice pedagogy in speech–language pathology" and "Perceptions of telepractice pedagogy in speech–language pathology: A quantitative analysis," as well as multiple publications on early diagnostic indicators of paediatric speech–language disorders.

**Konstantinos Priftis**, PhD, is a chartered psychologist and Associate Professor of Neuropsychology and Clinical Neuropsychology at the Department of General Psychology of the University of Padua, Italy. His main scientific interests are within the cognitive and clinical neuropsychology of spatial and mathematical cognition. He is the author of more than 65 publications in international, peer-reviewed journals (e.g., *Science*, *Nature*, *Brain*, *Journal of Cognitive Neuroscience*). The results of his studies have been mentioned in National Geographic blogs, *The Washington Post*, *The Guardian*, and *The New York Times*. Since the onset of the COVID-19 pandemic, he has studied the neuropsychological consequences of SARS-CoV-2 and COVID-19, with particular reference to spoken and written language disorders.

**Sarah Wallace**, OBE, is Consultant Speech and Language Therapist in Critical Care and Dysphagia at Wythenshawe Hospital in Manchester and Honorary Senior Lecturer at the University of Manchester. She holds national leadership roles with the Intensive Care Society (ICS), the National Tracheostomy Safety Project, and the Royal College of Speech and Language Therapists (RCSLT) as Specialist Advisor. She teaches and conducts research internationally, authoring numerous publications, policies, and guidelines. Throughout the pandemic, Sarah developed clinical research, guidance, and strategy for the RCSLT Covid-19 Advisory Group, SLP COVID-19 Global Group, and ICS National Rehabilitation Collaborative. She volunteers for Speech Therapy Cambodia. Sarah was recently awarded an RCSLT Fellowship for her contribution to the profession and received an OBE in the Queen's New Year's Honours List 2020 for services to the National Health Service in the UK.

**Elizabeth C. Ward** is the director of the Centre for Functioning and Health Research within Queensland Health and Professor in the School of Health and Rehabilitation Sciences, University of Queensland, Australia. She is a leading international researcher with key research interests in the areas of dysphagia management, head and neck cancer care, telepractice, and health services research. Liz has a strong passion for improving the quality of evidence for telepractice and has led the design and evaluation of multiple telepractice models in speech-language pathology, as well as cognate disciplines including occupational therapy, physiotherapy, and pharmacy.

# 1

# COVID-19

## A new challenge in speech-language pathology

*Bijoyaa Mohapatra and Ranjini Mohan*

### 1.1 Introduction

In December 2019, a highly pathogenic and often fatal virus emerged in Wuhan, China (Q. Li et al. 2020). By 2020, it had spread to Europe, North America, and nearly 120 countries around the world. Early reports indicated that the severe acute respiratory syndrome coronavirus 2 (SARS-CoV-2), currently termed the Coronavirus Disease 2019 (COVID-19), spread at an alarming rate via airborne droplets from an infected person (Fauci et al. 2020). Whilst early efforts to implement social distancing and contact tracing were somewhat effective, it became clear that COVID-19 was highly contagious and caused significant mortality (Centers for Disease Control and Prevention 2020, 2022). COVID-19 results in a multisystem infection, and its severity can range from asymptomatic or mild infections to serious illness and death (Alberti et al. 2020). COVID-19 can induce viral pneumonia with new lung infiltrates, severe dyspnea, and hypoxia in the respiratory system. A hyperinflammatory state may produce numerous organ dysfunction, – including involvement of lungs, liver, kidney, and gastrointestinal systems (Gupta et al. 2020) – and myocarditis and heart failure in patients who are extremely ill with COVID-19 (Goha et al. 2020). It can thus damage physical, cognitive, and psychological function in a variety of ways. Symptoms that are particularly relevant to rehabilitation needs are delirium, neurological manifestations such as Guillain–Barré syndrome (Alberti et al. 2020), encephalitis (Ye et al. 2020), stroke and its associated physical and cognitive sequelae, speech and swallowing disorders (Archer et al. 2021), and post-traumatic stress disorder in people admitted to intensive care units (ICUs) (Janiri et al. 2021).

Physicians, psychologists, and therapists from around the world are working to establish rehabilitation treatment for people with COVID-19 and are designing

DOI: 10.4324/9781003257318-1

programmes and specialised care to meet people's short- and long-term needs resulting from the infection. COVID-19 complications have led to the initiation and continuation of interdisciplinary rehabilitation during acute hospitalisations, providing patient and family self-care trainings after discharge from inpatient rehabilitation, outpatient rehabilitation care, at-home in-person therapy, or telerehabilitation services (Lew et al. 2020). Speech-language pathologists (SLPs) in acute and outpatient rehabilitation units target outcomes that are defined by clinical impairments and the needs of the patients (Mohapatra and Mohan 2020) and provide healthcare interventions that are intended to enhance or preserve function in these clinical populations.

As clinical observations and research regarding the implications of COVID-19 on infected individuals are increasing, its effects on those at risk of exposure are also coming to the forefront. Healthcare professionals directly exposed to those who are infected, especially those that perform aerosol-generating procedures (AGPs), are at increased risk of contracting the virus. This has led several groups of healthcare professionals, advocacy groups, and organisations to modify clinical practice standards to reduce the risk of exposure to the virus. Some of these guidelines for SLPs include the use of personal protective equipment (PPE), performing a risk assessment when evaluations involve AGPs during voice and swallow evaluations, and the use of telepractice platforms to provide services (Araújo et al. 2020; Freeman-Sanderson et al. 2021; Vergara et al. 2020). However, clinical practice during the pandemic with modified service standards has not always been smooth or consistent. In an initial survey by Chadd et al. (2021), 95.6% of SLPs claimed that the pandemic had affected their professional assignments, responsibilities, and duties and reported that there had been changes in ways of service delivery (remote delivery via telephone consultations) and, most typically, a drop in clinical caseload. Additionally, SLPs found that national guidance and policy and telerehabilitation were not accessible, which affected their service delivery (Vergara et al. 2020). Further work is therefore needed to address the barriers to implementation of COVID-safety accommodations in clinical practice.

Whilst the safety of healthcare professionals is a priority due to the high risk of exposure, international and local guidelines to protect the general public from infections are also being emphasised. Strategies to contain the spread of COVID-19 infection include confinement inside houses, reduced social contact with family and friends, use of personal protective equipment (PPE) measures, and discontinuation of health and social care. Recent findings have suggested that such restrictions have cumulatively led to sedentary lifestyle, newer health problems, and a greater influence on the quality of life of both affected and unaffected persons (van den Borst et al. 2021). Taken together, these concerns have the potential to worsen health, physical, and psychological function for individuals who have not been infected with COVID-19 as well.

In the following paragraphs, we offer an overview of the effects of the COVID-19 pandemic on speech, swallowing, and cognitive functions. We also discuss the role of SLPs in the rehabilitation of patients with COVID-19, new methods of clinical training and service delivery adopted during the COVID-19 pandemic, and anticipated challenges in continuing service delivery post-pandemic.

## 1.2 Assessment and management of speech-swallowing-cognitive consequences of COVID-19

### 1.2.1 Speech

Dysphonia is the most common speech disorder observed over the clinical course of COVID-19. In an epidemiological study of over 700 hospitalised patients with mild-to-moderate COVID-19, nearly 27% of cases were dysphonic (Lechien et al. 2022). Individuals who were dysphonic were also more symptomatic, with cough, chest pain, fatigue, diarrhea, nausea, and vomiting being more prevalent than in the non-dysphonic group. Amongst non-hospitalised patients with COVID-19, nearly 44% reported mild-to-moderate dysphonia along with vocal fatigue, cough, and dyspnea (Cantarella et al. 2022). There is also evidence of persistent dysphonia in some patients three months after hospital discharge (Leis-Cofiño et al. 2022). The etiology of dysphonia seen in COVID-19 patients may be multifold. It may be associated with inflammation and oedema of the laryngeal tissues (Lechien et al. 2020) and/or lung infection and muscle fatigue that impacts the efficiency of vocal production (Cantarella et al. 2022).

Critically ill patients with COVID-19 often require endotracheal intubation for mechanical ventilation. These patients often have dysphonia and dyspnea due to impairments in vocal fold movement and glottic and/or subglottic stenosis (Neevel et al. 2021). A multi-site observational study found that two-thirds of patients who required intubation displayed dysphonia upon extubation, which was predicted by intubation injury and pre-existing respiratory disease (Regan et al. 2021). Over a third of patients had persistent dysphonia at discharge.

Due to the high risk of exposure to the SARS-CoV-2 virus during voice assessment, SLPs may be at medium to high risk of contamination depending on the procedure they are involved in. For example, perceptual or acoustic assessment of voice in the hospital/office may offer medium risk of exposure, but laryngeal endoscopic evaluations pose a very high risk. Additionally, most voice rehabilitative exercises are AGPs that include breathing or semi-occluded voice therapy exercises (Cantarella et al. 2021). Therefore, SLPs follow Occupational Safety and Health Administration and CDC guidelines in the use of PPE, social distancing, and hand hygiene practices when in contact with those suspected of or confirmed with COVID-19 (Castillo-Allendes et al. 2021).

Treatment of voice disorders following intubation-related injuries in the ICU primarily involve vocal hygiene education, alternative-augmentative communication strategies, and referral to otolaryngologists upon discharge (Miles et al. 2022). If early voice therapy is deemed necessary in the ICU, SLPs perform a risk-benefit assessment to determine the best time to intervene. Due to the increased risk of vocal fatigue, sessions are kept short and of low intensity, and exercises that trigger cough are avoided to protect the clinicians. Patients with dysphonia upon discharge have received voice services in person as well as via telepractice (Castillo-Allendes et al. 2021). Few telerehabilitation models have been proposed for laryngology care. Strategies include perceptual voice analysis with sustained and dynamic vocalisation; ways to optimise telepractice through timely scheduling and pre-visit check-ins; record-keeping through vocal hygiene diaries; and tele-biofeedback of vocal performance and use of patient-reported outcome measures (Castillo-Allendes et al. 2021; Strohl et al. 2020). Research comparing voice therapy offered in person and via telepractice has revealed comparable outcomes (Kelchner 2013). However, evidence of their effectiveness in remediating dysphonia related to COVID-19 and SARS-CoV-2 infection is still needed.

### 1.2.2 Swallowing

Dysphagia is the most common COVID-19 outcome seen in patients across rehabilitation settings. ICU patients with COVID-19 display pooling of secretions, pharyngeal residue, and silent aspiration (Osbeck Sandblom et al. 2021). Prolonged intubation in ICU can increase the risk of laryngeal injury and dysphagia in more than 90% of cases (Brodsky et al. 2020). Post-extubation dysphagia is also associated with episodes of silent aspiration (Osbeck Sandblom et al. 2021) and pulmonary aspiration in more than one-third of patients (Laguna et al. 2022). Some patients needing prolonged mechanical ventilation may require a tracheostomy to facilitate weaning of ventilation, which also leads to dysphagia and pulmonary infections (Laguna et al. 2022) as well as longer time to initiate oral intake after extubation (Dawson et al. 2020).

Patients in general wards are also reported to have a high prevalence of oropharyngeal dysphagia (Dawson et al. 2020; Martin-Martinez et al. 2021). Acute respiratory distress syndrome (ARDS) associated with COVID-19 results in a compromised respiratory system, thus disrupting the coordination between swallowing, and breathing essential for safe swallowing (Mohan and Mohapatra 2020). Dysphagia is also complicated by sedation, altered consciousness, delirium, and fatigue in patients with severe COVID-19 (Dawson et al. 2020; Vergara et al. 2020).

Dysphagia screening and assessment are recommended for patients who are conscious and have stable respiratory status. Vergara et al. (2020) reviewed 19 international guidelines for dysphagia management and summarised the recommendations. Dysphagia assessments are considered AGPs due to the likelihood of coughing during food and liquid trials; therefore, SLPs are mandated to use PPE to reduce the risk of transmission of the virus and subsequent infection. Cough strength, gag reflex, and extensive oral cavity examinations need to be avoided, and at least a one- to two-metre distance maintained between patient and clinician when swallow examination involving respiratory rate, oral stasis, voice change, aspiration, and swallow function are undertaken. Standardised rating scales such as the International Dysphagia Diet Standardization Initiative Functional Diet Scale (Steele et al. 2018) and Functional Oral Intake Scale (Crary et al. 2005) are recommended to guide therapeutic planning (Vergara et al. 2020) alongside patient observations during mealtimes or clinical swallow exams. Other guidelines are that instrumental evaluations must only be performed when a potentially life-threatening underlying condition is suspected or the clinical assessment does not provide enough diagnostic information for treatment decisions to be made (Eyigör and Umay 2021; Schindler et al. 2021).

When required, videofluoroscopic swallowing studies are considered to be safer than fiberoptic endoscopic evaluation and pharyngoesophageal manometry (both require insertion of a flexible naso-endoscope that poses a greater risk of viral transmission to the SLP). Regardless of the instrument selected, a thorough risk-benefit assessment must be performed, and precautionary measures must be taken by the multidisciplinary team, such as using a PPE kit, promoting self-feeding in patients, encouraging social distancing when feasible, and conducting quick assessments to reduce exposure (Vergara et al. 2020).

Dysphagia rehabilitation also involves AGPs, and guidelines have recommended ceasing and/or postponing interventions that involve contact with the aerodigestive tract (Vergara et al. 2020). When treatment cannot be postponed, modifications to the frequency, duration, and type of interventions are recommended along with alterations to the environment. Patients intubated in the ICU may be on enteral or nasogastric tubes for nutrition and hydration (Mohan and Mohapatra 2020). Extubated patients and those in the general ward diagnosed with dysphagia may be recommended modified food and liquid diets along with behavioural modifications such as postural changes and altered delivery methods. Rehabilitative exercises that involve coughing (e.g., super-supraglottic swallow) or manipulation of the oral cavity (e.g., thermal-tactile stimulation, oral hygiene) are contraindicated during active infection, and the SLP may prescribe other selective exercises. Risk of transmission can be avoided by using PPE and by ensuring that patients engage in oral hygiene practices independently. For patients discharged from the hospital who need therapeutic follow-up, telerehabilitation is recommended (Aoyagi et al. 2021; Miles et al. 2022; Vergara et al. 2020).

### 1.2.3 Cognition

Cognitive problems are increasingly being recognised as a common complication of COVID-19. These problems are often considered either as collateral damage or a long-term consequence of COVID (Ritchie et al. 2020). Cognitive problems may be a direct consequence of structural brain damage to the cortex, an indirect effect of non-central nervous system (CNS) systemic impairment, or a psychological reaction of the CNS via an immune response in patients recovering from

COVID-19 (Kumar et al. 2021; Ritchie et al. 2020). Impaired cognitive function may also arise due to prolonged duration of hypoxia or mechanical ventilation (Mart and Ware 2020). In general, cognitive impairment is estimated to occur in 70%–100% of patients requiring mechanical ventilation and persists in approximately 20% of those five years later (Herridge et al. 2016; Wilcox et al. 2013). Often a consequence of ARDS, along with a host of other potential impairments, cognitive dysfunctions result in reduced quality of life (Denke et al. 2018).

In COVID-19 patients, cognitive deficits are seen in the areas of attention, memory, executive functions, and verbal fluency (Daroische et al. 2021; Rogers et al. 2020; Varatharaj et al. 2020). Impaired attention has been observed as a short-term consequence (Crunfli et al. 2021) and a long-term consequence of COVID-19 (Hampshire et al. 2021; Woo et al. 2020). When considering attention, sustained attention (Zhou et al. 2020) and divided attention (Jaywant et al. 2021) are mostly affected in these patients. Impaired memory is also reported to be present in COVID-19 patients, either as a short-term problem (Crunfli et al. 2021; Lu et al. 2020) or as a long-term outcome (Woo et al. 2020). Jaywant et al. (2021) evaluated the frequency, intensity, and profile of cognitive dysfunction in patients (n=57) who had been hospitalised for a long time with COVID-19 and required acute inpatient rehabilitation. They reported primary impairment in working memory (amongst 55% of the patients), followed by set shifting, divided attention, and processing speed abilities. In a systematic review, Rogers et al. (2020) reported neuropsychiatric symptoms such as confusion, depressed mood, anxiety, impaired memory, and insomnia, with confusion and agitation as prevalent factors in ICU patients and dysexecutive syndromes in patients at discharge. In a cross-specialty wide surveillance study of acute neurological and psychiatric complications of COVID-19 in the United Kingdom, Varatharaj et al. (2020) reported altered mental status and cerebrovascular incidents in different proportions amongst their patients. Of the data sets from 125 patients, nearly 46% had an ischemic stroke.

Other short- and long-term neurological issues include CNS problems (dizziness, headaches, mental state, ataxia, seizure) and peripheral nervous system damage (impaired sense of smell, taste, vision, nerve pain). These neuropsychiatric and behavioural symptoms may be associated with neurological injury such as hypoxia, stroke, and viral encephalitis that may result from COVID-19 (Arenivas et al. 2020). Together, these findings call attention to the existence of long-term cognitive sequelae in survivors of COVID-19, termed "Long COVID." In a large study that intended to capture the prevalence of Long COVID cognitive deficits in the early chronic phase, cognitive tests were hosted online to measure distinct aspects of human cognition including planning/reasoning, working memory, attention, and emotion-processing abilities in response to the COVID-19 pandemic (Hampshire et al. 2021). Respondents who had been hospitalised and those who had not been hospitalised but had biologically confirmed COVID-19 infection showed cognitive deficits. Respondents who received greater assistance for respiratory symptoms associated with COVID-19 (e.g., ventilators) performed worse on the cognitive tasks compared to those who stayed at home (Hampshire et al. 2021).

To gain a thorough understanding of the complex neurocognitive presentation of COVID-19, standardised neurological assessments should at least include tests assessing attention, executive functions, learning, memory as well as speed of information processing (Kumar et al. 2021). The Mini-Mental State Evaluation, Montreal Cognitive Assessment, Hamilton Rating Scale for Depression, and Functional Independence Measure may be used as cognitive screeners (Alemanno et al. 2021) and administered remotely since video teleconferencing shows good agreement with conventional face-to-face testing in persons with cognitive impairments and dementia (Cullum et al. 2014). Studies have used iPad-based online tools such as the Trail Making Test, Sign Coding Test, Continuous Performance Test, and Digital Span Test to evaluate the impacts of COVID-19 on cognitive functions in recovered patients (Zhou et al. 2020).

A coordinated and appropriately resourced approach to rehabilitation for the recovery phase is essential to manage both the long-term consequences of COVID-19 infection and to restore the functions lost as a result of the indirect effects of COVID. Unfortunately, evidence regarding cognitive rehabilitation outcomes in individuals with COVID-19 is lacking. Some institutions are referring patients with post-COVID cognitive symptoms to cognitive rehabilitation therapy (CRT), which includes cognitive training and psychological support (Zarrabian and Hassani-Abharian 2020). Mantovani et al. (2020) proposed methods and technologies for cognitive rehabilitation, including virtual reality, augmented reality, serious games, and telerehabilitation strategies (Mantovani et al. 2020). Simultaneously, caregiver education regarding probable cognitive, behavioural, and affective changes have been suggested. Other recommendations are to make remote and online information and education sessions available to monitor patients' well-being (Devita et al. 2021).

## 1.3 Impact of COVID-19 on speech language pathology service delivery

At the beginning of the COVID-19 pandemic, several groups compiled national and international guidelines in modifying assessment and intervention methods for individuals with cognitive-communication and swallowing disorders. Clinicians who engaged in AGPs such as endoscopic assessments of voice and swallowing, oral mechanism examinations, and tracheoesophageal prosthesis management had to follow strict protocols to minimise exposure and transmission risk (Anagiotos and Petrikkos 2021; Mick and Murphy 2020; Zimmermann and Nkenke 2020). Postponing procedures when possible, use of PPE, physical distancing, teleconsultation, and telerehabilitation were commonly recommended clinical practice guidelines across international healthcare groups (see Birgand et al. 2021; Chacon et al. 2021 for review of the guidelines). However, there is only limited evidence supporting the effectiveness of these guidelines, and further research is needed.

Prior to 2020, traditional speech-language pathology services were primarily provided face to face. In the early phase of the pandemic, SLPs ceased providing interventions due to school and business closures, and those that continued services provided them through telephone or videoconferencing (Chadd et al. 2021). The frequency and intensity of services and number of clients receiving services also reduced. The easily transmissible nature of the virus and various restrictions and precautions of the COVID-19 pandemic necessitated changes to service delivery to protect professionals and clients. Whilst the use of telepractice was not uncommon before COVID-19, the pandemic greatly accelerated the use of telepractice as a model of service delivery when governments waived the barriers of licensing restrictions and reimbursement (Bashshur et al. 2020; Kraljević et al. 2020).

According to surveys of SLPs across the world, there was a significant increase in the use of telepractice in the United States (ASHA Staff 2020; Campbell and Goldstein 2021); Croatia (Kraljević et al. 2020); Iceland (Crowe et al. 2021); and Saudi Arabia (Al Awaji et al. 2022), amongst others. Although telepractice use increased, there were still challenges in its implementation. Many clinicians reported unfamiliarity with the use of telepractice prior to the pandemic, resulting in lower self-reported proficiency in its use during the pandemic (Campbell and Goldstein 2021). In the United Kingdom, SLPs reported that they offered fewer services to clients owing to inconsistencies in local and national guidelines, lack of telepractice resources, or inappropriateness of the modality for certain clients (Chadd et al. 2021). Another survey of SLPs in the United States reported other barriers to implementation of telepractice during COVID-19 (Kollia and Tsiamtsiouris 2021). The most frequently cited barriers were related to equipment (internet interruptions, lack of access to online materials and technical support); training (lack of specialised training and resources); privacy (lack of dedicated telepractice rooms, concerns about patient privacy compliance); and case complexity (telepractice not appropriate for complex clients who need more physical cues and redirection) (Kollia and Tsiamtsiouris 2021). In spite of these barriers, the majority of SLPs reported that they would continue to use telepractice at higher than pre-pandemic levels (Campbell and Goldstein 2021; Kollia and Tsiamtsiouris 2021) due to the ease of use and perceived benefits.

In the field of communication sciences and disorders, telerehabilitation interventions are primarily provided synchronously using technology such as computers, webcams, tablets, and smartphones. However, in the field of telerehabilitation over the last two decades, virtual reality has been integrated into interventions to provide personalised rehabilitation or clinical care (Perez-Marcos 2018; Riva and Gamberini 2000; Tuena et al. 2020). Virtual reality allows the user to be immersed in, and interact within, a computer-generated environment. It has been used successfully as a part of rehabilitation in several clinical areas related to motor and cognitive rehabilitation in stroke and traumatic brain injury (Moreno et al. 2019; Wiley et al. 2020) as well as in those with mental health disorders (J. Li et al. 2014; McCann et al. 2014).

In the context of the COVID-19 pandemic, the use of virtual reality appears to be a promising avenue in telerehabilitation, although few studies have evaluated its benefits in the current scenario. Kolbe and colleagues (2021) explored user experience of virtual reality in an inpatient rehabilitation unit. Hospital staff and patients with COVID-19 participated in the experience that included guided meditation, natural environment exploration, and cognitive stimulation games (Kolbe et al. 2021). Both groups were highly satisfied with the experience, and patients perceived enhanced benefits for rehabilitation treatments and well-being. Varela-Aldás and others (2021) compared recall of items in a story using traditional face-to-face spaced retrieval and spaced retrieval within a virtual reality system amongst healthy adults and found the virtual reality group to perform better (Varela-Aldás et al. 2021). These studies and others suggest that virtual reality, augmented reality, and serious games (interactive computer applications with learning and educational goals) can be engaging and rewarding experiences with plausible therapeutic benefits that may be integrated into cognitive and neurorehabilitation. The use of virtual reality in cognitive and neurorehabilitation is still at the very nascent stages, and much work is needed to investigate the reliability, validity, effectiveness, and efficacy of these approaches post-COVID.

Overall, telepractice is an accepted form of service delivery that offers a timely alternative to face-to-face options during the pandemic. Clinically, institutions and companies must provide technical training to SLPs in the use of virtual modalities and address the barriers that clients and clinicians face in implementing effective telepractice sessions. Unfortunately, there is not enough evidence of the effectiveness of telerehabilitation for the majority of clients with COVID-19. Future studies must establish not only the feasibility of telerehabilitation approaches but must compare in-person and telepractice services on therapeutic outcomes related to cognition, speech, language, and swallowing during the COVID-19 pandemic. Additionally, there is a dearth of information regarding patient perspectives and preferences; preliminary evidence from paediatric settings suggest that clients and caregivers are accepting of telepractice approaches but still rate them to be less effective than in-person services (Lam et al. 2021). SLPs may need to be more proactive in helping clients transition to telepractice, communicate confidence in the effectiveness of telepractice, and take a more active role in offering technical support and troubleshooting (Lam et al. 2021).

## 1.4 Impact of COVID-19 on education and training in speech-language pathology

Just as clinicians were compelled to shift to remote and online services, higher education institutions were forced to switch to fully online teaching during the early phase of the COVID-19 pandemic to maintain continuity of education and reduce viral transmission across campuses. It is estimated that there were 1.22 billion online learners worldwide in 2020 (C. Li and Lalani 2020). Many educational institutions responded quickly to provide faculty and staff with resources and training to adapt teaching and learning into online and later, hybrid formats. Videoconferencing was made available to students and practicing clinicians via easy access and low-cost technology and platforms such as Zoom, Webex, Skype, and Microsoft Teams. However, there were still challenges in adapting some clinical learning experiences to a virtual format, especially in practicing hands-on clinical skills. Several schools, clinics, and rehabilitation centres that typically supported student training via university partnerships closed their organisations to student clinicians due to the need for COVID-19 safety precautions, limited PPE supplies, less time to supervise student clinicians, and increased caseloads (Byrnes et al. 2020). This required clinical educators to identify alternative opportunities to assist students in meeting their clinical hours and training requirements.

Health profession programmes incorporated alternative remote training opportunities such as clinical simulations (Reed et al. 2020; Volkers 2020). Clinical simulations generally include standardised patients, virtual patients, interactive computer experiences, and/or written case studies (American Speech-Language-Hearing Association n.d.). Several studies support the use of simulations in clinical education, for example, in dysphagia (Benadom and Potter 2011; Potter and Allen 2013) and tracheostomy (Estis et al. 2015). Other pedagogical avenues that were explored in clinical education were teletraining, telesupervision, and telepractice. Many educational institutions switched to telerehabilitation in providing speech-language-hearing services to clients, requiring immediate training for students as well as clients in adapting to this service model. Graduate students who received telepractice training reported greater knowledge and comfort with telepractice (Hatcher et al. 2022). Telesupervision that requires the use of technology to assist in clinical supervision or training (Rousmaniere 2014, p. 206) was implemented to provide hands-on and offline clinical feedback (Voniati et al. 2021). Whilst the long-term effects of the various new pedagogical adaptations in response to the pandemic will become clearer in the next few years, telerehabilitation appears to be a cost-effective and flexible service delivery model that can also be used in low- and middle-income countries (Khoza-Shangase et al. 2021).

## 1.5 Future challenges for the speech-language pathology discipline

The COVID-19 pandemic has given rise to a persistent, debilitating condition called Long COVID or chronic COVID syndrome (Baig 2020; Callard and Perego 2021; Nath 2020) that requires considerable attention amongst clinical and rehabilitation disciplines. About 10% of COVID-19 survivors develop Long

COVID, and an estimated five million individuals are confronting Long COVID around the world (Altmann and Boyton 2021). In adults with COVID-19, delirium is commonly observed amongst COVID patients in the ICU and in the long haul; delirium can also be present concurrently with cognitive deficits associated with stroke in some clinical populations. Rehabilitation in the chronic phase could include patient-centred cognitive interventions targeting specific cognitive deficits (e.g., attention), time-pressure management, divided attention tasks, and/or metacognitive strategy training. In addition to the direct impact of COVID-19 on neurocognitive abilities, the overall effects of quarantines, isolation from friends and family, and the stress of modified lifestyle impacts cognition. The effect of such stressors on cognition has been established in areas of risk perception (Renn 1997); working memory and attention (Haegen and Luminet 2015); executive functions such as decision-making and problem-solving (Ostell 1991); and emotional regulation (Lok and Bishop 1999). In the current scenario, effects of cognitive rehabilitation and cognitive enhancement for both affected and unaffected individuals at risk for functional cognitive deficits related to COVID must be explored further.

Providing SLP services necessitates complete communication between SLPs and patients, both children and adults. In children, specifically with articulation disorders, it becomes difficult to use a PPE kit when children are observing the SLP's speech articulators. SLPs may need to make physical contact with the clients or use specific toys during the session, significantly increasing the risk of disease transmission (Tohidast et al. 2020). As a result, in-person treatment may not be a viable option. The disruption of routine early intervention services for children with communication disorders during the critical period of speech and language development may pose a threat to future academic performance, social skill development, and job opportunities (Tohidast et al. 2020). Children with developmental delays, stuttering, and hearing impairment may be especially vulnerable to these problems since early treatment is critical for improved functional outcomes. Adults with cognitive-communication and/or swallowing disorders also experience inconsistencies in receiving speech-language pathology services during the pandemic. Once the pandemic wanes, we will need to identify ways to support those individuals who missed rehabilitation services for their speech, language, cognitive, or swallowing needs. There is a great need to facilitate inclusion of these clients into care pathways to ensure adequate quality of life.

The adverse consequences of communication problems in children and adults leads to physical, mental, social, and financial distress amongst parents and caregivers. The COVID-19 pandemic has presumably created additional issues for these families, furthering caregivers' physical and mental issues during the pandemic (Ornell et al. 2020). Because of the negative financial impacts of the pandemic, families are likely going to be under more financial tension (Baldwin and Tomiura 2020). These additional pressures exacerbate issues and worries in families with youngsters who were already experiencing a range of challenges and problems. Also, immediate onset of specific discourse and communication issues in children can result in increased anxiety amongst parents or give rise to comorbid conditions like cognitive deficits that can affect recovery in adults.

Whilst remote and online learning have promoted continued professional development and clinical training during the pandemic, there are many ambiguities that need to be explored. There is a need to determine systematically the effectiveness, benefits, shortcomings, and economic impacts of online learning outcomes in speech-language pathology. This would assist in integrating virtual modalities into clinical training even after the pandemic has ended. Specialised training in telepractice will provide students with a wider skill set to enter the workforce, allowing more clients to access speech-language pathology services (Hatcher et al. 2022).

Finally, the various challenges that SLPs face in implementing telepractice must be addressed immediately as it has been the most popular mode of service delivery during the pandemic. Concerted effort is needed by institutions, healthcare centres, advocacy groups, speech and hearing associations, and SLPs and audiologists to train professionals on telepractice in the current scenario. Further research is needed on the effectiveness of providing telerehabilitation over face-to-face interventions in clinical populations with varying needs post-COVID.

## 1.6 Summary

The COVID-19 pandemic has profoundly affected the lives of people around the world and has resulted in several health and economic implications. The disease presents with a myriad of problems including respiratory illnesses, fever, fatigue, muscle weakness, chest pain, palpitations, cognitive and mood problems, and swallowing problems. SLPs play an important role in managing patients at high or suspected risk of COVID-19. An SLP's role ranges from investigating symptoms to rehabilitation activities in acute and long-term care settings. A comprehensive programme for patients with COVID-19 demonstrates that early screening and assessment, individualised treatment goals for dysphagia, voice, and cognitive rehabilitation, and patient education are beneficial to patients with COVID-19. As patients become medically stable and recover from COVID-19, SLPs provide family training to support swallowing, cognition, communication management, neuropsychological support, and safe discharge, whilst ensuring patient independence.

With the emergence of Long COVID, suitable rehabilitation measures remain a key area of concern for patients recovering from COVID-19. Therefore, in the long haul, SLPs will continue to play an important role in the treatment and management of neuropsychological effects of the infection and contribute to improving patients' quality of life. Additionally, governing bodies and associations/boards must develop proper guidelines that outline training and services to improve telerehabilitation services during and after the pandemic. Clinical care and scientific efforts are needed to establish and strengthen an interdisciplinary task force to deal with current COVID-19 and tackle future consequences of the infection and pandemic.

## Note

The authors contributed equally to this chapter.

## References

Al Awaji, N. N., AlMudaiheem, A. A., & Mortada, E. M. (2022). Changes in speech, language and swallowing services during the Covid-19 pandemic: The perspective of speech-language pathologists in Saudi Arabia. *PloS One*, 17(1), e0262498. https://doi.org/10.1371/journal.pone.0262498.

Alberti, P., Beretta, S., Piatti, M., Karantzoulis, A., Piatti, M. L., Santoro, P., et al. (2020). Guillain-Barré syndrome related to COVID-19 infection. *Neurology-Neuroimmunology Neuroinflammation*, 7(4). doi:10.1212/NXI.0000000000000741.

Alemanno, F., Houdayer, E., Parma, A., Spina, A., Del Forno, A., Scatolini, A., et al. (2021). COVID-19 cognitive deficits after respiratory assistance in the subacute phase: A COVID-rehabilitation unit experience. *PloS One*, 16(2), e0246590. doi:10.1371/journal.pone.0246590.

Altmann, D. M., & Boyton, R. J. (2021). Decoding the unknowns in long covid. *BMJ*, 372. https://doi.org/10.1136/bmj.n132.

American Speech-Language-Hearing Association (n.d.). Certification standards for speech-language pathology frequently asked questions: Clinical simulation. www.asha.org/certification/certification-standards-for-slp-clinical-simulation/. Accessed 28 February 2022.

Anagiotos, A., & Petrikkos, G. (2021). Otolaryngology in the COVID-19 pandemic era: The impact on our clinical practice. *European Archives of Oto-Rhino-Laryngology*, 278(3), 629–636.

Aoyagi, Y., Inamoto, Y., Shibata, S., Kagaya, H., Otaka, Y., & Saitoh, E. (2021). Clinical manifestation, evaluation, and rehabilitative strategy of dysphagia associated with COVID-19. *American Journal of Physical Medicine and Rehabilitation*, 100(5), 424–431.

Araújo, B. C. L., de Melo Lima, T. R. C., de Gois-Santos, V. T., Santos, V. S., de Magalhães Simões, S., & Martins-Filho, P. R. (2020). Speech therapy practice in hospital settings and COVID-19 pandemic. *Revista da Associacao Medica Brasileira*, 66, 10–12.

Archer, S. K., Iezzi, C. M., & Gilpin, L. (2021). Swallowing and voice outcomes in patients hospitalized with COVID-19: An observational cohort study. *Archives of Physical Medicine and Rehabilitation*, 102(6), 1084–1090.

Arenivas, A., Carter, K. R., Harik, L. M., & Hays, K. M. (2020). COVID-19 neuropsychological factors and considerations within the acute physical medicine and rehabilitation setting. *Brain Injury*, 34(8), 1136–1137.

ASHA Staff (2020). COVID-19 impact on ASHA members: The personal and the professional. *The ASHA LeaderLive*, June–July 2020. https://leader.pubs.asha.org/do/10.1044/leader.AAG.25062020.28/full/. Accessed 28 February 2022.

Baig, A. M. (2020). Deleterious outcomes in long-hauler COVID-19: The effects of SARS-CoV-2 on the CNS in chronic COVID syndrome. *ACS Chemical Neuroscience*, 11(24), 4017–4020.

Baldwin, R., & Tomiura, E. (2020). Thinking ahead about the trade impact of COVID-19. In *Economics in the time of COVID-19* (pp. 59–71). London: Centre for Economic Policy Research.

Bashshur, R., Doarn, C. R., Frenk, J. M., Kvedar, J. C., & Woolliscroft, J. O. (2020). Telemedicine and the COVID-19 pandemic, lessons for the future. *Telemedicine Journal and E-Health*, 26(5), 571–573.

Benadom, E. M., & Potter, N. L. (2011). The use of simulation in training graduate students to perform transnasal endoscopy. *Dysphagia*, 26(4), 352–360.

Birgand, G., Mutters, N. T., Otter, J., Eichel, V. M., Lepelletier, D., Morgan, D. J., et al. (2021). Variation of national and international guidelines on respiratory protection for health care professionals during the COVID-19 pandemic. *JAMA Network Open*, 4(8), e2119257–e2119257. doi:10.1001/jamanetworkopen.2021.19257.

Brodsky, M. B., Pandian, V., & Needham, D. M. (2020). Post-extubation dysphagia: A problem needing multidisciplinary efforts. *Intensive Care Medicine*, 46(1), 93–96.

Byrnes, Y. M., Civantos, A. M., Go, B. C., McWilliams, T. L., & Rajasekaran, K. (2020). Effect of the COVID-19 pandemic on medical student career perceptions: A national survey study. *Medical Education Online*, 25(1), 1798088. doi:10.1080/10872981.2020.1798088.

Callard, F., & Perego, E. (2021). How and why patients made Long Covid. *Social Science and Medicine*, 268, 113426. https://doi.org/10.1016/j.socscimed.2020.113426.

Campbell, D. R., & Goldstein, H. (2021). Genesis of a new generation of telepractitioners: The COVID-19 pandemic and pediatric speech-language pathology services. *American Journal of Speech-Language Pathology*, 30(5), 2143–2154.

Cantarella, G., Aldè, M., Consonni, D., Zuccotti, G., Di Berardino, F., Barozzi, S., et al. (2022). Prevalence of dysphonia in non hospitalized patients with COVID-19 in Lombardy, the Italian epicenter of the pandemic. *Journal of Voice*, to appear.

Cantarella, G., Barillari, M. R., Lechien, J. R., & Pignataro, L. (2021). The challenge of virtual voice therapy during the COVID-19 pandemic. *Journal of Voice*, 35(3), 336–337.

Castillo-Allendes, A., Contreras-Ruston, F., Cantor-Cutiva, L. C., Codino, J., Guzman, M., Malebran, C., et al. (2021). Voice therapy in the context of the COVID-19 pandemic: Guidelines for clinical practice. *Journal of Voice*, 35(5), 717–727.

Centers for Disease Control and Prevention (2020). COVIDView: A weekly surveillance summary of U.S. COVID-19 activity. https://stacks.cdc.gov/view/cdc/86961. Accessed 28 February 2022.

Centers for Disease Control and Prevention (2022). Interim infection prevention and control recommendations for healthcare personnel during the coronavirus disease 2019 (COVID-19) pandemic. www.cdc.gov/coronavirus/2019-ncov/hcp/infection-control-recommendations.html. Accessed 28 February 2022.

Chacon, A. M., Nguyen, D. D., McCabe, P., & Madill, C. (2021). Aerosol-generating behaviours in speech pathology clinical practice: A systematic literature review. *PLoS One*, 16(4), e0250308. https://doi.org/10.1371/journal.pone.0250308.

Chadd, K., Moyse, K., & Enderby, P. (2021). Impact of COVID-19 on the speech and language therapy profession and their patients. *Frontiers in Neurology*, 12, 96. doi:10.3389/fneur.2021.629190.

Crary, M. A., Mann, G. D. C., & Groher, M. E. (2005). Initial psychometric assessment of a functional oral intake scale for dysphagia in stroke patients. *Archives of Physical Medicine and Rehabilitation*, 86(8), 1516–1520.

Crowe, K., Másdóttir, T., & Einarsdóttir, J. T. (2021). Service delivery and the use of tel-epractice during the COVID-19 pandemic in Iceland. *Perspectives of the ASHA Special Interest Groups*, 6(6), 1786–1799.

Crunfli, F., Carregari, V. C., Veras, F. P., Vendramini, P. H., Valença, A. G. F., Antunes, A. S. L. M., et al. (2021). SARS-CoV-2 infects brain astrocytes of COVID-19 patients and impairs neuronal viability. *MedRxiv*. https://doi.org/10.1101/2020.10.09.20207464.

Cullum, C. M., Hynan, L., Grosch, M., Parikh, M., & Weiner, M. (2014). Teleneuropsy-chology: Evidence for video teleconference-based neuropsychological assessment. *Journal of the International Neuropsychological Society*, 20(10), 1028–1033.

Daroische, R., Hemminghyth, M. S., Eilertsen, T. H., Breitve, M. H., & Chwiszczuk, L. J. (2021). Cognitive impairment after COVID-19 = A review on objective test data. *Frontiers in Neurology*, 1238. doi:10.3389/fneur.2021.699582.

Dawson, C., Capewell, R., Ellis, S., Matthews, S., Adamson, S., Wood, M., et al. (2020). Dysphagia presentation and management following coronavirus disease 2019: An acute care tertiary centre experience. *The Journal of Laryngology & Otology*, 134(11), 981–986.

Denke, C., Balzer, F., Menk, M., Szur, S., Brosinsky, G., Tafelski, S., et al. (2018). Long-term sequelae of acute respiratory distress syndrome caused by severe community-acquired pneumonia: Delirium-associated cognitive impairment and post-traumatic stress disorder. *Journal of International Medical Research*, 46(6), 2265–2283.

Devita, M., Bordignon, A., Sergi, G., & Coin, A. (2021). The psychological and cognitive impact of Covid-19 on individuals with neurocognitive impairments: Research top-ics and remote intervention proposals. *Aging Clinical and Experimental Research*, 33(3), 733–736.

Estis, J. M., Rudd, A. B., Pruitt, B., & Wright, T. (2015). Interprofessional simulation-based education enhances student knowledge of health professional roles and care of patients with tracheostomies and Passy-Muir® Valves. *Journal of Nursing Education and Practice*, 5(6), 123–128.

Eyigör, S., & Umay, E. (2021). Dysphagia management during COVID-19 pandemic: A review of the literature and international guidelines. *Turkish Journal of Physical Medi-cine and Rehabilitation*, 67(3), 267–274.

Fauci, A. S., Lane, H. C., & Redfield, R. R. (2020). Covid-19 – navigating the uncharted. *New England Journal of Medicine*, 382, 1268–1269.

Freeman-Sanderson, A., Ward, E. C., Miles, A., de Pedro Netto, I., Duncan, S., Inamoto, Y., et al. (2021). A consensus statement for the management and rehabilitation of com-munication and swallowing function in the ICU: A global response to COVID-19. *Archives of Physical Medicine and Rehabilitation*, 102(5), 835–842.

Goha, A., Mezue, K., Edwards, P., Nunura, F., Baugh, D., & Madu, E. (2020). COVID-19 and the heart: An update for clinicians. *Clinical Cardiology*, 43(11), 1216–1222.

Gupta, A., Madhavan, M. V., Sehgal, K., Nair, N., Mahajan, S., Sehrawat, T. S., et al. (2020). Extrapulmonary manifestations of COVID-19. *Nature Medicine*, 26(7), 1017–1032.

Haegen, M. V., & Luminet, O. (2015). Stress, psychosocial mediators, and cognitive mediators in parents of child cancer patients and cancer survivors: Attention and work-ing memory pathway perspectives. *Journal of Psychosocial Oncology*, 33(5), 504–550.

Hampshire, A., Trender, W., Chamberlain, S. R., Jolly, A. E., Grant, J. E., Patrick, F., et al. (2021). Cognitive deficits in people who have recovered from COVID-19. *EClinical-Medicine*, 101044. doi:10.1016/j.eclinm.2021.101044.

Hatcher, A., Frost, K., Weiler, B., & Bland, L. (2022). A survey of speech-language pathol-ogy graduate students' perceptions of telepractice pre- and posttraining during the COVID-19 pandemic. *Perspectives of the ASHA Special Interest Groups*, 7(1), 268–275.

Herridge, M. S., Moss, M., Hough, C. L., Hopkins, R. O., Rice, T. W., Bienvenu, O. J., et al. (2016). Recovery and outcomes after the acute respiratory distress syndrome (ARDS) in patients and their family caregivers. *Intensive Care Medicine*, 42(5), 725–738.

Janiri, D., Carfì, A., Kotzalidis, G. D., Bernabei, R., Landi, F., Sani, G., et al. (2021). Post-traumatic stress disorder in patients after severe COVID-19 infection. *JAMA Psychiatry*, 78(5), 567–569.

Jaywant, A., Vanderlind, W. M., Alexopoulos, G. S., Fridman, C. B., Perlis, R. H., & Gunning, F. M. (2021). Frequency and profile of objective cognitive deficits in hospitalized patients recovering from COVID-19. *Neuropsychopharmacology*, 46(13), 2235–2240.

Kelchner, L. (2013). Telehealth and the treatment of voice disorders: A discussion regarding evidence. *Perspectives on Voice and Voice Disorders*, 23(3), 88–94.

Khoza-Shangase, K., Moroe, N., & Neille, J. (2021). Speech-language pathology and audiology in South Africa: Clinical training and service in the era of COVID-19. *International Journal of Telerehabilitation*, 13(1), e6376. https://doi.org/10.5195/ijt.2021.6376.

Kolbe, L., Jaywant, A., Gupta, A., Vanderlind, W. M., & Jabbour, G. (2021). Use of virtual reality in the inpatient rehabilitation of COVID-19 patients. *General Hospital Psychiatry*, 71, 76–81.

Kollia, B., & Tsiamtsiouris, J. (2021). Influence of the COVID-19 pandemic on telepractice in speech-language pathology. *Journal of Prevention & Intervention in the Community*, 49(2), 152–162.

Kraljević, J. K., Matić, A., & Dokoza, K. P. (2020). Telepractice as a reaction to the COVID-19 crisis: Insights from Croatian SLP settings. *International Journal of Telerehabilitation*, 12(2), 93–103.

Kumar, S., Veldhuis, A., & Malhotra, T. (2021). Neuropsychiatric and cognitive sequelae of COVID-19. *Frontiers in Psychology*, 12, 553. doi:10.3389/fpsyg.2021.577529.

Laguna, L. B., Marcos-Neira, P., de Lagrán Zurbano, I. M., Marco, E. M., Guisasola, C. P., Soria, C. D. V., et al. (2022). Dysphagia and mechanical ventilation in SARS-COV-2 pneumonia: It's real. *Clinical Nutrition*. doi:10.1016/j.clnu.2021.11.018.

Lam, J. H. Y., Lee, S. M. K., & Tong, X. (2021). Parents' and students' perceptions of telepractice services for speech-language therapy during the COVID-19 pandemic: Survey study. *JMIR Pediatrics and Parenting*, 4(1), e25675. doi:10.2196/25675.

Lechien, J. R., Chiesa-Estomba, C. M., Cabaraux, P., Mat, Q., Huet, K., Harmegnies, B., et al. (2022). Features of mild-to-moderate COVID-19 patients with dysphonia. *Journal of Voice*. doi:10.1016/j.jvoice.2020.05.012.

Lechien, J. R., Chiesa-Estomba, C. M., De Siati, D. R., Horoi, M., Le Bon, S. D., Rodriguez, A., et al. (2020). Olfactory and gustatory dysfunctions as a clinical presentation of mild-to-moderate forms of the coronavirus disease (COVID-19): A multicenter European study. *European Archives of Oto-Rhino-Laryngology*, 277(8), 2251–2261.

Leis-Cofiño, C., Arriero-Sánchez, P., González-Herranz, R., Arenas-Brítez, Ó., Hernández-García, E., & Plaza, G. (2022). Persistent dysphonia in hospitalized COVID-19 patients. *Journal of Voice*. doi:10.1016/j.jvoice.2021.07.001.

Lew, H. L., Oh-Park, M., & Cifu, D. X. (2020). The war on COVID-19 pandemic: Role of rehabilitation professionals and hospitals. *American Journal of Physical Medicine and Rehabilitation*, 99(7), 571–572.

Li, C., & Lalani, F. (2020). The COVID-19 pandemic has changed education forever. This is how. www.weforum.org/agenda/2020/04/coronavirus-education-global-covid19-online-digital-learning. Accessed 1 March 2022.

Li, J., Theng, Y.-L., & Foo, S. (2014). Game-based digital interventions for depression therapy: A systematic review and meta-analysis. *Cyberpsychology, Behavior, and Social Networking*, 17(8), 519–527.

Li, Q., Guan, X., Wu, P., Wang, X., Zhou, L., Tong, Y., et al. (2020). Early transmission dynamics in Wuhan, China, of novel coronavirus – infected pneumonia. *New England Journal of Medicine*, 382(13), 1199–1207.

Lok, C.-F., & Bishop, G. D. (1999). Emotion control, stress, and health. *Psychology and Health*, 14(5), 813–827.

Lu, Y., Li, X., Geng, D., Mei, N., Wu, P.-Y., Huang, C.-C., et al. (2020). Cerebral microstructural changes in COVID-19 patients – an MRI-based 3-month follow-up study. *EClinicalMedicine*, 25, 100484. doi:10.1016/j.eclinm.2020.100484.

Mantovani, E., Zucchella, C., Bottiroli, S., Federico, A., Giugno, R., Sandrini, G., et al. (2020). Telemedicine and virtual reality for cognitive rehabilitation: A roadmap for the COVID-19 pandemic. *Frontiers in Neurology*, 11, 926. doi:10.3389/fneur.2020.00926.

Mart, M. F., & Ware, L. B. (2020). The long-lasting effects of the acute respiratory distress syndrome. *Expert Review of Respiratory Medicine*, 14(6), 577–586.

Martin-Martinez, A., Ortega, O., Viñas, P., Arreola, V., Nascimento, W., Costa, A., et al. (2021). COVID-19 is associated with oropharyngeal dysphagia and malnutrition in hospitalized patients during the spring 2020 wave of the pandemic. *Clinical Nutrition*. doi:10.1016/j.clnu.2021.06.010.

McCann, R. A., Armstrong, C. M., Skopp, N. A., Edwards-Stewart, A., Smolenski, D. J., June, J. D., et al. (2014). Virtual reality exposure therapy for the treatment of anxiety disorders: An evaluation of research quality. *Journal of Anxiety Disorders*, 28(6), 625–631.

Mick, P., & Murphy, R. (2020). Aerosol-generating otolaryngology procedures and the need for enhanced PPE during the COVID-19 pandemic: A literature review. *Journal of Otolaryngology-Head & Neck Surgery*, 49(1), 1–10.

Miles, A., McRae, J., Clunie, G., Gillivan-Murphy, P., Inamoto, Y., Kalf, H., et al. (2022). An international commentary on dysphagia and dysphonia during the COVID-19 pandemic. *Dysphagia*. doi:10.1007/s00455-021-10396-z.

Mohan, R., & Mohapatra, B. (2020). Shedding light on dysphagia associated with COVID-19: The what and why. *OTO Open*, 4(2), 2473974X20934770.

Mohapatra, B., & Mohan, R. (2020). Speech-language pathologists' role in the multidisciplinary management and rehabilitation of patients with Covid-19. *Journal of Rehabilitation Medicine. Clinical Communications*, 3, 1000037. doi:10.2340/20030711-1000037.

Moreno, A., Wall, K. J., Thangavelu, K., Craven, L., Ward, E., & Dissanayaka, N. N. (2019). A systematic review of the use of virtual reality and its effects on cognition in individuals with neurocognitive disorders. *Alzheimer's & Dementia: Translational Research & Clinical Interventions*, 5, 834–850.

Nath, A. (2020). Long-haul COVID. *Neurology*, 95(13), 559–560.

Neevel, A. J., Smith, J. D., Morrison, R. J., Hogikyan, N. D., Kupfer, R. A., & Stein, A. P. (2021). Postacute COVID-19 laryngeal injury and dysfunction. *OTO Open*, 5(3). doi:10.1177/2473974X211041040.

Ornell, F., Schuch, J. B., Sordi, A. O., & Kessler, F. H. P. (2020). "Pandemic fear" and COVID-19: Mental health burden and strategies. *Revista Brasileira de Psiquiatria*, 42(3), 232–235.

Osbeck Sandblom, H., Dotevall, H., Svennerholm, K., Tuomi, L., & Finizia, C. (2021). Characterization of dysphagia and laryngeal findings in COVID-19 patients treated in the ICU – An observational clinical study. *PloS One*, 16(6), e0252347. doi:10.1371/journal.pone.0252347.

Ostell, A. (1991). Coping, problem solving and stress: A framework for intervention strategies. *British Journal of Medical Psychology*, 64(1), 11–24.

Perez-Marcos, D. (2018). Virtual reality experiences, embodiment, videogames and their dimensions in neurorehabilitation. *Journal of Neuroengineering and Rehabilitation*, 15(1), 1–8.

Potter, N. L., & Allen, M. (2013). Clinical swallow exam for dysphagia: A speech pathology and nursing simulation experience. *Clinical Simulation in Nursing*, 9(10), e461–e464. doi:10.1016/j.ecns.2012.08.001.

Reed, D. S., Hill, M. D., Justin, G. A., Giles, G. B., Santamaria, J. A., Hobbs, S. D., et al. (2020). Finding focus in crisis: Resident-driven graduate medical education at a military training facility during the COVID-19 pandemic. *Military Medicine*, 185(11–12), 469–471.

Regan, J., Walshe, M., Lavan, S., Horan, E., Gillivan Murphy, P., Healy, A., et al. (2021). Post-extubation dysphagia and dysphonia amongst adults with COVID-19 in the Republic of Ireland: A prospective multi-site observational cohort study. *Clinical Otolaryngology*, 46(6), 1290–1299.

Renn, O. (1997). Mental health, stress and risk perception insights from psychological research. In J. V. Lake, G. R. Bock, & G. Cardew (Eds.), *Health impacts of large releases of radionuclides* (pp. 205–225). Chichester, West Sussex: Wiley.

Ritchie, K., Chan, D., & Watermeyer, T. (2020). The cognitive consequences of the COVID-19 epidemic: Collateral damage? *Brain Communications*, 2(2), fcaa069. doi:10.1093/braincomms/fcaa069.

Riva, G., & Gamberini, L. (2000). Virtual reality in telemedicine. *Telemedicine Journal and e-Health*, 6(3), 327–340.

Rogers, J. P., Chesney, E., Oliver, D., Pollak, T. A., McGuire, P., Fusar-Poli, P., et al. (2020). Psychiatric and neuropsychiatric presentations associated with severe coronavirus infections: A systematic review and meta-analysis with comparison to the COVID-19 pandemic. *The Lancet Psychiatry*, 7(7), 611–627.

Rousmaniere, T. (2014). Using technology to enhance clinical supervision and training. In C. E. Watkins, Jr. & D. L. Milne (Eds.), *The Wiley international handbook of clinical supervision* (pp. 204–237). Chichester, West Sussex: Wiley-Blackwell.

Schindler, A., Baijens, L. W., Clave, P., Degen, B., Duchac, S., Dziewas, R., et al. (2021). ESSD commentary on dysphagia management during COVID pandemia. *Dysphagia*, 36(4), 764–767.

Steele, C. M., Namasivayam-MacDonald, A. M., Guida, B. T., Cichero, J. A., Duivestein, J., Hanson, B., et al. (2018). Creation and initial validation of the international dysphagia diet standardisation initiative functional diet scale. *Archives of Physical Medicine and Rehabilitation*, 99(5), 934–944.

Strohl, M. P., Dwyer, C. D., Ma, Y., Rosen, C. A., Schneider, S. L., & Young, V. N. (2022). Implementation of telemedicine in a laryngology practice during the COVID-19 pandemic: Lessons learned, experiences shared. *Journal of Voice*. doi:10.1016/j.jvoice.2020.06.017.

Tohidast, S. A., Mansuri, B., Bagheri, R., & Azimi, H. (2020). Provision of speech-language pathology services for the treatment of speech and language disorders in children during the COVID-19 pandemic: Problems, concerns, and solutions. *International Journal of Pediatric Otorhinolaryngology*, 138, 110262. doi:10.1016/j.ijporl.2020.110262.

Tuena, C., Pedroli, E., Trimarchi, P. D., Gallucci, A., Chiappini, M., Goulene, K., et al. (2020). Usability issues of clinical and research applications of virtual reality in older people: A systematic review. *Frontiers in Human Neuroscience*, 14, 93. https://doi.org/10.3389/fnhum.2020.00093.

van den Borst, B., Peters, J. B., Brink, M., Schoon, Y., Bleeker-Rovers, C. P., Schers, H., et al. (2021). Comprehensive health assessment 3 months after recovery from acute coronavirus disease 2019 (COVID-19). *Clinical Infectious Diseases*, 73(5), e1089–e1098. doi:10.1093/cid/ciaa1750.

Varatharaj, A., Thomas, N., Ellul, M. A., Davies, N. W., Pollak, T. A., Tenorio, E. L., et al. (2020). Neurological and neuropsychiatric complications of COVID-19 in 153 patients: A UK-wide surveillance study. *The Lancet Psychiatry*, 7(10), 875–882.

Varela-Aldás, J., Buele, J., Ramos Lorente, P., García-Magariño, I., & Palacios-Navarro, G. (2021). A virtual reality-based cognitive telerehabilitation system for use in the COVID-19 pandemic. *Sustainability*, 13(4), 2183. https://doi.org/10.3390/su13042183.

Vergara, J., Skoretz, S. A., Brodsky, M. B., Miles, A., Langmore, S. E., Wallace, S., et al. (2020). Assessment, diagnosis, and treatment of dysphagia in patients infected with SARS-CoV-2: A review of the literature and international guidelines. *American Journal of Speech-Language Pathology*, 29(4), 2242–2253.

Volkers, N. (2020). What COVID-19 teaches about online learning. *The ASHA LeaderLive*, June–July 2020. https://leader.pubs.asha.org/do/10.1044/leader.ftr1.25062020.46/full/. Accessed 17 March 2022.

Voniati, L., Kilili-Lesta, M., & Christoupoulou, M. C. (2021). Speech-language therapy clinical services, student education, and practical training in the time of COVID-19: The rise of telepractice, telesupervision, and distance learning in Cyprus. *Perspectives of the ASHA Special Interest Groups*, 6(4), 955–963.

Wilcox, M. E., Brummel, N. E., Archer, K., Ely, E. W., Jackson, J. C., & Hopkins, R. O. (2013). Cognitive dysfunction in ICU patients: Risk factors, predictors, and rehabilitation interventions. *Critical Care Medicine*, 41(9), S81–S98.

Wiley, E., Khattab, S., & Tang, A. (2020). Examining the effect of virtual reality therapy on cognition post-stroke: A systematic review and meta-analysis. *Disability and Rehabilitation: Assistive Technology*, 17(1), 50–60.

Woo, M. S., Malsy, J., Pöttgen, J., Seddiq Zai, S., Ufer, F., Hadjilaou, A., et al. (2020). Frequent neurocognitive deficits after recovery from mild COVID-19. *Brain Communications*, 2(2), fcaa205. doi:10.1093/braincomms/fcaa205.

Ye, M., Ren, Y., & Lv, T. (2020). Encephalitis as a clinical manifestation of COVID-19. *Brain, Behavior, and Immunity*, 88, 945–946.

Zarrabian, S., & Hassani-Abharian, P. (2020). COVID-19 pandemic and the importance of cognitive rehabilitation. *Basic and Clinical Neuroscience*, 11(2), 129–132.

Zhou, H., Lu, S., Chen, J., Wei, N., Wang, D., Lyu, H., et al. (2020). The landscape of cognitive function in recovered COVID 19 patients. *Journal of Psychiatric Research*, 129, 98–102.

Zimmermann, M., & Nkenke, E. (2020). Approaches to the management of patients in oral and maxillofacial surgery during COVID-19 pandemic. *Journal of Cranio-Maxillofacial Surgery*, 48(5), 521–526.

# 2

# THE IMPACT OF THE COVID-19 PANDEMIC ON CHILDREN'S SPEECH AND LANGUAGE DEVELOPMENT

*Sara A. Charney, Stephen M. Camarata, and Alexander Chern*

## 2.1 Introduction

COVID-19 has spread rapidly throughout the world since the first known case emerged in December 2019. Preventative strategies including mask wearing, social distancing, and virtual meetings have been incorporated as a part of everyday life to reduce the risk of infection. On 3 April 2020, new guidelines set by federal health officials were announced, recommending masks for all people over 2 years of age who were in a public setting, travelling, or around others in the same household who might be infected (Dwyer and Aubrey 2020). The COVID-19 pandemic has brought about many unintended, disruptive, and long-lasting consequences to society that should be considered. This is particularly important for creating future educational and developmental scaffolds in children who have experienced masking and other COVID-19 restrictions and to inform responses to future pandemic events.

For example, the COVID-19 pandemic has had a significant adverse impact on education. On 27 February 2020, the first school was shut down in the United States due to a coronavirus scare after an employee's relative tested positive for the virus. By 25 March 2020, all public school buildings were closed (Education Week 2020). The pandemic had a similar effect on the rest of the world – the majority of schools worldwide were fully closed by mid-March 2020 (UNESCO 2021), although there were notable exceptions such as Sweden (Vogel 2020).

Subsequently, when school start dates quickly approached in the fall of 2020, school administrators, teachers, and parents were forced to weigh the pros and cons of in-person classes. Many in-person classes were initially cancelled in favor

DOI: 10.4324/9781003257318-2

of virtual meetings to minimise spread of infection amongst schoolchildren and teachers. Ultimately, the school year opened with a mix of education plans in an attempt to keep children and teachers safe, ranging from in-person classes to remote schooling to hybrid models. During this time, preventative strategies continued in the school setting. On 15 September 2020, the Centers for Disease Control and Prevention (CDC) released indicators for dynamic school decision-making, offering five key mitigation strategies including consistent and correct use of masks, social distancing, hand hygiene, cleaning and disinfection, and contact tracing collaboration with local health departments (Centers for Disease Control and Prevention 2020).

Increasing concerns have also been raised regarding the potential short-term and long-term consequences of the COVID-19 pandemic on communication and social skills in children (Charney et al. 2021; Curtin et al. 2021; Epstein 2021; Hazlett 2021; Lewkowicz 2021). Broadly, there is a question as to whether precautionary practices such as masking and restricted learning opportunities may have unintentional and presently unknown consequences on children during their most critical time of development. This chapter highlights the potential impact of the pandemic on paediatric speech and language development, discusses specific vulnerable populations, and outlines possible mitigation strategies.

## 2.2 Impact of the COVID-19 pandemic on social interaction and language development

### 2.2.1 Transactional basis of speech, language, and social development

From the moment a neonate encounters other humans, especially parents, a nuanced entrainment process between parent and child is initiated (Camarata 2017). In essence, child initiations trigger teaching responses from parents and other adults that are incidentally attuned to the child's developmental level and yield ever more complex exemplars that support learning (Lense and Camarata 2020). For example, Camarata has described how this transactional process incidentally guides speech development. Parents and other communication partners rarely provide direct feedback on the details of speech production such as tongue placement, voicing, manner of production (such as frication), or other articulatory details (Camarata 1993, 2021). Rather, a child's immature production (e.g., "ba") is followed by a correct form ("bottle"). That is, when the child looks at a bottle and says, "Ba," the parent will typically reply by saying, "Bottle." Although seemingly simplistic, the parent response actually includes rich phonological feedback that children subsequently integrate into their own speech (e.g., the progression from "ba" to "baba" to "bada" to "bado" to "bottle"). It is perhaps noteworthy that this type of entrained speech production is also seen in nonhuman primates (e.g., marmosets) (Takahashi et al. 2016).

A voluminous literature indicates that these ubiquitous adult-child learning transactions underlie social and emotional development (Sameroff 2009), in addition to social communication (pragmatics), morphology, syntax, and semantics. Setting aside the structural elements of these social and linguistic domains, it is useful to focus on the visual and proximity elements of transactional learning to illuminate the potential impacts of COVID-19 preventative strategies such as masking (visual) and social distancing (proximity) on social interaction and language development. In terms of proximity, social distancing of two metres reduces access to visual and auditory cues. That is, details of facial expressions coupled with the co-occurring auditory signal are less salient with increasing distance when one modality is attenuated (Van der Stoep et al. 2016). Similarly, Erber (1974) reported that lip-reading becomes increasingly difficult at distances greater than five feet. This situation is exacerbated by use of opaque masking that further obscures visual and auditory cues.

### 2.2.2 Impact on speech development

To further illustrate the impact of visual and auditory cues on speech development, the authors would like to draw the attention of the reader to the transactions that support development of "ba" into "bottle," namely, the acquisition of a medial consonant (i.e., a voiceless alveolar stop, "t"). To be sure, the allophonic version is likely to be an alveolar tap in the intervocalic context of "bottle," but for the purposes of this example, the key feature is place of articulation rather than manner or voice. That is, the consonant is articulated with the tongue tip lifted and placed behind the teeth on the alveolar ridge.

A parent does not explicitly instruct the toddler who is saying "baba" for "bottle" that the medial consonant is alveolar rather than bilabial and that he or she needs to make the "t" sound with the tongue raised behind the teeth. Note that differential auditory discrimination of bilabial (e.g., "b"), alveolar (e.g., "d"), and velar stops (e.g., "g") is difficult and is not fully mastered in toddlers or preschoolers (Hicks and Ohde 2005). Instead, transactional learning in close proximity (normal conversational distance) in unmasked children and adults yields substantial visual cues (that are synchronised with the auditory signal) regarding place of articulation. A parent talking to the toddler can readily see that the medial consonant in "baba" was produced at the lips rather than with a raised tongue. Similarly, the child can "see" that the medial consonant is not bilabial but rather is produced with a raised tongue.

Although processing these visual cues is incidental and not conscious, it nonetheless contributes to speech development in the context of phonological transactions. Moreover, modifications of the speech architecture yield different acoustic features that are ultimately shaped into adult speech articulation. The attenuation of access to this information in typical development and, perhaps more so in atypical development (e.g., in children with hearing loss), illustrates the potential impact of masking and social distancing on speech development. This may be extended more broadly to language and social development as the myriad of subtle visual and auditory information is less available.

### 2.2.3 Peer interactions

The aforementioned speech development example illustrates how limiting access to visual cues has a deleterious impact on speech reading (lip-reading). However, preventative COVID-19 strategies may also limit socialisation, as restricting social encounters inherently reduces opportunities for peer interactions and social learning. It may be startling to realise that children born in the spring of 2020 are now nearly two years of age and have had extremely limited encounters with other children. But it is perhaps even more startling to realise that 2-year-olds in spring 2020 are now nearly four years of age, 3-year-olds are nearly five, and so on. It is difficult to overemphasise the amount of social and peer development that occurs during the preschool years. As with transactional learning between parents and children, peer-to-peer learning is foundational to play skills, group dynamics, learning, and healthy social development. Toddlers start off by playing by themselves and will observe other children playing. However, by the end of preschool years, children will have learnt relatively elaborate (albeit somewhat primitive by adolescent standards) collaborative play (Smith and Connolly 1972; Cohen 2018). They also have relatively sophisticated conversational skills and coordinate play routines and social exchanges in the context of peer interactions (Bukowski et al. 2011).

It is not surprising that the development of peer interaction is predicated upon hours and hours of peer interactions at home (play groups), on the playground, and at school, all of which were greatly reduced during the COVID-19 pandemic. The first level of reduction is in simple proximity. Children need to be in close proximity (less than six feet) in order to observe and engage in social play (Bukowski et al. 2011). The second level is the reduced access to facial expressions (e.g., smiles) from masks even when in close proximity.

Although the focus of this section is on peer development in preschoolers, there is emerging evidence that such preventative strategies have also had an adverse impact on peer development in adolescents. It is well-known that peer interactions are very important in teens and much of this interaction occurs in school and other in-person activities (e.g., attending movies, participating in sports, hanging out). In addition to yielding friendships and forming more complex social networks, these peer interactions are also developmental in nature as well because teens continue to learn nuances of social interaction and how to form and sustain relationships. Although it is beyond the scope of this chapter to review in detail how preventative strategies have had a devastating impact on teens, it is clear that dramatically reducing peer interaction is associated with dramatic increases in adverse mental health sequelae in this group.

### 2.2.4 Distance and hybrid education: negative impact on learning opportunities

Thus far, this chapter has focused on the narrow impacts of masking and social distancing on child speech, language, and social development, but there is an emerging literature on the impact of distance and hybrid education on preschool and school-age children. As described previously, this policy has dramatically reduced peer engagement and learning simply because children have not been together in person to nearly the same level as seen pre-pandemic. However, it is important to bear in mind that, as with communication development, optimal teaching is transactional because effective learning is developmental and teaching feedback that is attuned to a child's skill level is highly effective, especially in preschool, kindergarten, and primary grades.

Clearly, student-teacher attunement is much more difficult in distance and hybrid learning. Teacher monitoring of student engagement, attention, and lesson comprehension is problematic via virtual teaching platforms (e.g., Zoom or Google Meet). In a foundational way, seeing each student as an array on a screen is quite different than in an in-person, unmasked classroom. Even in masked, in-person teaching settings, it is far easier to scan the classroom for student engagement and attention than in a distance teaching environment, even when the latter is conducted without masks. This perspective on the advantages of in-person teaching has recently been supported by larger-than-expected drops in achievement across multiple grades, especially in early school years. This was seen in a recent systematic review of learning loss conducted by Donnelly and Patrinos (2021), which discussed several early studies that provide evidence of the impact of the COVID-19 pandemic on learning loss amongst students across a range of subjects, grade levels, and geographical regions.

### 2.3 Disproportionate impact of the pandemic on vulnerable populations

Preventative strategies aimed at reducing spread and risk of infection could potentially impact communication and speech and language development for all children. Given the disruptions in speech, language, and social cues resulting from mask wearing and social distancing and concomitant reductions in peer interactions, it is predictable that children from vulnerable populations are even more likely to be adversely affected.

### 2.3.1  Children with hearing loss

Children with hearing loss may be disproportionately affected by the COVID-19 pandemic. Hearing loss is a highly prevalent and undertreated condition that affects people of all ages (Lin et al. 2011; Chern and Golub 2019). In 2019, the CDC reported the prevalence of hearing loss to be 1.7 per every 1,000 babies screened (Centers for Disease Control and Prevention 2021a). Although masks have been deemed necessary in helping to prevent the spread of the COVID-19 virus, they create a barrier to visual cues and contribute to an unfavorable auditory environment, particularly for those with hearing loss.

Audiovisual integration is crucial for speech and language development in children. Masks create a physical barrier to visual cues provided through lip movements, cues that children with hearing loss especially depend on for both speech understanding and language learning. Around 4 months of age, infants tend to focus more on the speaker's eyes. However, by 6 months of age, they begin to shift their attention to the speaker's mouth. This is also when infants begin to enter the canonical babbling stage, in which they begin duplicating the lip and tongue movements of the speakers around them (Lewkowicz and Hansen-Tift 2012). In one eye-tracking study, the authors found a positive correlation between speech-reading accuracy and proportion of time that children from 5 to 8 years of age spent looking at the speaker's mouth during speech. They also found that children demonstrated a tendency to focus their attention on the speaker's mouth whilst speaking but watch the eyes when the speaker was not talking. Deaf children were more likely to employ this communicative pattern (also known as social tuning) than hearing children (Worster et al. 2018).

Masks not only provide a visual barrier but are also known to degrade the speech signal by serving as a low-pass filter, attenuating high frequencies that are important for speech perception. One study reported that the level of attenuation ranges from 3–4 decibels (dB) for simple medical masks and nearly 12 dB for N95 masks (Goldin et al. 2020). This especially impacts children with hearing loss, who already have difficulty with speech understanding compared to their normal hearing peers. One study found that under conditions involving background noise, speech understanding improved for those with severe to profound hearing loss when the speaker was wearing a transparent surgical mask as compared to an opaque mask. In contrast, those with normal hearing to moderate hearing loss performed equally as well between the cloth and transparent mask conditions (Atcherson et al. 2017). These findings demonstrate the fact that visual cues are particularly beneficial for individuals with hearing loss or for normal-hearing individuals in challenging auditory environments where sound is attenuated (i.e., mask wearing) or where there is significant background noise (Atcherson et al. 2017; Saunders et al. 2021).

Due to the need for social distancing during the COVID-19 pandemic, virtual (i.e., online) education has become much more prevalent. Although this has provided access to education where it would not have otherwise taken place (Lockee 2021), virtual education is not without its challenges, especially for children with hearing loss (Sher et al. 2020; Charney et al. 2021; Gordon et al. 2021; Schafer et al. 2021) and other vulnerable populations. So-called "Zoom fatigue" is a phenomenon that has been described as a general feeling of mental fatigue or exhaustion associated with overuse of virtual communication platforms, such as videoconferencing. This term was popularised during the beginning of the COVID-19 pandemic when the online videoconferencing software Zoom was commonly used for people to communicate whilst they were social distancing and staying home. The physical manifestations of "Zoom fatigue" may be similar to those of burnout, which include muscle tension, headaches, insomnia, and inattention (Salvagioni et al. 2017; White 2021). These symptoms are attributed to increased listening effort from difficulties interpreting non-verbal cues, poor audio/visual quality, audiovisual dyssynchrony, and/or overlapping speakers in large meetings whilst on virtual platforms (Sklar 2020).

Studies have shown that in a challenging listening environment (e.g., hearing loss, virtual meetings), individuals sustain a greater cognitive load and may more rapidly deplete their cognitive reserve, resulting in listening-related fatigue whilst learning (Bess et al. 2020; Hornsby et al. 2021). Research has demonstrated that individuals with hearing loss devote more cognitive resources to auditory processing at the expense of other cognitive processes, such as working memory (Pichora-Fuller and Singh 2006; Tun et al. 2009; Chern and Golub 2019; Sharma et al. 2021). Moreover, poor audio and video quality associated with videoconferencing further increases the necessity for visual cues. Studies have demonstrated that listeners rely more heavily on lip-reading as environmental and background noise increases (Vatikiotis-Bateson et al. 1998; Lansing and McConkie 2003). These difficult listening environments can disproportionately affect individuals with hearing loss, who already have difficulty with auditory perception, and can have downstream effects on learning (Bess et al. 2020; Hornsby et al. 2021).

Effective social communication (e.g., gestures, facial expressions) may also be inhibited by a virtual platform in which the head is framed in the centre of the screen, reducing access to "body language" and other subtle nonverbal cues. This setup may contribute to Zoom fatigue through the perceived need for over-exaggerated gestures (e.g., head nodding, thumbs up) to demonstrate what would have otherwise been more naturally and easily communicated in an in-person setting (Ramachandran 2021). This can be exacerbated further when members of a Zoom meeting choose to turn their cameras off. One study found that between three conditions (camera on without a mask, camera on with a mask, and camera off), speech understanding in typical-hearing individuals was worse in both the masked and camera-off conditions compared to the camera on with no mask condition (Giovanelli et al. 2021). Thus, individuals with hearing loss may be more greatly affected in these virtual settings, as they rely more heavily on lip reading and other gestures for comprehension compared to their normal hearing peers. Moreover, such limitations of remote learning (e.g., suboptimal audiovisual environment, decreased peer-learning opportunities, and social interactions) may be particularly problematic for young children with hearing loss who inherently have difficulty acquiring accurate phonological representations. Phonological representations, or mental representations of sounds that comprise words in spoken language, support not only speech and language development but literacy as well. It is well known that phonological encoding predicts later literacy development. Therefore, short-term adverse effects on speech and language development in hearing loss may be later associated with reading-related learning disabilities (Ehri et al. 2001).

### 2.3.2 Children with autism spectrum disorder

COVID restrictions present a distinct problem for children with autism spectrum disorder (ASD). All of the transactional impacts described previously are compounded by the reduced motivation for social communication that is a core feature of ASD (Camarata, 2014; American Psychiatric Association, 2013). Specifically, children with ASD require more salient cues and immediately contingent cues that are crucial for speech, language, and social learning in ASD (Koegel et al. 2016). Perhaps even more importantly, children with ASD also have a preference for predictability and routines.

Programmes that accommodate these needs in order to include children with ASD in the regular education setting can be completely undone by mask wearing, wherein teachers' and peers' faces are obscured and when the colours and patterns on the mask are in constant flux. It is not unusual for children with ASD to require weeks or even months of systematic, incremental behavioural support to interact with parents, teachers, and peers. Thus, COVID restrictions can have a disparate adverse impact on these students. It is also noteworthy that peer-assisted learning, social intervention, and other in-person learning opportunities are reduced or lost altogether. Children with ASD show a preference for engaging with screens and computers more than people, often stimming on these devices. Distance and hybrid learning then can prove especially debilitating because children with ASD are less likely to cooperate with didactic screen learning and will often prefer to activate favorite videos or video games when computer time is not restricted. As a result, Zoom learning and other forms of hybrid or distance learning may not only lead to reduced learning but actually derail gains made pre-pandemic.

### 2.3.3 Children from families with lower socioeconomic status

There is growing evidence that the learning of children from lower socioeconomic backgrounds has been disproportionately affected by the pandemic. One systematic review included studies showing significant disparate impact on loss of learning opportunities amongst vulnerable subgroups (Donnelly and Patrinos 2021). Another systematic review suggested that there was a negative effect of school closures on student achievement, particularly in younger students and those from families of lower socioeconomic status (Hammerstein et al. 2021). Researchers and education policymakers have speculated that this disparate impact arises from a cascade of risk factors associated with poverty that intensify the inhibitory learning effects arising from distance and hybrid learning. Access to newer computers that can support Zoom streaming, fast internet, and other infrastructure is often less available in addition to other well-known risk factors that were not the result of COVID-19 (e.g., reduced access to literacy materials, food insecurity).

The actual sources and causal linkages to these factors are not currently known, but there does appear to be a consistent, replicated finding that children from more disadvantaged backgrounds showed greater losses in achievement during COVID-19. This was most evident in preschool and early school-age children. Schnoor (2021) reported that minority students were likely to have parents who were considered essential workers and were unable to work at home. As a result, these parents were unable to provide the necessary supervision and support for their children to effectively engage in remote learning. Approximately 60% of low-income students (compared to 90% of high-income students) were regularly logging on for instruction. In schools with a predominantly Black and Hispanic student body, only 60% to 70% of students were regularly logging on for virtual learning. Minority students were more likely to experience learning loss compared to their white peers. The author suggested that this may have long-term academic, social, and economic effects on these individuals. Moreover, Schnoor suggests that remote learning has disrupted existing services and support systems originally aimed to help students stay in school and do well. These include cultivating relationships with faculty and engaging in after-school activities (Schnoor 2021). Clearly, the social and learning milieu associated with COVID-19 mitigation has had negative impacts on the educational outcomes of those in most need of educational supports.

## 2.4 Potential mitigation strategies

At the time of writing, there is no evidence that preventative strategies such as face mask usage or social distancing prevent or delay speech and language development in children (American Academy of Pediatrics 2022). However, not enough time has elapsed to make definitive conclusions, as longitudinal studies are needed to examine the impact of COVID-19 on paediatric speech and language development. Meanwhile, proactive measures and strategies can be implemented to mitigate any potential negative consequences of the pandemic on developing communication skills in children.

As mentioned previously, use of transparent masks has been shown to provide added visual cues to improve speech understanding, particularly for those with hearing loss (Atcherson et al. 2017). However, these transparent masks have also been shown to have the most attenuation of higher frequency sounds (i.e., greater than 8 dB) compared to other (i.e., surgical and cloth) masks (Corey et al. 2020). Consonants such as "s," "f," and "t" have higher frequencies. These sounds are essential for speech intelligibility and may be missed with use of such masks (Vitela et al. 2015). Optimising the visual and auditory environment is essential when attempting to remedy these attenuation effects, particularly in the classroom setting. The addition of personal amplification devices with headsets or lapel microphones when wearing clear/transparent masks can be a useful strategy to help offset any decrease in volume and intelligibility that may result from use of masks.

With the increase in remote learning and utilisation of virtual platforms (e.g., Zoom or Google Meet), new obstacles have emerged. This may include a distorted visual image or auditory signal as a result of disrupted internet connection and/or suboptimal equipment. Knowledge and awareness of all tools and strategies to help mitigate these potential barriers within virtual classrooms have become essential. Fortunately, most modern devices have built-in, high-quality microphones; however, there are additional ways of optimising the listening environment.

For instance, choosing a quiet environment to avoid disruptive background noise and utilising the mute function in group settings to avoid excess noise and/or participants speaking over each other may help enhance the overall virtual meeting experience. Employing the personal chat or "raise hand" functions when asking questions or commenting in real time is another viable strategy. Others have proposed following a pre-virtual meeting checklist to help set ground rules and expectations to ensure a mutual understanding of how the meeting will proceed. For example, participants may be asked to test audio and video prior to the meeting, turn on video (when appropriate), and utilise certain features (i.e., the chat function) to facilitate ease of communication. A designated chat moderator responsible for troubleshooting technical issues and addressing individual questions that arise may also be helpful (Ohnigian et al. 2021). Learners can opt to use headphones or other means of amplification, which may particularly benefit those with hearing loss. However, it is important that children with hearing loss still obtain appropriate treatment (i.e., hearing aids), as they may struggle in various in-person environments, such as those with background noise.

Interruptions and associated technical difficulties are frequent in the virtual meeting setting. As such, use of closed captioning can help prevent miscommunication. In recent years, auto-generated transcriptions in various media outlets (e.g., movie theaters) have become increasingly prevalent to promote inclusivity of individuals who are deaf or hard of hearing. Under Title III of the Americans with Disabilities Act (ADA) that went into effect in January 2017, movie theaters are required to have, maintain, and offer the equipment necessary to provide closed captioning and audio descriptions at moviegoers' requests (Department of Justice 2016).

Such optimisation of the audiovisual environment can help minimise the cognitive fatigue associated with these virtual platforms. Other strategies include taking more frequent breaks and employing smaller group sessions (i.e., breakout rooms). Promoting a safe learning environment (i.e., with psychological safety and community) by allowing time to welcome learners and ask them to introduce themselves may help participants become more comfortable in a virtual meeting setting. Ultimately, educators can leverage virtual platforms to create successful learning sessions for children. Multimedia learning has been known to promote student engagement and active learning of educational content (Davis and Norman 2016; Roberts 2018). Over a virtual platform, utilising supplemental videos, diagrams, and drawings may be even more crucial for effective education. This can provide access to speech and language learning opportunities to children as in-person education remains more limited during the COVID-19 pandemic. If these tools are utilised creatively and functionally, virtual learning can ultimately augment and elevate in-person speech and language education for children (Lockee 2021; Ohnigian et al. 2021).

Individuals involved in the speech and language development of children – including parents, teachers, and clinicians (speech-language pathologists, audiologists, otolaryngologists, paediatricians, etc.) – can employ these preventative strategies and bring awareness to the potential impact of the COVID-19 pandemic on communication. Medical providers and educators hold much of the responsibility in educating parents on these strategies. Parents have a crucial role in optimising the remote learning experience for children at home and providing early speech and language stimulation. When parents are at home with children, seeking to promote a healthy social environment can stimulate communication growth. For example, encouraging children to engage frequently with older siblings may result in a more expanded vocabulary, improved pragmatics, and other forms of language development. A proactive approach will help mitigate any potential negative impact of the pandemic on communication skills of children and may ultimately positively influence early childhood education and development through cultivation of novel learning modalities.

## 2.5 Future directions

With the advent of new variants of the virus such as the Delta and Omicron variants, it becomes increasingly unlikely that the SARS-CoV-2 virus will be completely eradicated. Indeed, scientists expect COVID-19 ultimately to become endemic. Although the virus will continue to circulate, people will gain enough immunity through vaccination and natural infections that there will be decreased transmissibility and significantly less COVID-19-associated hospitalisations and death (Feldscher 2021; Phillips 2021). Moreover, remote learning through virtual platforms will likely remain a fixture in child education. Although currently there are many limitations and difficulties associated with remote learning, technology will continue to improve such that virtual learning can eventually enhance the overall educational experience during the early years of speech and language development.

One such improvement is already underway and includes the option for closed captioning. Virtual meeting platforms such as Zoom and Google Meet have begun to provide options for auto-generated closed captions, which may help mitigate the challenging audiovisual environment for users, particularly those with hearing loss. When the auditory environment is optimised in these platforms, children with hearing loss may also benefit, as they have more consistent visual access to the speaker's mouth, can utilise headphones (or other assistive devices), and are able to adjust volume as needed.

During the COVID-19 pandemic, telehealth played a large role in helping patients avoid direct physical contact and minimise the risk of transmission of the infection whilst simultaneously maximising continuity of and access to healthcare. Telehealth has also ensured delivery of paediatric speech and language services during the pandemic. Pre-pandemic, this mode of delivery allowed access to speech and language services for those who live in rural areas, have limited transportation, or have other socioeconomic barriers to care. However, these same groups may also lack the internet and/or computer access required for telehealth. Telehealth can continue to mitigate the potential effect of COVID-19 on paediatric speech and language development and will prove beneficial during future healthcare crises.

The long-term impact of the COVID-19 pandemic on paediatric speech and language development is currently unknown. Recent COVID-19 publications include those examining the effect of masks on speech comprehension (Kolesnik et al. 2021; Marler and Ditton 2021), the effect of the pandemic on outpatient speech and language therapy (Tohidast et al. 2020), and the impact of the pandemic on infant and toddler development (Imboden et al. 2022). Other manuscripts have examined the impact of COVID-19 on individuals with hearing loss, notably difficulties with communication (Gordon et al. 2021; Schafer et al. 2021) and access to hearing healthcare (Pattisapu et al. 2020; Jenks et al. 2022). However, many of these publications are commentaries that speculate on the effect of COVID-19. Studies are needed to establish if the COVID-19 pandemic will have any long-term impact on paediatric speech and language development. Although at the time of writing this chapter, there were no studies that demonstrated such an impact, more time needs to elapse before researchers can conduct these longitudinal studies. Studies could usefully examine the impact of virtual learning (and associated decrease of in-person learning) on speech and language development, decreased social interactions on pragmatic and social communication development, and masks on decreased audiovisual integration (from lack of visual cues) and its effect on speech and language learning.

## 2.6 Summary

The long-term impact of the COVID-19 pandemic on the development of speech and language in children is currently unknown. Schools were closed for more than 168 million children worldwide for nearly an entire year due to COVID-19 lockdowns (UNICEF 2021). Approximately 1 in 7 (or 214 million) children globally missed over three fourths of their in-person learning in schools (UNESCO 2021). Widespread reduction of in-person education, social distancing measures, mask-wearing mandates, and virtual platforms for meetings and education were implemented for reducing risk of infection and containing the pandemic. Use of preventative strategies and increased awareness of possible communication difficulties in children, particularly in vulnerable populations, may mitigate potential negative consequences of these measures.

## References

American Academy of Pediatrics (2022). Do masks delay speech and language development? www.healthychildren.org/English/health-issues/conditions/COVID-19/Pages/Do-face-masks-interfere-with-language-development.aspx. Accessed 14 January 2022.

American Psychiatric Association (2013). *Diagnostic and statistical manual of mental disorders* (5th ed.). doi: 10.1176/appi.books.9780890425596.

Atcherson, S. R., Mendell, L. L., Baltimore, W. J., Patro, C., Lee, S., Pousson, M., & Spann, M. J. (2017). The effect of conventional and transparent surgical masks on speech understanding in individuals with and without hearing loss. *Journal of the American Academy of Audiology*, 28(1), 58–67.

Bess, F. H., Davis, H., Camarata, S., & Hornsby, B. W. Y. (2020). Listening-related fatigue in children with unilateral hearing loss. *Language, Speech, and Hearing Services in Schools*, 51(1), 84–97.

Bukowski, W. M., Buhrmester, D., & Underwood, M. K. (2011). Peer relations as a developmental context. In M. K. Underwood & L. H. Rosen (Eds.), *Social development: Relationships in infancy, childhood, and adolescence* (pp. 153–179). New York: Guilford Press.

Camarata, S. M. (1993). The application of naturalistic conversation training to speech production in children with speech disabilities. *Journal of Applied Behavior Analysis*, 26(2), 173–182.

Camarata, S. M. (2014). Early identification and early intervention in autism spectrum disorders: Accurate and effective? *International Journal of Speech-Language Pathology*, 16(1), 1–10. doi: 10.3109/17549507.2013.859732.

Camarata, S. M. (2017). *The intuitive parent: Why the best thing for your child is you*. New York: Penguin Random House.

Camarata, S. M. (2021). Naturalistic recast intervention. In A. L. Williams, S. McLeod, & R. J. McCauley (Eds.), *Interventions for speech sound disorders in children* (2nd ed., pp. 337–362). Baltimore: Brookes.

Centers for Disease Control and Prevention (2020). CDC releases indicators for dynamic school decision-making infographic. www.cdc.gov/media/releases/2020/p0915-dynamic-school-decision-making-infographic.html. Accessed 14 January 2022.

Centers for Disease Control and Prevention (2021a). Data and statistics about hearing loss in children. www.cdc.gov/ncbddd/hearingloss/data.html. Accessed 14 January 2022.

Centers for Disease Control and Prevention (2021b). Science brief: Community use of masks to control the spread of SARS-CoV-2. www.cdc.gov/coronavirus/2019-ncov/science/science-briefs/masking-science-sars-cov2.html. Accessed 14 January 2022.

Charney, S. A., Camarata, S. M., & Chern, A. (2021). Potential impact of the COVID-19 pandemic on communication and language skills in children. *Otolaryngology – Head and Neck Surgery*, 165(1), 1–2.

Chern, A., & Golub, J. S. (2019). Age-related hearing loss and dementia. *Alzheimer Disease and Associated Disorders*, 33(3), 285–290.

Cohen, D. (2018). *The development of play*. London: Routledge.

Corey, R. M., Jones, U., & Singer, A. C. (2020). Acoustic effects of medical, cloth, and transparent face masks on speech signals. *The Journal of the Acoustical Society of America*, 148(4), 2371–2375.

Curtin, S., Werker, J., & Yeung, H. (2021). Face-mask use and language development: Should I be worried? The International Congress of Infant Studies. https://infantstudies.org/face-mask-use-and-language-development-should-i-be-worried/. Accessed 14 January 2022.

Davis, G., & Norman, M. (2016). Principles of multimedia learning – center for teaching and learning. https://ctl.wiley.com/principles-of-multimedia-learning/. Accessed 14 January 2022.

Department of Justice (2016). Nondiscrimination on the basis of disability by public accommodations movie theaters; Movie captioning and audio description. www.ada.gov/regs2016/movie_rule.htm. Accessed 14 January 2022.

Donnelly, R., & Patrinos, H. A. (2021). Learning loss during Covid-19: An early systematic review. *Prospects*, 1–9. doi:10.1007/s11125-021-09582-6.

Dwyer, C., & Aubrey, A. (2020). CDC now recommends Americans voluntarily wear cloth masks in public. www.npr.org/sections/coronavirus-live-updates/2020/04/03/826219

824/president-trump-says-cdc-now-recommends-americans-wear-cloth-masks-in-public. Accessed 14 January 2022.

Education Week (2020). The coronavirus spring: The historic closing of U.S. schools (a timeline). www.edweek.org/leadership/the-coronavirus-spring-the-historic-closing-of-u-s-schools-a-timeline/2020/07. Accessed 14 January 2022.

Ehri, L. C., Nunes, S. R., Willows, D. M., Schuster, B. V., Yaghoub-Zadeh, Z., & Shanahan, T. (2001). Phonemic awareness instruction helps children learn to read: Evidence from the national reading panel's meta-analysis. *Reading Research Quarterly*, 36(3), 250–287.

Epstein, V. (2021). Masks and baby's speech development: As it turns out, it matters. https://parenting.kars4kids.org/masks-and-babys-speech-development-as-it-turns-out-it-matters/. Accessed 14 January 2022.

Erber, N. P. (1974). Effects of angle, distance, and illumination on visual reception of speech by profoundly deaf children. *Journal of Speech and Hearing Research*, 17(1), 99–112.

Feldscher, K. (2021). What will it be like when COVID-19 becomes endemic? www.hsph.harvard.edu/news/features/what-will-it-be-like-when-covid-19-becomes-endemic/. Accessed 14 January 2022.

Giovanelli, E., Valzolgher, C., Gessa, E., Todeschini, M., & Pavani, F. (2021). Unmasking the difficulty of listening to talkers with masks: Lessons from the COVID-19 pandemic. *i-Perception*, 12(2), 1–11.

Goldin, A., Weinstein, B., & Shiman, N. (2020). How do medical masks degrade speech reception? *The Hearing Review*, 27(5), 8–9.

Gordon, K. A., Daien, M. F., Negandhi, J., Blakeman, A., Ganek, H., Papsin, B., & Cushing, S. L. (2021). Exposure to spoken communication in children with cochlear implants during the COVID-19 lockdown. *JAMA Otolaryngology-Head & Neck Surgery*, 147(4), 368–376.

Hammerstein, S., König, C., Dreisörner, T., & Frey, A. (2021). Effects of COVID-19-related school closures on student achievement – A systematic review. *Frontiers in Psychology*, 12, 746289. doi:10.3389/fpsyg.2021.746289.

Hazlett, A. (2021). Do masks hurt speech development? It depends on the child. https://undark.org/2021/09/20/do-masks-hurt-speech-development-it-depends-on-the-kid/. Accessed 14 January 2022.

Hicks, C. B., & Ohde, R. N. (2005). Developmental role of static, dynamic, and contextual cues in speech perception. *Journal of Speech, Language, and Hearing Research*, 48(4), 960–974.

Hornsby, B. W. Y., Davis, H., & Bess, F. H. (2021). The impact and management of listening-related fatigue in children with hearing loss *Otolaryngologic Clinics of North America*, 54(6), 1231–1239.

Imboden, A., Sobczak, B. K., & Griffin, V. (2022). The impact of the COVID-19 pandemic on infant and toddler development. *Journal of the American Association of Nurse Practitioners*. doi:10.1097/jxx.0000000000000653.

Jenks, C. M., DeSell, M., & Walsh, J. (2022). Delays in infant hearing detection and intervention during the COVID-19 pandemic: Commentary. *Otolaryngology-Head and Neck Surgery*, 1945998211067728. doi:10.1177/01945998211067728.

Koegel, L. K., Ashbaugh, K., & Koegel, R. L. (2016). Pivotal response treatment. In R. Lang, T. B. Hancock, & N. N. Singh (Eds.), *Early intervention for young children with autism spectrum disorder* (pp. 85–112). Switzerland: Springer International Publishing AG.

Kolesnik, K., Bryan, D., Harley, W., Segeritz, P., Guest, M., Rajagopal, V., & Collins, D. J. (2021). Respiration mask waveguide optimisation for maximised speech intelligibility. *The Journal of the Acoustical Society of America*, 150(3), 2030–2039.

Lansing, C. R., & McConkie, G. W. (2003). Word identification and eye fixation locations in visual and visual-plus-auditory presentations of spoken sentences. *Perception and Psychophysics*, 65(4), 536–552.

Lense, M. D., & Camarata, S. (2020). PRESS-play: Musical engagement as a motivating platform for social interaction and social play in young children with ASD. *Music and Science*, 3. doi:10.1177/2059204320933080.

Lewkowicz, D. J. (2021). Masks can be detrimental to babies' speech and language development. www.scientificamerican.com/article/masks-can-be-detrimental-to-babies-speech-and-language-development1/. Accessed 15 January 2022.

Lewkowicz, D. J., & Hansen-Tift, A. M. (2012). Infants deploy selective attention to the mouth of a talking face when learning speech. *Proceedings of the National Academy of Sciences of the United States of America*, 109(5), 1431–1436.

Lin, F. R., Niparko, J. K., & Ferrucci, L. (2011). Hearing loss prevalence in the United States. *Archives of Internal Medicine*, 171(20), 1851–1852.

Lockee, B. B. (2021). Online education in the post-COVID era. *Nature Electronics*, 4(1), 5–6.

Marler, H., & Ditton, A. (2021). "I'm smiling back at you": Exploring the impact of mask wearing on communication in healthcare. *International Journal of Language and Communication Disorders*, 56(1), 205–214. doi:10.1111/1460-6984.12578.

Ohnigian, S., Richards, J. B., Monette, D. L., & Roberts, D. H. (2021). Optimizing remote learning: Leveraging Zoom to develop and implement successful education sessions. *Journal of Medical Education and Curricular Development*, 8, 238212052110207. doi:10.1177/23821205211020760.

Pattisapu, P., Evans, S. S., Noble, A. R., Norton, S. J., Ou, H. C., Sie, K. C. Y., & Horn, D. L. (2020). Defining essential services for deaf and hard of hearing children during the COVID-19 pandemic. *Otolaryngology-Head and Neck Surgery*, 163(1), 91–93. doi:10.1177/0194599820925058.

Phillips, N. (2021). The coronavirus is here to stay – here's what that means. www.nature.com/articles/d41586-021-00396-2. Accessed 15 January 2022.

Pichora-Fuller, M. K., & Singh, G. (2006). Effects of age on auditory and cognitive processing: Implications for hearing aid fitting and audiologic rehabilitation. *Trends in Amplification*, 10(1), 29–59.

Ramachandran, V. (2021). Four causes for "Zoom fatigue" and their solutions. https://news.stanford.edu/2021/02/23/four-causes-zoom-fatigue-solutions/. Accessed 15 January 2022.

Roberts, D. (2018). The engagement agenda, multimedia learning and the use of images in higher education lecturing: Or, how to end death by PowerPoint. *Journal of Further and Higher Education*, 42(7), 969–985.

Salvagioni, D. A. J., Melanda, F. N., Mesas, A. E., González, A. D., Gabani, F. L., & Andrade, S. M. (2017). Physical, psychological and occupational consequences of job burnout: A systematic review of prospective studies. *PLoS One*, 12(10). doi:10.1371/JOURNAL.PONE.0185781.

Sameroff, A. (2009). The transactional model. In A. Sameroff (Ed.), *The transactional model of development: How children and contexts shape each other* (pp. 3–21). Washington, DC: American Psychological Association.

Saunders, G. H., Jackson, I. R., & Visram, A. S. (2021). Impacts of face coverings on communication: An indirect impact of COVID-19. *International Journal of Audiology*, 60(7), 495–506.

Schafer, E. C., Dunn, A., & Lavi, A. (2021). Educational challenges during the pandemic for students who have hearing loss. *Language, Speech, and Hearing Services in Schools*, 52(3), 889–898.

Schnoor, A. (2021). Impact of COVID-19 school lockdowns on low-income and minority children. https://sites.suffolk.edu/jhbl/2021/02/01/impact-of-covid-19-school-lockdowns-on-low-income-and-minority-children/. Accessed 15 January 2022.

Sharma, R. K., Chern, A., & Golub, J. S. (2021). Age-related hearing loss and the development of cognitive impairment and late-life depression: A scoping overview. *Seminars in Hearing*, 42(1), 10–25. doi:10.1055/s-0041-1725997.

Sher, T., Stamper, G. C., & Lundy, L. B. (2020). COVID-19 and vulnerable population with communication disorders. *Mayo Clinic Proceedings*, 95(9), 1845–1847.

Sklar, J. (2020). "Zoom fatigue" is taxing the brain. Here's why that happens. www.nationalgeographic.com/science/2020/04/coronavirus-zoom-fatigue-is-taxing-the-brain-here-is-why-that-happens/. Accessed 15 January 2022.

Smith, P. K., & Connolly, K. (1972). Patterns of play and social interaction in pre-school children. In N. B. Jones (Ed.), *Ethological studies of child behaviour* (pp. 65–96). New York: Cambridge University Press.

Takahashi, D. Y., Fenley, A. R., & Ghazanfar, A. A. (2016). Early development of turn-taking with parents shapes vocal acoustics in infant marmoset monkeys. *Philosophical Transactions of the Royal Society B: Biological Sciences*, 371(1693). doi:10.1098/rstb.2015.0370.

Tohidast, S. A., Mansuri, B., Bagheri, R., & Azimi, H. (2020). Provision of speech-language pathology services for the treatment of speech and language disorders in children during the COVID-19 pandemic: Problems, concerns, and solutions. *International Journal of Pediatric Otorhinolaryngology*, 138, 110262. doi:10.1016/j.ijporl.2020.110262.

Tun, P. A., McCoy, S., & Wingfield, A. (2009). Aging, hearing acuity, and the attentional costs of effortful listening. *Psychology and Aging*, 24(3), 761–766.

UNESCO (2021). COVID 19 and school closures: One year of education disruption. https://data.unicef.org/resources/one-year-of-covid-19-and-school-closures/#:~:text=Children cannot afford another year of school closures.,at pre-primary%2C primary%2C lower and upper secondary levels. Accessed 15 January 2022.

UNICEF (2021). COVID-19: Schools for more than 168 million children globally have been completely closed for almost a full year, says UNICEF. www.unicef.org/press-releases/schools-more-168-million-children-globally-have-been-completely-closed. Accessed 15 January 2022.

Van der Stoep, N., Van der Stigchel, S., Nijboer, T. C., & Van der Smagt, M. J. (2016). Audiovisual integration in near and far space: Effects of changes in distance and stimulus effectiveness. *Experimental Brain Research*, 234(5), 1175–1188.

Vatikiotis-Bateson, E., Eigsti, I. M., Yano, S., & Munhall, K. G. (1998). Eye movement of perceivers during audiovisual speech perception. *Perception and Psychophysics*, 60(6), 926–940.

Vitela, A. D., Monson, B. B., & Lotto, A. J. (2015). Phoneme categorization relying solely on high-frequency energy. *The Journal of the Acoustical Society of America*, 137(1), EL65–EL70. doi:10.1121/1.4903917.

Vogel, G. (2020). How Sweden wasted a "rare opportunity" to study coronavirus in schools. www.science.org/content/article/how-sweden-wasted-rare-opportunity-study-coronavirus-schools. Accessed 15 January 2022.

White, T. (2021). Zoom fatigue: Symptoms, causes, coping tips, healthline. www.health line.com/health/zoom-fatigue. Accessed 15 January 2022.

Worster, E., Pimperton, H., Ralph-Lewis, A., Monroy, L., Hulme, C., & MacSweeney, M. (2018). Eye movements during visual speech perception in deaf and hearing children. *Language Learning*, 68(Suppl 1), 159–179.

# 3

# TELEPRACTICE IN CHILD SPEECH-LANGUAGE PATHOLOGY DURING COVID-19

*Megan Overby*

## 3.1 Introduction

Paediatric speech-language disorders are a significant global issue. For example, in Australia at least 474,000 schoolchildren (Commonwealth of Australia Community Affairs References Committee 2014) and 20% of preschoolers (Reilly et al. 2010) are reported to have communication impairment. In the United States, more than one million children receive school-based speech-language services (American Speech-Language-Hearing Association (ASHA) 2020a), whilst in China, at least 3% of 3-year-olds have speech and language development delay (Fan et al. 2021; Jiang 2020). Speech-language services are crucial to the well-being of these children who, without appropriate and timely intervention, may experience adverse educational consequences, poor social outcomes, and/or reduced quality of life as sequelae to their disorder(s) (Tohidast et al. 2020; Johnson et al. 1999). These negative consequences are pervasive. For example, 50%–100% of children with preschool speech-language disorder have later academic difficulties (see Lewis et al. [2000] for review). Childhood speech impairment may have emotional and social consequences that limit the child's interactions and participation with others across the lifespan (Hitchcock et al. 2015; McCormack et al. 2009). If left untreated during childhood, some disorders may worsen or develop into chronic, lifelong communication difficulties (Rosenbaum and Simon 2016).

Prior to COVID-19, the majority of children with speech-language impairment received services for these communication difficulties through a traditional, in-person delivery model (Kollia and Tsiamtsiouris 2021). A speech-language pathologist (SLP) would deliver services in person in the child's home or in an office based in a clinic, hospital, or private practice setting. Only 1.6%–9% of

DOI: 10.4324/9781003257318-3

global paediatric speech-language services were provided via telepractice delivery (ASHA 2020b; Fong et al. 2020; Tucker 2012), which is the delivery of speech-language services via telecommunications technology (ASHA n.d.) inclusive of, for example, phone calls or computer-based technologies such as interactive video-conferencing over a digital network connection (Grogan-Johnson et al. 2011). Traditional in-person delivery of services was typically preferred over telepractice by both SLPs and children's caregivers (Khoza-Shangase et al. 2021).

There were many reasons why telepractice was not as commonly used as in-person service delivery when providing speech-language services to children before the pandemic. SLPs lacked the requisite skills needed to troubleshoot frequent technology-based problems (e.g., audio or visual breakdowns) encountered in telepractice (McGill and Fiddler 2021; Overby and Baft-Neff 2017). Clinicians needed to acquire skill and experience in adapting in-person materials to telepractice instruction (Overby 2018). Telepractice was further hampered by a lack of reliable technology infrastructure and by technology-based problems such as limited access to the internet in rural areas, outdated infrastructure (e.g., slow connectivity), and/or shared internet amongst family members or housing units (McGill and Fiddler 2021; Mohan et al. 2017).

Academic training in telepractice applications was also largely lacking. In the United States and territories, only 36%–41% of surveyed graduate programmes reported offering such training to graduate students (Grogan-Johnson et al. 2015), and only 7.2% of 293 SLP surveyed telepractitioners had any telepractice training in graduate school (ASHA 2016) (see Figure 3.1). Before the pandemic, many clinicians did not adopt telepractice because they anticipated this type of service delivery would lack the intimacy needed to establish client rapport (Freckmann et al. 2017), which is especially important when working with children. Other perceived obstacles to telepractice included the absence of tactile cueing or direct manipulation of the client's articulators (Coufal et al. 2018; Freckmann et al. 2017) and limited funding for technology, personnel, and training (Sanchez et al. 2019; Tucker 2012).

## 3.2  Paediatric telepractice growth during COVID-19

However, after the declaration of the pandemic in March 2020, many SLPs had to shift the bulk of their paediatric speech-language services from an in-person format to a telepractice form of service delivery. Clinic offices were suddenly closed, and at various times, government regulations prohibited in-person contact except for essential workers. This meant that telepractice was now a crucial and important option for providing paediatric clinical services in a safe and socially responsible manner, despite the aforementioned concerns and perceived obstacles to its widespread implementation.

In the United States, telepractice had been used by only 5.1% of school-based SLPs before the pandemic, but 91.5% of these SLPs switched to telepractice by

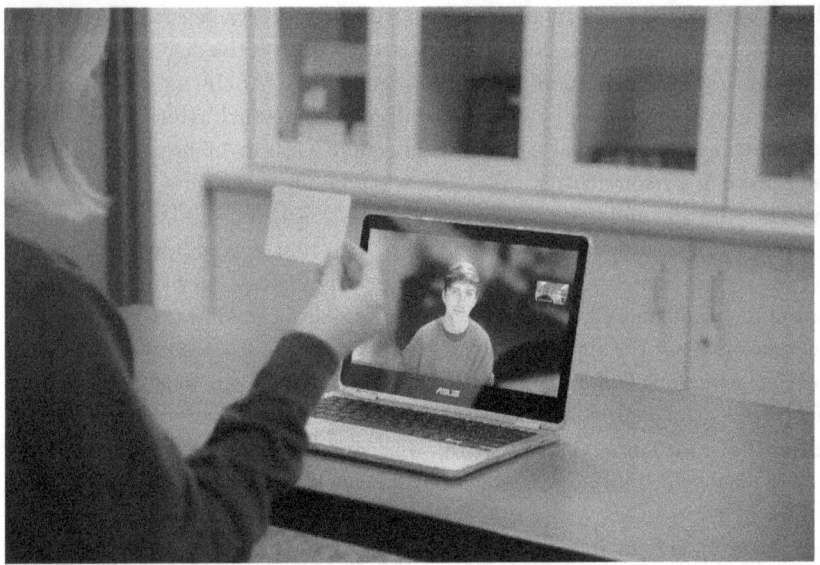

**FIGURE 3.1**   Student clinician in telepractice

October 2020 (ASHA 2020b). Similarly, approximately 80% of paediatric SLPs in India (N=255) and Croatia (N=84) were using telepractice at the start of the COVID-19 pandemic (Aggarwal et al. 2021; Kraljevic et al. 2020). Despite such increases, telepractice adoption in some areas of the world was not robust (Fong et al. 2020) and, in some cases, was even absent (Kraljevic et al. 2020). For instance, in Turkey, a survey of SLPs (N=82) reported they were not providing any therapy at all to child clients during the pandemic, and nearly all (99%) of the SLPs had not had any telepractice education (Aktürk and Toğram 2021). In Western Kenya, most therapy continued to be in person, though services were significantly curtailed, and alternative delivery options are just now being considered (Gibson et al. 2020).

The switch to telepractice during COVID-19 appears to have occurred where telepractice was already well established or accepted by SLPs as a viable service model, technology infrastructure could be quickly expanded, and/or government agencies and business endeavors coordinated to overcome technology-based barriers and licensing regulations (Campbell and Goldstein 2021a; Fong et al. 2020; McGill and Fiddler 2021). In addition, recent technology advancements in mobile communication devices, improvements in synchronous electronic communication (particularly in the availability of many options for Health Insurance Portability and Accountability Act compliant videoconferencing), and the increased availability of high-speed broadband connectivity created new opportunities and expanded opportunities for telepractice adoption (Campbell and Goldstein 2021a).

For at least some paediatric SLPs, telepractice will continue to be a major form of service delivery to children with speech-language needs, even after the pandemic crisis is over. In a recent survey of 293 SLPs (93% in the United States; 7% outside the United States), only 8% of participants indicated they would not provide telepractice services beyond the pandemic (Campbell and Goldstein 2021b), and similar trends have been reported by SLPs in Quebec (Macoir et al. 2021), India (Aggarwal et al. 2021), and Australia (Filbay et al. 2021). Telepractice is increasingly being covered by insurance providers, suggesting there may be a financial incentive by third-party payers to cover at least some of the costs of telepractice-based services. In coming years, the COVID-19 pandemic may become endemic (Hunter 2020), implying an ongoing need for telepractice as a major service delivery option for SLPs.

## 3.3 Paediatric telepractice implementation during COVID-19

The increase in telepractice as a service delivery method during COVID-19 led researchers to study the ways in which telepractice was now being implemented. A study of 1,109 school-based SLPs in the United States found that the most frequent form (66.9%) of telepractice service during the pandemic was preparing packets for parents to work with their children (Tambyraja et al. 2021). The authors speculated that provision of packets may have allowed clinicians to successfully address therapy objectives when parents cancelled sessions or when video-conferencing technology proved too difficult; attend to the particulars of the child's Individualized Education Plan (IEP); and meet the requirements of Free and Appropriate Education. Tambyraja and colleagues found that the second most common (63.8%) implementation of telepractice service delivery by school-based SLPs was the provision of individual or group telepractice services using computer-based technologies, the most frequent of which were Zoom (66.6%) and Google Hangouts (40.9%). Laptops or desktops were the most common (72%) hardware used during the pandemic. Participants used, on average, at least three types of technology, and the number of technologies used was positively correlated with a clinician's years of experience. Similar findings were reported in a survey of 259 SLPs in the United States (Campbell and Goldstein 2021a), in which Zoom was reported to be the most frequently used (78%) platform, followed by FaceTime (21%).

Similar findings were also found by Aggarwal and colleagues (2021) about SLPs' use of telepractice in India during the pandemic. Eighty-four surveyed clinicians, 85% of whom provided services to children, reported that the most common (82%) platform used was the WhatsApp video calling feature, although SLPs often used more than a single platform. The authors explain that WhatsApp is ubiquitous in India because it is free and easy to use and is a common way for healthcare providers to communicate with clients and the public. Zoom was the second most common platform used, possibly because it offers a free 40-minute video call. Facebook was used least often because clinicians had to either access their personal account or create a new professional-only one. Therapy sessions were typically in an individual setting. A facilitator was utilised for 44% of the sessions to ensure the session went as planned. (A facilitator is an adult [often a parent or caregiver] who can assist the client in following the clinician's directions, provide tactile cueing, offer the client emotional support, and/or ensure the client attends the session.)

In Iceland, 30 SLPs (most of whom provided paediatric services) were surveyed about the platforms used to provide telepractice services during COVID-19 (Crowe et al. 2021). Similar to findings from other researchers, most SLPs used more than one platform. The most commonly used platform in Iceland was Kara Connect, though seven others were also used (Zoom, Microsoft Teams, Skype, Facebook Messenger, video conference via Saga [an electronic medical-records software], Webex, and Google Meet). The choice of platform depended on what was provided by the SLPs' workplace.

According to Campbell and Goldstein (2021a), some paediatric SLPs reported using additional devices such as another computer, tablet, or cellphone when delivering services by telepractice and may have used external microphones and/or headphones as well (see Figure 3.2). Some (41%) client families also used multiple devices (computers, tablets, etc.). Despite the use of multiple devices

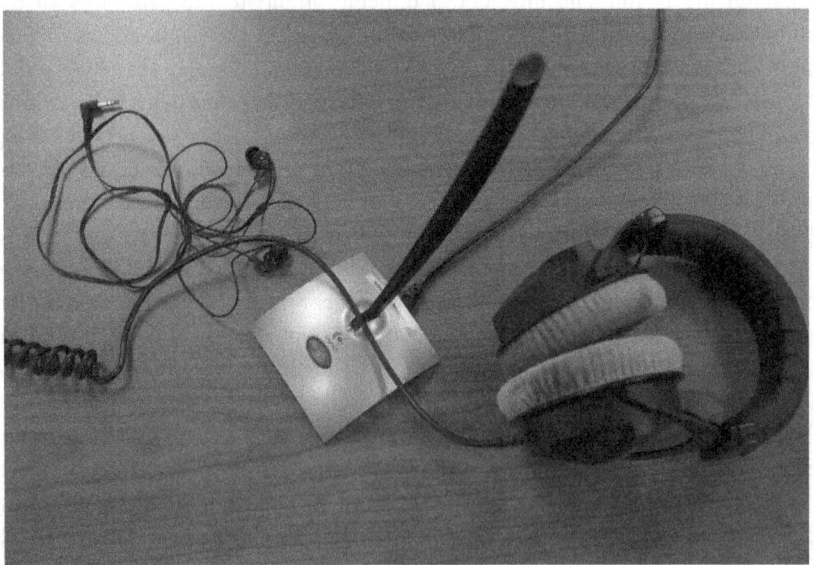

**FIGURE 3.2**   External components in telepractice (earbuds, external mic, and professional headphones)

and platforms by clinicians and client families, lack of reliable and consistent connectivity was a common experience for SLPs and clients alike.

During the pandemic, many parents were able to be remotely trained to help provide speech-language services to their child (United States Government Accountability Office (GAO) 2020). Although parent engagement increased for some children with parents being more directly involved with their child's therapy, there were disparities with some children not receiving consistent parental support at home (Halls-Mill et al. 2021). In telepractice, an SLP might instruct a parent on the level of cueing to provide when producing a word or how to provide assistance in tactile cueing and manipulate the child's mouth to aid in speech sound production.

Parent satisfaction with training programmes provided by telepractice during COVID-19 was broadly encouraging. In Iran, 336 caregivers of children with autism spectrum disorder participated in a two-month long online training course to acquire the education, practical advice, and guidance for implementing individualised learning plans for their child during the COVID-19 lockdown (Samadi et al. 2020). Training included structured teaching approaches, behavioural management, and environmental modifications appropriate to the caregiver's child. At the end of the training, 61% of the caregivers rated online training courses positively, whereas only 7.4% of them had expressed a positive view of online training courses at the start of the course. In Hong Kong, parents were also moderately satisfied with the efficacy of telepractice for their children during COVID-19 (Lam et al. 2021). Based on a 5-point Likert scale from 1 (i.e., strongly disagree) to 5 (i.e., strongly agree), the mean rating of telepractice efficacy during COVID-19 by parents (N=85) of children with speech-language impairment was 3.48. Parents nevertheless believed telepractice to be less effective than in-person delivery.

Clinician satisfaction with online parental training programmes during COVID-19 was also encouraging. A study of 106 clinicians from the United States and Canada revealed a majority of the clinicians successfully adapted the Lidcombe Program (Harris et al. 2002) for children who stutter from the traditional in-person delivery format to telepractice (Santayana et al. 2021), supporting prior research on the practicality and viability of a videoconference-based Lidcombe Program service delivery model (e.g., O'Brian et al. 2014). A majority (73%) of clinicians said observing the parents in treatment sessions (a component of the Lidcombe Program) was easy, and 64% said they experienced no difficulty demonstrating to parents via videoconferencing how to implement the Lidcombe Program treatment.

Parent conferences with the child's SLP appeared to be facilitated by telepractice technology. For example, under the Individuals with Disabilities Act (2004), the team responsible for implementing the child's IEP must meet at least once a year to review the IEP and make needed changes based on the child's progress and current needs (United States Department of Education 2021). Because these meetings were conducted by phone or videoconferencing during the pandemic, they were more efficient for parents than the pre-pandemic in-person meetings were (GAO 2020). Parents could now attend these meetings from their home or office. In addition, using the phone or videoconferencing meant that both parents could now participate in conference, whereas only one parent might have been able to do so before the pandemic due to scheduling and/or childcare concerns.

School districts responded to the pandemic in several ways, including encouraging SLPs to working collaboratively with general education teachers so as not to give the student excessive or duplicative work or overwhelm the families (GAO 2020). For example, a math teacher might be encouraged to give the child fewer math assignments so as to allow more time for related services such as speech-language pathology. However, some districts provided more resources and support to general education teachers than to SLPs, leaving SLPs with little consistent direction (Sylvan et al. 2020). Other school districts worked with SLPs to modify the child's IEP goals to be more manageable within a telepractice format, whilst some school districts considered good faith efforts by the child's SLP to provide therapy services to be sufficient. Some school districts provided mobile Wi-Fi hotspots, free laptops, and other devices to families of children with speech-language needs, whilst encouraging clinicians to use a variety of telepractice strategies such as texting and emailing.

Other benefits of widespread adoption of telepractice included providing services to children who were geographically remote or who had difficulty obtaining in-person therapy due to travel time to the SLP's office or school. Teenage clients were more apt to participate in therapy when not in their peer environment (Crowe et al. 2021), and some SLPs regarded their increased skills and knowledge in telepractice application as an unexpected benefit of the COVID-19 public health situation (Sylvan et al. 2020). Another major advantage of telepractice was the perceived improved safety of this type of service delivery format, which allowed SLPs to work with their clients without fear of transmission of the COVID-19 virus (Kollia and Tsiamtsiouris 2021).

## 3.4 Barriers to paediatric telepractice during COVID-19

Despite the successes of telepractice and the rapid technological improvements experienced in many parts of the world during COVID-19, there were barriers to implementing this form of service delivery. Some barriers, such as poor technical support or outdated infrastructure (see McGill and Fiddler [2021] for review), which had been present before the pandemic, continued to interfere with telepractice use. For example, some SLPs reported ongoing concerns with audio quality (Halls-Mill et al. 2021) as well as areas of limited connectivity, access to technology, and families' discomfort with this method of service delivery (Campbell and Goldstein 2021a). Although Tambyraja et al. (2021) found that many (45.3%) school districts provided their SLP employees with the necessary hardware to conduct telepractice, 34.5% of their survey of 1,109 participants were provided with no resources at all from their school district. Similarly, a survey of 145 SLPs in the United States, 60% of whom were based in schools, revealed that a dearth of appropriate equipment and materials was the most frequently encountered barrier by SLPs to reliable and accessible telepractice services during the pandemic (Kollia and Tsiamtsiouris 2021).

Online assessment of speech-language needs was challenging because appropriate online assessment tools are limited, and toys and objects normally used for in-person therapy did not easily translate to telepractice use (Kollia and Tsiamtsiouris 2021). Using digital assessment tools often requires the purchase of a user license as well as two devices (e.g., iPads), and so use of these tools may be costly for an SLP or organisation (Curcio et al. 2020). Furthermore, though digital in form, most of these assessments are intended for in-person evaluations and are not normed for telepractice administration. Curcio and colleagues recommend that a hybrid approach (i.e., a combination of in-person and telepractice delivery formats) to assessment is probably best practice during the pandemic, though masking and social distancing should be enforced during the in-person portion of the assessment.

In addition to a lack of technology infrastructure support, some school districts failed to provide sufficient guidance and/or district policy to SLPs initiating telepractice (GAO 2020). School districts were generally unprepared to assist SLPs, having no contingency plan for a health emergency and little understanding of the job requirements and demands (Sylvan et al. 2020). Similar problems were reported by SLPs in Iceland, where it was said that the most frequent source of support was from colleagues, with only 10 out of 30 SLPs stating they received support or advice from their employers (Crowe et al. 2021). When schools closed and went to online or remote learning, there was often no consistent school policy to assist SLPs about how speech-language services were to be delivered in this new environment, leaving scheduling and implementation up to the individual clinician. Some schools with remote learning also shortened their school day, making it difficult for clinicians to provide all the services described in the child's IEP within the time allotted for teaching. Some clinicians found the lack of consistent school policy supporting telepractice led to confusion and workload increases (Halls-Mill et al. 2021). Sometimes, a school-level administrator was the primary decision maker about the platforms to be used for telepractice, whilst in other cases, SLPs received direction from central administration. Because some SLPs work in different schools, and sometimes in different school districts, these differences in schools' decision-making policy sometimes resulted in duplicative work or workload inefficiencies.

Other barriers to providing therapy during COVID-19 included children's limitations with home Wi-Fi access (70.4%), poor attendance (68.8%) at therapy sessions, and low levels of children's engagement during therapy (64.9%) (Tambyraja et al. 2021). Similar findings were reported by Campbell and Goldstein

(2021a). Even if a child's family did have Wi-Fi access, there may have been data limits or a need to share resources (e.g., hardware, internet connectivity) with other family members. These barriers were notable for SLPs trying to provide telepractice speech-language services to children for whom English was not the child's primary language, children with complex needs, and/or children from a low socioeconomic background (GAO 2020; Young and Robinson 2020). Because families with limited English proficiency and/or low socioeconomic status experienced a disproportionate impact of lack of access to broadband, internet, computers, and other digital technologies during the pandemic, it was challenging to explain to family members how to navigate remote technology even when translators were available (Young and Robinson 2020). Consequently, many families with limited English or who were from a low socioeconomic background could not provide their child with needed speech-language at-home practice. Despite these reported challenges, there are comparatively little data available about telepractice efficacy for many limited English or diverse communities (Staley et al. 2020), and future study of the appropriate use of telepractice to these often underserved populations is critical. Additional information is specifically needed about the acceptability and efficacy of telepractice and unique barriers experienced within limited English and diverse communities.

Accessing speech-language services by telepractice was especially difficult for children with complex needs (GAO 2020; Halls-Mill et al. 2021; Young and Robinson 2020). This was due to the inability to provide needed appropriate positioning of the child (which may have been difficult for parents to attain and maintain), little access to augmentative and alternative communication devices that they used in school to help them communicate, and/or the specific IEP goals written for implementation within a school environment. Children with complex needs often needed physical (hands-on) cueing, which was not possible in telepractice service delivery unless a parent or facilitator were capable of this task (Kollia and Tsiamtsiouris 2021). In addition, because some parents of children with complex communication also had to coordinate other therapy sessions for their child (e.g., occupational therapy, physical therapy), they experienced a significant degree of difficulty scheduling telepractice sessions for their child's communication needs.

Similar problems were reported in providing telepractice services to at-risk children. These were children who were not eligible for IEP-based special education direct services but had been receiving in-person, prevention-based SLP services via consultation with the child, the child's family, or the child's teacher. However, after the pandemic was declared, SLPs found some districts discouraged clinicians from providing prevention-based services or supporting at-risk children (Sylvan et al. 2020). Although some SLPs continued to serve these children through consultation with teachers and/or providing parents with packets of therapy-related material, many SLPs did not have the resources or time to continue their same pre-pandemic level of involvement with this population.

Some parents felt overwhelmed by the number of programme-related responsibilities they were expected to undertake during the pandemic, which ranged from helping the clinician monitor and maintain their child's behaviour during therapy to assisting the SLP to achieve particular objectives within the therapy session (GAO 2020). Low levels of parent engagement and no-shows for therapy during the pandemic meant some of the efforts and planning by SLPs could not be realised, adversely impacting student progress and creating additional workload/ time pressures for clinicians. Some parents may have had difficulty participating in therapy because they lacked sufficient flexibility in their schedules, having to work from home and/or care for other children at home (Tambyraja et al. 2021). However, Tambyraja and colleagues also found that more experienced SLPs had more engaged students in therapy who were more likely to attend therapy sessions than did SLPs with less experience.

According to ASHA (2020b), approximately half (56%) of SLPs consider telepractice to be challenging. For some SLPs, large caseload size and time pressures during the pandemic interfered with successful implementation of telepractice (Farquharson et al. 2021). Many SLPs have experienced higher workloads but, despite feeling underappreciated at times, still advocated for their clients and for needed resources (Sylvan et al. 2020). SLPs with larger caseloads had more difficulty with no-shows and therapy cancellations, in successfully contacting parents, and with managing Wi-Fi technology issues than did SLPs with smaller caseload sizes. Although caseload size is often a significant predictor of SLPs' job satisfaction (e.g., Blood et al. 2002; Caesar and Wolf Nelson 2008), SLPs' job satisfaction during COVID-19 revealed that time pressures, not caseload size, were significantly related to job satisfaction (Farquharson et al. 2021). Farquharson and colleagues further reported that whilst many SLPs (48%) described a decline in job satisfaction during the pandemic, a nearly equal percentage (45%) reported no change in job satisfaction.

If telepractice is to continue to evolve in post-pandemic times, additional research is needed about the barriers and the potential solutions to this form of service delivery (Campbell and Goldstein 2021b). More training in telepractice will aid acceptance of this form of service delivery (Fong et al. 2020) and potentially aid SLPs in developing more proficient telepractice skills (Hao et al. 2021; Kollia and Tsiamtsiouris 2021; Tohidast et al. 2020). Additional consideration will need to be given to expanding third-party repayment for telepractice services, consistent regulations for licensure, and establishing recommended technology standards for telepractice (Campbell and Goldstein 2021; Tohidast et al. 2020).

## 3.5 Summary

Due to advancements in technology, the current state of telepractice delivery for paediatric speech-language services is different from how it was before the pandemic (Campbell and Goldstein 2021a). Problems such as limited internet access and slow connectivity remain but are less serious than they used to be. The prevalence and easy access to multiple videoconferencing platforms have meant that telepractice can now be implemented in many parts of the world. In addition, platform options are now so efficient that users incur little expense. Consequently, many SLPs using telepractice now frequently use more than one computer-based technology and/or device.

Parent involvement in their child's speech-language therapy process increased notably as a result of increased telepractice adoption, and parent conferences were facilitated due to the ease of scheduling. However, some parents felt overwhelmed by the burden of additional programme-related responsibilities, and some parents were unavailable to assist their child because of work demands. School districts were largely unprepared to assist SLPs in the implementation of telepractice and often did not offer clinicians important technological support or guidance, though many districts made efforts to provide families with free laptops or teacher consultation services.

Even though SLPs' knowledge and skills increased from expanded telepractice adoption, telepractice was challenging to deliver to at-risk children as well as children who had complex communication needs, limited English, and/or who came from a low socioeconomic background. For many SLPs, the increase in telepractice as a service delivery option meant an increase in the perceived time pressures associated with their job. Despite the problems encountered with telepractice during the pandemic, it is likely that high levels of telepractice use will continue into the future.

## References

Aggarwal, K., Patel, R., & Ravi, R. (2021). Uptake of telepractice among speech-language therapists following COVID-19 pandemic in India. *Speech, Language and Hearing*, 24(4), 228–340.

Aktürk, S., & Toğram, B. (2021). Investigation of services provided by speech and language pathologists during COVID-19 pandemic: Turkey sample. Conference poster. https://14thcongress.logopedists.gr/posters/178Poster.pdf. Accessed 28 December 2021.

American Speech-Language-Hearing Association (2016). 2016 SIG 18 telepractice services survey results. www.asha.org/siteassets/practice-portal/telepractice/2016-telepractice-survey.pdf. Accessed 28 December 2021.

American Speech-Language-Hearing Association (2020a). ASHA: How to help children with speech and language disorders in virtual and modified in-person classroom settings. www.asha.org/News/2020/How-to-Help-Children-With-Speech-and-Language-Disorders-in-Virtual-and-Modified-In-Person-Classroom-Settings/. Accessed 28 December 2021.

American Speech-Language-Hearing Association (2020b). COVID-19 tracker survey. www.asha.org/research/memberdata/covid-19-tracker-survey/. Accessed 28 December 2021.

American Speech-Language Hearing Association (n.d.). Teletpractice. www.asha.org/practice-portal/professional-issues/telepractice/. Accessed 28 December 2021.

Blood, G. W., Ridenour, J. S., Thomas, E. A., Qualls, C. D., & Hammer, C. S. (2002). Predicting job satisfaction among speech-language pathologists working in public schools. *Language, Speech, and Hearing Services in Schools*, 33(4), 282–290.

Caesar, L. G., & Wolf Nelson, N. (2008). Perceptions of job stress and satisfaction among school-based SLPs: Challenges versus rewards. *SIG 13 Perspectives on Swallowing and Swallowing Disorders (Dysphagia)*, 9(4), 126–134.

Campbell, D., & Goldstein, H. (2021a). Evolution of telehealth technology, evaluations, and therapy: Effects of the COVID-19 pandemic on pediatric speech-language pathology services. *American Journal of Speech-Language Pathology*, 1–16. https://doi.org/10.1044/2021_AJSLP-21-00069.

Campbell, D., & Goldstein, H. (2021b). Genesis of a new generation of telepractitioners: The COVID-19 pandemic and pediatric speech-language pathology services. *American Journal of Speech-Language Pathology*, 30(5), 2143–2154.

Commonwealth of Australia Community Affairs References Committee (2014). Prevalence of different types of speech, language and communication disorders and speech pathology services in Australia. Parliament of Australia. www.aph.gov.au/Parliamentary_Business/Committees/Senate/Community_Affairs/Speech_Pathology/Report. Accessed 28 December 2021.

Coufal, K., Parham, D., Jakubowitz, M., Howell, C., & Reyes, J. (2018). Comparing traditional service delivery and telepractice for speech sound production using a functional outcome measure. *American Journal of Speech-Language Pathology*, 27(1), 82–90.

Crowe, K., Másdóttir, T., & Einarsdóttir, J. (2021). Service delivery and the use of telepractice during the COVID-19 pandemic in Iceland. *Perspectives of the ASHA Special Interest Groups: SIG 17 Global Issues in Communication Sciences and Related Disorders*, 6(6), 1786–1799.

Curcio, S., Nixon, S., & Robinson, T. (2020). Conducting speech-language evaluations in an outpatient pediatric setting during the COVID-19 pandemic. *Journal of the National Black Association for Speech-Language and Hearing*, 15(2), 77–79.

Fan, S., Zhang, Y., Qin, J., Song, X., Wang, M., & Ma, J. (2021). Family environmental risk factors for developmental speech delay in children in Northern China. *Scientific Reports*, 11, 3924. https://doi.org/10.1038/s41598-021-83554-w.

Farquharson, K., Tambyraja, S., & Coleman, J. (2021). Change in school-based speech-language pathologists' job satisfaction during COVID-19 school closures: Applying the conservation of resources theory. *Language, Speech, and Hearing Services in Schools*, 1–12. https://doi.org/10.1044/2021_LSHSS-21-00079.

Filbay, S., Hinman, R., Lawford, B., Fry, R., & Bennell, K. (2021). Telehealth by allied health practitioners during the COVID19 pandemic: An Australian wide survey of clinicians and clients. The University of Melbourne. https://healthsciences.unimelb.edu.au/__data/assets/pdf_file/0009/3775923/Telehealth-by-allied-health-practitioners-during-the-COVID-19-pandemic-Report-April-2021.pdf. Accessed 28 December 2021.

Fong, R., Tsai, C. F., & Yiu, O. Y. (2020). The implementation of telepractice in speech language pathology in Hong Kong during the COVID-19 pandemic. *Telemedicine Journal and e-Health*, 27(1), 30–38.

Freckmann, A., Hines, M., & Lincoln, M. (2017). Clinicians' perspectives of therapeutic alliance in face-to-face and telepractice speech-pathology sessions. *International Journal of Speech-Language Pathology*, 19(3), 287–296.

Gibson, R., Rochus, D., Musasizi, D., Alouch, F., & Staley, B. (2020). The impact of COVID-19 on speech-language pathology practices in Western Kenya. *Perspectives of the ASHA Special Interest Groups: SIG 17 Global Issues in Communication Sciences and Related Disorders*, 5(6), 1801–1804.

Grogan-Johnson, S., Gabel, R., Taylor, J., Rowan, L., Alvares, R., & Schenker, J. (2011). A pilot exploration of speech sound disorder intervention delivered by telehealth to school-age children. *International Journal of Telerehabilitation*, 3(1), 31–42.

Grogan-Johnson, S., Meehan, R., McCormick, K., & Miller, N. (2015). Results of a national survey of preservice telepractice training in graduate speech-language pathology and audiology programs. *Contemporary Issues in Communication Science & Disorders*, 42, 122–137.

Halls-Mill, S., Johnson, L., Gross, M., Latham, D., & Everhart, N. (2021). Providing telepractice in schools during a pandemic: The experiences and perspectives of speech-language pathologists. *Language, Speech, and Hearing Services in Schools*, 1–17. https://doi.org/10.1044/2021_LSHSS-21-00023.

Hao, Y., Zhang, S., Conner, A., & Lee, N. Y. (2021). The evolution of telepractice use during the COVID-19 pandemic: Perspectives of pediatric speech-language pathologists. *International Journal of Environmental Research and Public Health*, 18(22), 12197. https://doi.org/10.3390/ijerph182212197.

Harris, V., Onslow, M., Packman, A., Harrison, E., & Menzies, R. (2002). An experimental investigation of the impact of the Lidcombe Program on early stuttering. *Journal of Fluency Disorders*, 27(3), 203–214.

Hitchcock, E. R., Harel, D., & Byun, T. M. (2015). Social, emotional, and academic impact of residual speech errors in school-aged children: A survey study. *Seminars in Speech and Language*, 36(4), 283–294.

Hunter, P. (2020). The spread of the COVID-19 coronavirus. *EMBO Reports*, 21, e50334 https://doi.org/10.15252/embr.202050334.

Jiang, Y. (2020). Factors related to delayed language development in children. *International Medicine and Guidance News*, 26, 166–169.

Johnson, C. J., Beitchman, J. H., Young, A., Escobar, M., Atkinson, L., Wilson, B., & Wang, M. (1999). Fourteen-year follow-up of children with and without speech/language impairments. *Journal of Speech, Language, and Hearing Research*, 42(3), 744–760.

Khoza-Shangase, K., Moroe, N., & Neille, J. (2021). Speech-language pathology and audiology in South Africa: Clinical training and service in the era of COVID-19. *International Journal of Telerehabilitation*, 13(1), 1–31.

Kollia, B., & Tsiamtsiouris, J. (2021). Influence of the COVID-19 pandemic on telepractice in speech-language pathology. *Journal of Prevention & Intervention in the Community*, 49(2), 152–162.

Kraljevic, J., Matic, A., & Pavicic Dokoza, K. (2020). Telepractice as a reaction to the COVID-19 crisis: Insights from Croatian SLP settings. *International Journal of Telerehabilitation*, 12(2), 93–104.

Lam, J., Lee, S., & Tong, X. (2021). Parents' and students' perceptions of telepractice services for speech-language therapy during the COVID-19 pandemic: Survey study. *Journal of Medical Internet Research Pediatrics and Parenting*, 4(1), 1–8.

Lewis, B. A., Freebairn, L. A., & Taylor, H. G. (2000). Academic outcomes in children with histories of speech sound disorders. *Journal of Communication Disorders*, 33(1), 11–30.

Macoir, J., Desmarais, C., Martel-Sauvageau, V., & Monetta, L. (2021). Proactive changes in clinical practice as a result of the COVID-19 pandemic: Survey on use of telepractice by Quebec speech-language pathologists. *International Journal of Language & Communication Disorders*, 56(5), 1086–1096.

McCormack, J., McLeod, S., McAllister, L., & Harrison, L. J. (2009). A systematic review of the association between childhood speech impairment and participation across the lifespan. *International Journal of Speech-Language Pathology*, 11(2), 155–170.

McGill, M., & Fiddler, K. (2021). A user's guide for understanding and addressing telepractice technology challenges via ZOOM. *Perspectives of the ASHA Special Interest Groups: SIG 18 Telepractice*, 6(2), 494–499.

Mohan, H. S., Anjum, A., & Rao, P. K. (2017). A survey of telepractice in speech-language pathology and audiology in India. *International Journal of Telerehabilitation*, 9(2), 69–80.

O'Brian, S., Smith, K., & Onslow, M. (2014). Webcam delivery of the Lidcombe program for early stuttering: A phase I clinical trial. *Journal of Speech, Language, and Hearing Disorders*, 57(3), 825–830.

Overby, M. (2018). Stakeholders' qualitative perspectives of effective telepractice pedagogy in speech-language pathology. *International Journal of Language and Communication Disorders*, 53(1), 101–112.

Overby, M., & Baft-Neff, A. (2017). Perceptions of telepractice pedagogy in speech-language pathology: A quantitative analysis. *Journal of Telemedicine and Telecare*, 23(5), 550–557.

Reilly, S., Wake, M., Ukoumunne, O. C., Bavin, E., Prior, M., Cini, E., Conway, L., Eadie, P., & Bretherton, L. (2010). Predicting language outcomes at 4 years of age: Findings from early language in Victoria study. *Pediatrics*, 126(6), 1530–1537.

Rosenbaum, S., & Simon, P. (Eds.). (2016). *Speech and language disorders in children: Implications for the social security administrations supplemental security income program*. Washington, DC: National Academies Press.

Samadi, S., Bakhshalizadeh-Moradi, S., Khandani, F., Foladgar, M., Poursaid-Mohammad, M., & McConkey, R. (2020). Using hybrid telepractice for supporting parents of children with ASD during the COVID-19 lockdown: A feasibility study in Iran. *Brain Sciences*, 10(11), 892–906.

Sanchez, D., Reiner, J. F., Sadlon, R., Price, O. A., & Long, M. W. (2019). Systematic review of school telehealth evaluations. *Journal of School Nursing*, 35(1), 61–76.

Santayana, G., Carey, B., & Shenker, R. (2021). No other choice: Speech-language pathologists' attitudes toward using telepractice to administer the Lidcombe Program during a pandemic. *Journal of Fluency Disorders*, 70, 1–12. https://doi.org/10.1016/j.jfludis.2021.105879.

Staley, B., O'Boyle, J., Armstrong, E., Coonan, E., Taylor, L., & Dutton, J. (2020). The impact of COVID-19 on professional practice in the Northern Territory, Australia. *Perspectives of the ASHA Special Interest Groups: SIG 17 Global Issues in Communication Sciences and Related Disorders*, 5(6), 1789–1792.

Sylvan, L., Goldstein, E., & Crandall, M. (2020). Capturing a moment in time: A survey of school-based speech-language pathologists' experiences in the immediate aftermath of the COVID-19 public health emergency. *Perspectives of the ASHA Special Interest Groups: SIG 16 School-Based Issues*, 5(6), 1735–1749.

Tambyraja, S., Farquharson, K., & Coleman, J. (2021). Speech-language teletherapy services for school-aged children in the United States during the COVID-19 pandemic. *Journal of Education for Students Placed at Risk*, 26(2), 91–111.

Tohidast, S. A., Mansuri, B., Bagheri, R., & Azimi, H. (2020). Provision of speech-language pathology services for the treatment of speech and language disorders in children during the COVID-19 pandemic: Problems, concerns, and solutions. *International Journal of Pediatric Otorhinolaryngology*, 138, 110262. https://doi.org/10.1016/j.ijporl.2020.110262.

Tucker, J. K. (2012). Perspectives of speech-language pathologists on the use of telepractice in schools: Quantitative survey results. *International Journal of Telerehabilitation*, 4(2), 61–72.

United States Department of Education (2021). Individuals with disabilities education act (2004). https://sites.ed.gov/idea/. Accessed 28 December 2021.

United States Government Accountability Office (2020). Distance learning: Challenges providing services to K-12 English learners and students with disabilities during COVID-19. www.gao.gov/assets/gao-21-43.pdf. Accessed 28 December 2021.

Young, L., & Robinson, T. (2020). Challenges and quasi solutions while working through the COVID-19 pandemic: Speech-language pathology in a public setting. *Journal of the National Black Association for Speech-Language and Hearing*, 15(2), 88–90.

# 4

# NEUROLINGUISTIC DEFICITS AND OTHER COGNITIVE DISORDERS IN ADULTS WITH SEVERE COVID-19 INFECTION

*Konstantinos Priftis*

## 4.1 Introduction: SARS-CoV-2/COVID-19 and the nervous system

Severe acute respiratory syndrome coronavirus 2 (SARS-CoV-2), and the resulting coronavirus disease 2019 (COVID-19) has caused a pandemic. At the time of writing, more than 555,000,000 cases have been reported worldwide, resulting in more than 6,300,000 deaths (World Health Organization n.d.). COVID-19 is mainly characterised by signs of pulmonary dysfunction (see, e.g., Hu et al. 2021; Layne et al. 2022). Nevertheless, there is now convincing evidence that the nervous system can also be affected (Misra et al. 2021; Paterson et al. 2020; Varatharaj et al. 2020). In fact, different neurological disorders have been reported in patients with COVID-19. These disorders include hypo/anosmia, hypo/ageusia, the Guillain-Barré syndrome, stroke, and encephalitis/encephalopathy. Confusion, agitation, dementia-like signs, and psychotic signs have also been reported after COVID-19 (Paterson et al. 2020; Varatharaj et al. 2020).

Misra et al. (2021) performed a systematic review of the neurological consequences of COVID-19. Data from 145,721 patients were analysed. Of these patients, 89% were hospitalised. The authors estimated that up to one-third of the included patients with COVID-19 showed at least one neurological sign. The most common neurological signs were fatigue (estimated prevalence 32%), myalgia (estimated prevalence 20%), hypo/ageusia (estimated prevalence 21%), hypo/anosmia (estimated prevalence 19%), and headache (estimated prevalence 13%). With respect to neurological diagnoses, the most common was stroke (2%). Regarding the oldest subgroup of patients (> 60 years), the estimated prevalence of acute confusion/delirium was 34%, and the presence of any neurological deficits was associated with mortality.

DOI: 10.4324/9781003257318-4

The etiology of COVID-19 is certainly multifactorial, but the exact patho-physiological mechanisms that lead to the neurological and psychiatric consequences of COVID-19 are not yet clear. The following neuropathological mechanisms have been described (for a review, see Balcom et al. 2021; see also Daroische et al. 2021):

1. *Neurotropism and neuroinvasion.* SARS-CoV-2 can reach the CNS indirectly (e.g., blood-brain barrier) and/or directly by means of axonal transmission through olfactory neurons (Alomari et al. 2020; Brann et al. 2020; Briguglio et al. 2020; Butowt and Bilinska 2020; Meinhardt et al. 2021).
2. *Cerebrovascular deficits* including ischemic and hemorrhagic strokes (Gulko et al. 2020; Lee et al. 2021).
3. *Host neuroimmune responses* including cytokine storm and endothelial damage (Alipoor et al. 2021; Mortaz et al. 2020).

Regardless of the pathophysiological mechanism at work, when the function of the CNS is disrupted by SARS-CoV-2, several neuropsychological disorders can arise. The rest of this chapter examines the prevalence and manifestation of these disorders in people with COVID-19.

## 4.2 COVID-19 and neuropsychological disorders

### 4.2.1 Non-neurolinguistic disorders

In non-neurolinguistic disorders, cognitive domains such as attention, executive functions, and memory may be compromised. Alnefeesi et al. (2021) reviewed the effects of COVID-19 on cognition during the acute and recovery phases. Patients with specific neurological diseases presumably attributed to COVID-19 (e.g., stroke, encephalitis/encephalopathy) were also included in this review. After pooling the samples from the included studies (total sample n=644), Alnefeesi et al. reported prevalence estimates of cognitive impairment ranging between 43% and 66.8% in hospitalised patients with COVID-19. The results showed that delirium was the most common impairment, characterised by deficits in working memory and attention.

In fact, a considerable increase in IL-6, TNFα, and IL-1β cytokines is known to affect working memory and attention (Alnefeesi et al. 2021). Given that deficits in working memory and attention are the core aspects of delirium, cytokines can be considered as key mediators between COVID-19 and associated cognitive impairments. Nonetheless, Alnefeesi et al. suggested that the role of iatrogenic factors (e.g., pharmacological treatment of COVID-19) and pre-morbid factors (e.g., dementia) should be further considered to better explain the causal link between COVID-19 and cognitive dysfunction.

In the majority of studies reviewed by Alnefeesi et al. (2021), cognitive dysfunction was not specifically, systematically, and objectively assessed by means of standardised neuropsychological tests. To fill this gap, Daroische et al. (2021) reviewed the effects of COVID-19 on objectively assessed cognitive dysfunction. Twelve studies were selected in which patients were administered standardised neuropsychological tests. Neuropsychological assessment took place beginning from a few days after the onset of COVID-19 up to six months post-onset. There was also considerable variability regarding the severity of COVID-19 signs and symptoms, with some studies including severely affected patients who received mechanical ventilation for several days. By contrast, in other studies, outpatients were tested who showed only mild signs and symptoms of COVID-19.

Daroische et al. (2021) reported that patients with recent SARS-CoV-2 infection could show a variety of cognitive dysfunction. All studies that included measures of global cognitive function reported the presence of impairment, ranging from 15% to 80% of patients. In seven studies, attention and executive functions were impaired (Almeria et al. 2020; Beaud et al. 2021; Negrini et al. 2021; Ortelli et al. 2021; Raman et al. 2021; Woo et al. 2020; Zhou et al. 2020). In three out of four studies employing memory measures, long-term memory deficits were reported (Alemanno et al. 2021; Beaud et al. 2021; Negrini et al. 2021), whereas in two studies, short-term memory deficits were reported (Alemanno et al. 2021; Zhou et al. 2020). Finally, the presence of visuospatial impairment was reported in two out of four studies employing such measures (Beaud et al. 2021; Raman et al. 2021).

Daroische et al. (2021) concluded that patients with COVID-19 could be affected by global cognitive impairment and/or impairment of specific cognitive functions such as attention and executive functions. On the contrary, the results of studies investigating short-/long-term memory or visuospatial functions seem to require further elaboration and new studies are required. Nonetheless, the presence of cognitive dysfunction in patients with COVID-19 might have been underestimated for at least two reasons. First, Daroische et al. excluded patients with COVID-19 who were also affected by neurological dysfunction such as stroke, delirium, and acute encephalopathies. Second, only group studies were included, whereas potentially interesting single cases and case series were excluded from the review.

In a recent study by García-Sánchez et al. (2022), 63 patients received a complete neuropsychological battery after 187 days on average from the diagnosis of SARS-CoV-2 infection. The patients were referred for neuropsychological evaluation because of subjective cognitive complaints. A comprehensive battery of neuropsychological tests was used. The battery comprised measures of general cognitive status, attention, short-/long-term memory, language, processing speed, visuoperceptual and visuoconstructive functions, and executive functions. The results showed that multiple-domain deficits (60.3%) were more frequent than single-domain deficits (39.7%). Attention deficits were the most common cognitive disorder reported (61.9% of the sample), followed by executive deficits (43% of the sample).

## 4.2.2 Neurolinguistic disorders

Neurolinguistic disorders refer to impairment of language processing in all modalities. This includes the production and comprehension of spoken language (aphasia), reading (alexia), and writing (agraphia). This section examines what is known about these disorders in adults with COVID-19.

### 4.2.2.1 Literature search

Neurolinguistic impairments in patients with COVID-19 have been less often investigated in previous studies than non-neurolinguistic impairments. For example, Daroische et al. (2021) found only one study – Almeria et al. (2020) – in which specific neurolinguistic tasks were used. Almeria et al. reported a patient who showed difficulties in confrontation naming on the Boston Naming Test (Kaplan et al. 2001).

To further investigate the relations between COVID-19 and neurolinguistic disorders, the author performed a literature search on Pubmed and Google Scholar. Two disease-related terms were used in the search (i.e., either SARS-CoV-2 or COVID-19). These terms were combined each time with one of the following neurolinguistic terms: "aphasia"; "alexia" (dyslexia); "agraphia" (dysgraphia); or "language disorders." Twenty-three patients who showed signs of neurolinguistic disorders have been reported in the literature. Patients showed signs of neurolinguistic disorders before, during, or after the patients had been diagnosed with COVID-19 (see Table 4.1). All patients were tested within single-case studies or in cohort studies. By contrast, there were no prospective group studies.

### 4.2.2.2 Time onset of neurolinguistic disorders

The onset of neurolinguistic disorders preceded the diagnosis of SARS-CoV-2 in 11/23 cases (48%). Thus, neurolinguistic disorders might constitute, in some cases, the initial signs of COVID-19. Therefore, neuropsychological assessment can sometimes play a key role in the diagnosis of the disease. In one case, the onset of neurolinguistic disorders was simultaneous with the diagnosis of SARS-CoV-2 (1/23: 4%). The diagnosis of neurolinguistic disorders followed that of SARS-CoV-2 in the remaining 11/23 cases (48%). When the onset of linguistic disorders followed the diagnosis of SARS-CoV-2, 4/11 (36%) of these patents were negative on swab tests at the time of language assessment, but the earlier presence of SARS-CoV-2 was documented through the presence of antibodies. Four of these 11 patients (36%) were still positive. Finally, no information was reported on the remaining 3/11 (28%) of the patients.

**TABLE 4.1** Neurolinguistic disorders and neurological data of patients affected by SARS-CoV-2

| Patient ID number | Author(s) (year) | Study type (single case or cohort) | Lesion cause | Lesion site(s) documented by structural neuroimaging and/or EEG | Language disorder | Language assessment | Subtype of language disorder | Onset of neurolinguistic disorder (before, during, after SARS-CoV-2 diagnosis) | Recovery of language disorder | Other cognitive/behavioural disorders present |
|---|---|---|---|---|---|---|---|---|---|---|
| 1 | Ali et al. (2021) | Single case | Ischemic stroke | Territory of the left middle cerebral artery; bilaterally: territory of anterior cerebral arteries | Aphasia | NIHSS (Lyden et al. 1999) | N/R | Before | Fully recovered | Confusion, agitation, aggressiveness |
| 2 | Beretta et al. (2021) | Single case | Encephalitis | Left insula, middle frontal gyrus, inferior parietal lobule, and superior temporal gyrus; bilaterally: cingulate gyrus | Aphasia | GCS (Teasdale and Jennett 1974) | N/R | Before | Fully recovered | Confusion |

(Continued)

**TABLE 4.1** (Continued)

| Patient ID number | Author(s) (year) | Study type (single case or cohort) | Lesion cause | Lesion site(s) documented by structural neuroimaging and/or EEG | Language disorder | Language assessment | Subtype of language disorder | Onset of neurolinguistic disorder (before, during, after SARS-CoV-2 diagnosis) | Recovery of language disorder | Other cognitive/behavioural disorders present |
|---|---|---|---|---|---|---|---|---|---|---|
| 3 | Biag et al. (2021) | Single case | Ischemic stroke | Territory of the left middle cerebral artery, basal nuclei, insula | Severe aphasia, mild dysarthria | NIHSS (Lyden et al. 1999) | Expressive aphasia | Before | Improved | N/R |
| 4 | Bessa et al. (2020) | Single case | Ischemic stroke | Territory of the left middle cerebral artery extending to the deep nuclei | Aphasia | NIHSS (Lyden et al. 1999) | Conduction aphasia | After (negativised at the moment of neurolinguistic disorders onset) | Improved | N/R |
| 5 | Castillo-Pinto et al. (2022) | Single case | Ischemic stroke | Territory of the left middle cerebral artery | Mild aphasia, dysarthria | NIHSS (Lyden et al. 1999) | N/R | Before | N/R | N/R |
| 6 | Cotelli et al. (2020) | Single case | No evidence of focal or diffused brain lesions | Absent | Foreign accent syndrome | N/R | Lost regional accent | After (negativised at the moment of neurolinguistic disorders onset) | Unchanged | Absent |

| | | | | | | | | | | |
|---|---|---|---|---|---|---|---|---|---|---|
| 7 | Betül Gunduz and Ozsahin (2021) | Single case | Ischemic stroke | Left pons | Aphasia | N/R | Motor aphasia | Before | Passed away | N/R |
| 8 | Finsterer and Scorza (2021) | Single case | Hemorrhagic stroke | Left temporal | Aphasia | N/R | Sensori–motor aphasia | After (not reported whether the patient was still positive) | Fully recovered | Absent |
| 9 | Kudo et al. (2021) | Single case | Encephalopathy | Left supramarginal gyrus; bilaterally: frontal cortices | Aphasia, agraphia | N/R | Amnestic aphasia, N/R for agraphia | After (still positive at the moment of neurolinguistic disorders onset) | Aphasia improved; Agraphia N/R | N/R |
| 10 | Lameijer et al. (2020) | Cohort (Patient 3) | Ischemic stroke | Territory of the left middle cerebral artery | Aphasia | N/R | Global aphasia | After (still positive at the moment of neurolinguistic disorders onset) | Improved | Apathy |
| 11 | Lameijer et al. (2020) | Cohort (Patient 4) | Ischemic stroke | bilaterally: territories of the middle and posterior cerebral arteries | Severe aphasia | N/R | N/R | After (still positive at the moment of neurolinguistic disorders onset) | Unchanged | N/R |

(Continued)

**TABLE 4.1** (Continued)

| Patient ID number | Author(s) (year) | Study type (single case or cohort) | Lesion cause | Lesion site(s) documented by structural neuroimaging and/or EEG | Language disorder | Language assessment | Subtype of language disorder | Onset of neurolinguistic disorder (before, during, after SARS-CoV-2 diagnosis) | Recovery of language disorder | Other cognitive/behavioural disorders present |
|---|---|---|---|---|---|---|---|---|---|---|
| 12 | De Almeida Lima et al. (2020) | Single case | Ischemic stroke | Territory of the left middle cerebral artery | Aphasia, dysarthria | N/R | N/R | Before | N/R | N/R |
| 13 | Morrison et al. (2020) | Single case | Unknown | Absent | Aphasia, stuttering | N/R | Anomic aphasia | Before | N/R | N/R |
| 14 | Muccioli et al. (2020) | Single case | Encephalo-pathy | Left frontal lobe; bilaterally: parietal and posterior periventricular white matter | Aphasia | N/R | Anomia, agrammatism, and sporadic semantic paraphasia | Before | Fully recovered | Inattention, dysexecutive syndrome, agitation, confusion |
| 15 | Nagamine (2021) | Single case | Ischemic stroke | Left insula | Foreign accent syndrome | N/R | Speaking in a regional accent | After (not reported whether the patient was still positive at the moment of neurolinguistic disorders onset) | N/R | N/R |

| 16 | Pensato et al. (2020) | Single case | Encephalo-pathy | Absent | Aphasia | N/R | Expressive aphasia with phonological and neological paraphasias; comprehension preserved | Before | Fully recovered | Ideomotor slowing, agitated delirium |
|----|----|----|----|----|----|----|----|----|----|----|
| 17 | Perrin et al. (2020) | Cohort (Patient 2) | Encephalo-pathy | White matter hyperintensities in middle cerebellar peduncles, an acute mm-scale cytotoxic oedema on the posterior left frontal bilateral diffuse slowing on EEG | Aphasia | N/R | Mixed fluent and non-fluent aphasia | After (still positive at the moment of neurolinguistic disorders onset) | Improved | Anterograde amnesia, dysexecutive syndrome, apraxia, confusion, agitation |

*(Continued)*

**TABLE 4.1** (Continued)

| Patient ID number | Author(s) (year) | Study type (single case or cohort) | Lesion cause | Lesion site(s) documented by structural neuroimaging and/or EEG | Language disorder | Language assessment | Subtype of language disorder | Onset of neurolinguistic disorder (before, during, after SARS-CoV-2 diagnosis) | Recovery of language disorder | Other cognitive/behavioural disorders present |
|---|---|---|---|---|---|---|---|---|---|---|
| 18 | Priftis et al. (2020) | Single case | Ischemic stroke | Left temporo-parieto-insular, extending to the homo-lateral semioval centre | Agraphia, aphasia | ENPA (Capasso and Miceli 2001) | Pure peripheral agraphia, mild conduction aphasia | After (negativised at the moment of neurolinguistic disorders onset) | Highly improved | Absent |
| 19 | Priftis et al. (2021) | Single case | Ischemic stroke | Left occipito-temporal extending to the white matter | Alexia | ENPA (Capasso and Miceli 2001) | Pure alexia (i.e., alexia without agraphia) | After (negativised at the moment of neurolinguistic disorders onset) | Fully recovered | Absent |
| 20 | Rettenmaier et al. (2021) | Single case | Encephalo-pathy | Thalamus bilaterally | Aphasia | N/R | Non-fluent aphasia | Before | Improved | N/R |

| 21 | Scharpf et al. (2021) | Single case | Ischemic stroke | Penumbra in the territory of the left middle cerebral artery | Aphasia | N/R | Global aphasia | After (not reported whether the patient was still positive at the moment of neurolinguistic disorders onset) | Deceased | N/R |
|----|-----------------------|-------------|-----------------|-------------------------------------------------------------|---------|-----|----------------|------------------------------------------------------------------------------------------------------------|----------|-----|
| 22 | Sharifi-Razavi et al. (2021) | Cohort | Ischemic stroke | Left basal nuclei | Aphasia | N/R | Broca's aphasia | Before | Unchanged | N/R |
| 23 | Valencia Sanchez et al. (2021) | Cohort (Patient 5) | Encephalo-pathy | Diffuse slowing, triphasic waves, and intermittent rhythmic deltaactivity, bilateral frontal regions | Aphasia | N/R | N/R | During | Fully recovered | Delirium |

*Legend*: N/R=not reported; Absent: no evidence after formal or informal assessment

### 4.2.2.3 Neurological causes and neuroanatomical localisation of the lesions

The causes and sites of brain lesions were documented by structural or functional neuroimaging, including electroencephalography (EEG). For two patients, there was no direct evidence of brain disease or lesion. For the remaining 21 patients, two neurological causes were reported as underlying the onset of neurolinguistic disorders: stroke and encephalitis/encephalopathy (see Table 4.1). Most of the patients were affected by stroke (14/21, 67%), followed by those affected by encephalitis/encephalopathy (7/21, 33%).

Of the 14 patients affected by stroke, 13 patients (93%) were affected by ischemic stroke, whereas one patient (7%) was affected by hemorrhagic stroke. In most cases affected by ischemic stroke, the lesions were in the territory of the left middle cerebral artery. SARS-CoV-2 cannot be directly considered as a cause of ischemic stroke. Nevertheless, there is now substantial evidence suggesting that SARS-CoV-2 may be considered a risk factor for ischemic stroke. In fact, the risk of ischemic stroke in patients affected by SARS-CoV-2 appears to be double the same risk observed in patients affected by SARS-CoV-1 (Fridman et al. 2020). The same holds when patients affected by SARS-CoV-2 are compared with those affected by severe sepsis. Furthermore, the risk of ischemic stroke in patients affected by SARS-CoV-2 appears to be eight times higher than the same risk in patients affected by influenza (Fridman et al. 2020). Finally, some recent results have suggested that the effects of ischemic strokes in patients affected by SARS-CoV-2 are more severe and disabling than those of patients not affected by SARS-CoV-2 (Ntaios et al. 2020).

Although the seven patients affected by encephalopathy/encephalitis had widespread unilateral or bilateral lesions (see Table 4.1), the most frequently damaged brain areas were the frontal lobes. The mechanisms through which SARS-CoV-2 is related to the onset of encephalitis/encephalopathy are not yet completely clear (for a review, see Balcolm et al. 2021). With reference to encephalitis, SARS-CoV-2 seems to be related to the following causes: viral neuroinvasion (see, e.g., Meinhardt et al. 2021); disrupted blood-brain barrier (see, e.g., Alexopoulos et al. 2020); or autoimmunological reactions (see, e.g., Cao et al. 2020). With regard to encephalopathy, SARS-CoV-2 appears to be associated with metabolic dysfunction (see, e.g., Antony and Haneef 2020) or the presence of hypoxia/ischemia/cerebral microthrombi (see, e.g., Lee et al. 2021; for a review, see Balcolm et al. 2021).

### 4.2.2.4 Assessment of neurolinguistic disorders

The quality of neurolinguistic assessment was rather low in most of the reviewed studies. In fact, in most cases (16/23, 70%; see Table 4.1), no standardised single tests or batteries were administered to the patients. Thus, in the majority of studies, the diagnosis of neurolinguistic disorders was probably based only on general and potentially vague clinical impressions. Therefore, those diagnoses might have been rather unspecific and probably lacked both sensitivity and specificity.

In the remaining cases (7/23, 30%), some diagnostic tools were used. In Beretta et al. (2021), a patient was tested with the Glasgow Coma Scale (GCS; Teasdale and Jennett 1974). Note, however, that neurolinguistic assessment by means of the GCS is limited to oral comprehension of a very restricted number of spoken commands. Four more patients (Ali et al. 2021; Biag et al. 2021; Bessa et al. 2020; Castillo-Pinto et al. 2022) were tested by means of the National Institutes of Health Stroke Scale (NIHSS; Lyden et al. 1999). The NIHSS does include some more specific linguistic tasks than the GCS. Nevertheless, the number and structure of language tasks in the NIHSS remain very limited. Therefore, the NIHSS cannot be considered a suitable diagnostic instrument to perform a comprehensive and detailed neurolinguistic assessment with reference to classic or modern models of language processing.

Priftis et al. (2020, 2021) conducted the only two studies in which a specific test battery was used to assess neurolinguistic disorders (i.e., *Esame neuropsicologico per l'afasia (ENPA)/Neuropsychological Exam for Aphasia;* Capasso and Miceli 2001). This is a comprehensive and standardised neurolinguistic battery inspired by modern (psycho)linguistic and neuropsychological models of language processing. The battery includes different levels of language processing: spoken/written single words; spoken/written single non-words; and spoken/written sentences. Through the ENPA, the following input/output components of language processing can be investigated: oral fluency, oral repetition, oral comprehension, oral production, written comprehension, and written production. Finally, the revealed neurolinguistic disorders can be further classified according to damage at various levels of (psycho)linguistic processing (e.g., phonetic, phonemic, graphemic, morphological, lexical, syntactic, and semantic).

## 4.2.2.5 Neurolinguistic disorders and their subtypes

Twenty patients were affected by oral neurolinguistic disorders such as aphasia with or without speech disorders (e.g., dysarthria, stuttering; see Table 4.1). Regarding the reported aphasia subtypes, eight patients were affected by non-fluent aphasias (reported diagnostic labels: expressive, motor, sensorimotor, global, Broca's, non-fluent). Four patients were affected by fluent aphasias (reported diagnostic labels: conduction, amnestic, anomic). Furthermore, a patient was reported to be affected by a mixed form of fluent and non-fluent aphasia, which was not further specified, making it difficult to interpret this rather unusual aphasic pattern (Perrin et al. 2020). No specific subtypes of neurolinguistic disorders were reported for the rest of the aphasic patients.

Two non-aphasic patients were affected by a peculiar speech disorder called foreign accent syndrome (FAS; Cotelli et al. 2020; Nagamine 2021). FAS is a very rare speech disorder in which affected patients start speaking with a new accent that sounds as if it were foreign. In other cases, patients can start speaking with a new regional accent, or they can lose their regional accent (Cotelli et al. 2020; Nagamine 2021).

Written language disorders were present in three patients, two of whom were also affected by aphasia. A patient who was affected by amnestic aphasia presented with agraphia, which was not further classified according to possible diagnostic subtypes (Kudo et al. 2021). Another patient with mild signs of conduction aphasia presented with agraphia without alexia. This is a subtype of peripheral agraphia, in which patients can read perfectly but cannot write (Priftis et al. 2020). Finally, one patient presented with alexia without agraphia. This is a subtype of peripheral alexia, in which patients are still able to write but cannot read, even words and sentences that patients are able to write (Priftis et al. 2021).

### 4.2.2.6 Comorbidity of neurolinguistic and non-neurolinguistic disorders

For most patients, the co-presence of non-neurolinguistic disorders (i.e., other cognitive and behavioural disorders) was not tested or was absent when tested. Although some patients were also affected by non-neurolinguistic disorders (e.g., amnesia, apraxia, dysexecutive syndromes, agitation), no clear and systematic pattern emerged (see Table 4.1). Neurolinguistic disorders thus can be the only clear evidence of cognitive dysfunction in some patients affected by COVID-19.

### 4.2.2.7 Recovery of neurolinguistic disorders

In most patients, neurolinguistic disorders were fully recovered or at least improved in the subacute or chronic phase. It remains largely unclear, however, whether full recovery or improvement was due to spontaneous evolution, medical treatment of the disease, and/or neurolinguistic rehabilitation.

## 4.3 Summary

In the present chapter, evidence for neuropsychological disorders in patients with COVID-19 has been reviewed. Concerning non-neurolinguistic disorders, the most frequently encountered disorders assessed by objective and standardised neuropsychological tests affected attention and executive functions and, to a lesser degree, memory. Neuropsychological findings are consistent with the results of neuroimaging studies that have revealed potential involvement of the frontal lobes together with other areas in patients with COVID-19 (see, e.g., Hosp et al. 2021; Kas et al. 2021).

The focus of the chapter was, however, on neurolinguistic disorders in patients with COVID-19. The review of the literature revealed the presence of

23 patients with COVID-19 who were affected by neurolinguistic disorders. Most patients were affected by spoken-language and speech disorders (i.e., aphasias, dysarthria, stuttering or foreign accent syndrome), whereas one patient showed only a written-language disorder (i.e., alexia) (Priftis et al. 2021). Finally, two patients were affected both by spoken- and written-language disorders (i.e., aphasia and agraphia) (Kudo et al. 2021; Priftis et al. 2020). As structural and/ or functional neuroimaging revealed, all but two patients with neurolinguistic disorders had lesions attributed to stroke or encephalitis/encephalopathy. Neurolinguistic disorders depended on the affected areas of the brain. As in the case of non-neurolinguistic disorders, the frontal lobes might be mainly involved because most of the reported neurolinguistic disorders consisted in non-fluent aphasias, which are typically the result of damage to the prerolandic (i.e., frontal) brain regions.

Some important limitations, however, were present in the reviewed studies on neurolinguistic disorders. These are summarised as follows:

1.  In most studies, neurolinguistic disorders were diagnosed only on the basis of informal clinical impressions. Indeed, diagnostic tools were used in only a few studies. Of these studies, only two made use of a specific tool (ENPA) for the assessment of neurolinguistic disorders (Priftis et al. 2020, 2021). Thanks to this tool, all possible spoken and written language disorders were investigated in two patients with COVID-19. All possible input and output components of (psycho)linguistic processing were investigated at various levels (i.e., phonetic, phonemic, graphemic, morphological, lexical, syntactic, and semantic). If standardised, comprehensive batteries for the assessment of neurolinguistic disorders are not used in future prospective studies, the prevalence, types, and subtypes of language processing impairment in COVID-19 cannot be fully investigated and diagnosed. The possible contribution of non-linguistic disorders should also be more fully taken into account.
2.  Some of the supposed aphasic signs reviewed in this chapter might have been the result of non-linguistic disorders such as delirium. In these cases, differential neuropsychological assessment is required to disentangle the contribution of neurolinguistic and non-neurolinguistic factors.
3.  No prospective group studies were present in the literature.

In conclusion, there is some evidence that patients with COVID-19 can present with neurolinguistic disorders. Prospective cohorts and group studies employing specific and standardised neuropsychological tools of (psycho)linguistic processing are required to shed light on the epidemiology and diagnostic taxonomy of neurolinguistic disorders present in patients with COVID-19. Finally, treatment of correctly diagnosed neurolinguistic disorders should be promptly provided to all affected patients to help them communicate with other people whilst involved in their everyday life activities.

## Acknowledgements

This chapter is dedicated to the beloved memories of Antonio Di Bono and Antonio Loguercio. I shall always keep going on guided by your values and principles.

## References

Alemanno, F., Houdayer, E., Parma, A., Spina, A., Del Forno, A., Scatolini, A., et al. (2021). COVID-19 cognitive deficits after respiratory assistance in the subacute phase: A COVID-rehabilitation unit experience. *PloS One*, 16(2), e0246590. https://doi.org/10.1371/journal.pone.0246590.

Alexopoulos, H., Magira, E., Bitzogli, K., Kafasi, N., Vlachoyiannopoulos, P., Tzioufas, A., et al. (2020). Anti-SARS-CoV-2 antibodies in the CSF, blood-brain barrier dysfunction, and neurological outcome: Studies in 8 stuporous and comatose patients. *Neurology® Neuroimmunology & Neuroinflammation*, 7(6), e893. https://doi.org/10.1212/NXI.0000000000000893.

Ali, L., Jamoussi, H., Kouki, N., Fray, S., Echebbi, S., Ben Ali, N., et al. (2021). COVID-19 infection and recurrent stroke in young patients with protein S deficiency: A case report. *The Neurologist*, 26(6), 276–280.

Alipoor, S. D., Mortaz, E., Varahram, M., Garssen, J., & Adcock, I. M. (2021). The immunopathogenesis of neuroinvasive lesions of SARS-CoV-2 infection in COVID-19 patients. *Frontiers in Neurology*, 12, 697079. https://doi.org/10.3389/fneur.2021.697079.

Almeria, M., Cejudo, J. C., Sotoca, J., Deus, J., & Krupinski, J. (2020). Cognitive profile following COVID-19 infection: Clinical predictors leading to neuropsychological impairment. *Brain, Behavior, & Immunity – Health*, 9, 100163. https://doi.org/10.1016/j.bbih.2020.100163.

Alnefeesi, Y., Siegel, A., Lui, L. M. W., Teopiz, K. M., Ho, R. C. M., Lee, Y., et al. (2021). Impact of SARS-CoV-2 infection on cognitive function: A systematic review. *Frontiers in Psychiatry*, 11, 699582. www.frontiersin.org/article/10.3389/fpsyt.2020.621773.

Alomari, S. O., Abou-Mrad, Z., & Bydon, A. (2020). COVID-19 and the central nervous system. *Clinical Neurology and Neurosurgery*, 198, 106116. https://doi.org/10.1016/j.clineuro.2020.106116.

Antony, A. R., & Haneef, Z. (2020). Systematic review of EEG findings in 617 patients diagnosed with COVID-19. *Seizure*, 83, 234–241.

Balcom, E. F., Nath, A., & Power, C. (2021). Acute and chronic neurological disorders in COVID-19: Potential mechanisms of disease. *Brain*, 144(12), 3576–3588.

Beaud, V., Crottaz-Herbette, S., Dunet, V., Vaucher, J., Bernard-Valnet, R., Du Pasquier, R., et al. (2021). Pattern of cognitive deficits in severe COVID-19. *Journal of Neurology, Neurosurgery, and Psychiatry*, 92(5), 567–568.

Beretta, S., Stabile, A., Balducci, C., Di Francesco, J. C., Patruno, A., Rona, R., et al. (2021). COVID-19-associated immune-mediated encephalitis mimicking acute-onset Creutzfeldt-Jakob disease. *Annals of Clinical and Translational Neurology*, 8(12), 2314–2318.

Bessa, P. B., Brito, A. K. B., Pereira, F. R., Silva, S. Q. E., Almeida, T. V. R., & Almeida, A. P. (2020). Ischemic stroke related to HIV and SARS-CoV-2 co-infection: A case report. *Revista Da Sociedade Brasileira de Medicina Tropical*, 53, e20200692. https://doi.org/10.1590/0037-8682-0692-2020.

Betül Gunduz, Z., & Ozsahin, A. (2021). Acute ischemic stroke in young adult: Atrial fibrillation, hyperthyroidism, and COVID-19 collaboration. *SAGE Open Medical Case Reports*, 9, 2050313X2110486. https://doi.org/10.1177/2050313X211048632.

Biag, E., Solis, K., Abd Elazim, A., & Hussein, O. (2021). COVID-19 associated wake-up stroke treated with DWI/FLAIR mismatch guided intravenous alteplase: A case report. *The Neurologist*, 26(6), 271–273.

Brann, D. H., Tsukahara, T., Weinreb, C., Lipovsek, M., Van den Berge, K., Gong, B., et al. (2020). Non-neuronal expression of SARS-CoV-2 entry genes in the olfactory system suggests mechanisms underlying COVID-19-associated anosmia. *Science Advances*, 6(31), eabc5801. https://doi.org/10.1126/sciadv.abc5801.

Briguglio, M., Bona, A., Porta, M., Dell'Osso, B., Pregliasco, F. E., & Banfi, G. (2020). Disentangling the hypothesis of host dysosmia and SARS-CoV-2: The bait symptom that hides neglected neurophysiological routes. *Frontiers in Physiology*, 11, 671. https://doi.org/10.3389/fphys.2020.00671.

Butowt, R., & Bilinska, K. (2020). SARS-CoV-2: Olfaction, brain infection, and the urgent need for clinical samples allowing earlier virus detection. *ACS Chemical Neuroscience*, 11(9), 1200–1203.

Cao, A., Rohaut, B., Le Guennec, L., Saheb, S., Marois, C., Altmayer, V., et al. & CoCo-Neurosciences study group (2020). Severe COVID-19-related encephalitis can respond to immunotherapy. *Brain*, 143(12), e102. https://doi.org/10.1093/brain/awaa337.

Capasso, R., & Miceli, G. (2001). *Esame neuropsicologico per l'afasia*. Milan, Italy: Springer-Verlag.

Castillo-Pinto, C., Lamotte, G., Mehta, A., Sonti, R., Di Maria, G., Ruiz, D., et al. (2022). Healthcare worker with large vessel acute ischemic stroke likely related to mild SARS-CoV-2 infection. *The Neurohospitalist*, 12(1), 48–56.

Cotelli, M. S., Cotelli, M., Manelli, F., Bonetti, G., Rao, R., Padovani, A., et al. (2020). Effortful speech with distortion of prosody following SARS-CoV-2 infection. *Neurological Sciences*, 41(12), 3767–3768.

Daroische, R., Hemminghyth, M. S., Eilertsen, T. H., Breitve, M. H., & Chwiszczuk, L. J. (2021). Cognitive impairment after COVID-19-a review on objective test data. *Frontiers in Neurology*, 12, 699582. https://doi.org/10.3389/fneur.2021.699582.

de Almeida Lima, A. N., Santos Leite Pessoa, M., Franco Costa Lima, C., Picasso de Araújo Coimbra, P., & Bezerra Holanda, J. L. (2020). Images in vascular medicine: Acute peripheral artery occlusion and ischemic stroke in a patient with COVID-19. *Vascular Medicine*, 25(5), 482–483.

Finsterer, J., & Scorza, F. A. (2021). Intracerebral bleeding after Janus-kinase inhibitor baricitinib for COVID-19. *Brain Hemorrhages*, 2(4), 151–152.

Fridman, S., Bres Bullrich, M., Jimenez-Ruiz, A., Costantini, P., Shah, P., Just, C., et al. (2020). Stroke risk, phenotypes, and death in COVID-19: Systematic review and newly reported cases. *Neurology*, 95(24), e3373–e3385. https://doi.org/10.1212/WNL.0000000000010851.

García-Sánchez, C., Calabria, M., Grunden, N., Pons, C., Arroyo, J. A., Gómez-Anson, B., et al. (2022). Neuropsychological deficits in patients with cognitive complaints after COVID-19. *Brain and Behavior*, e2508. https://doi.org/10.1002/brb3.2508.

Gulko, E., Oleksk, M. L., Gomes, W., Ali, S., Mehta, H., Overby, P., et al. (2020). MRI brain findings in 126 patients with covid-19: Initial observations from a descriptive literature review. *American Journal of Neuroradiology*, 41(12), 2199–2203.

Hosp, J. A., Dressing, A., Blazhenets, G., Bormann, T., Rau, A., Schwabenland, M., et al. (2021). Cognitive impairment and altered cerebral glucose metabolism in the subacute stage of COVID-19. *Brain*, 144(4), 1263–1276.

Hu, B., Guo, H., Zhou, P., & Shi, Z.-L. (2021). Characteristics of SARS-CoV-2 and COVID-19. *Nature Reviews Microbiology*, 19(3), 141–154.

Kaplan, E., Goodglass, H., & Weintraub, S. (2001). *Boston naming test* (2nd ed.). Philadelphia: Lippincott Williams & Wilkins.

Kas, A., Soret, M., Pyatigoskaya, N., Habert, M.-O., Hesters, A., Le Guennec, L., et al. (2021). The cerebral network of COVID-19-related encephalopathy: A longitudinal voxel-based 18F-FDG-PET study. *European Journal of Nuclear Medicine and Molecular Imaging*, 1–15. https://doi.org/10.1007/s00259-020-05178-y.

Kudo, T., Hayashi, Y., Kunieda, K., Yoshikura, N., Kimura, A., Otsuki, M., et al. (2021). Persistent intrathecal interleukin-8 production in a patient with SARS-CoV-2-related encephalopathy presenting aphasia: A case report. *BMC Neurology*, 21(1), 426. https://doi.org/10.1186/s12883-021-02459-3.

Lameijer, J. R. C., van Houte, J., van Berckel, M. M. G., Canta, L. R., Yo, L. S. F., Nijziel, M. R., et al. (2020). Severe arterial thromboembolism in patients with Covid-19. *Journal of Critical Care*, 60, 106–110.

Layne, S. P., Walters, K.-A., Kash, J. C., & Taubenberger, J. K. (2022). More autopsy studies are needed to understand the pathogenesis of severe COVID-19. *Nature Medicine*, 1–2. https://doi.org/10.1038/s41591-022-01684-8.

Lee, M.-H., Perl, D. P., Nair, G., Li, W., Maric, D., Murray, H., et al. (2021). Microvascular injury in the brains of patients with Covid-19. *The New England Journal of Medicine*, 384(5), 481–483.

Lyden, P., Lu, M., Jackson, C., Marler, J., Kothari, R., Brott, T., et al. (1999). Underlying structure of the National Institutes of health stroke scale: Results of a factor analysis. *Stroke*, 30, 2347–2354.

Meinhardt, J., Radke, J., Dittmayer, C., Franz, J., Thomas, C., Mothes, R., et al. (2021). Olfactory transmucosal SARS-CoV-2 invasion as a port of central nervous system entry in individuals with COVID-19. *Nature Neuroscience*, 24(2), 168–175.

Misra, S., Kolappa, K., Prasad, M., Radhakrishnan, D., Thakur, K. T., Solomon, T., et al. (2021). Frequency of neurologic manifestations in COVID-19: A systematic review and meta-analysis. *Neurology*, 97(23), e2269–e2281. https://doi.org/10.1212/WNL.0000000000012930.

Morrison, N., Levy, J., Shoshany, T., Dickinson, A., & Whalen, M. (2020). Stuttering and word-finding difficulties in a patient with COVID-19 presenting to the emergency department. *Cureus*, 12(11), e11774. https://doi.org/10.7759/cureus.11774.

Mortaz, E., Tabarsi, P., Varahram, M., Folkerts, G., & Adcock, I. M. (2020). The immune response and immunopathology of COVID-19. *Frontiers in Immunology*, 11, 2037. https://doi.org/10.3389/fimmu.2020.02037.

Muccioli, L., Pensato, U., Cani, I., Guerra, L., Provini, F., Bordin, G., et al. (2020). COVID-19-related encephalopathy presenting with aphasia resolving following tocilizumab treatment. *Journal of Neuroimmunology*, 349, 577400. https://doi.org/10.1016/j.jneuroim.2020.577400.

Nagamine, T. (2021). Foreign accent syndrome associated with left insula infarction after COVID-19 pneumonia. *Canadian Journal of Emergency Medicine*, 23(6), 858–859.

Negrini, F., Ferrario, I., Mazziotti, D., Berchicci, M., Bonazzi, M., de Sire, A., et al. (2021). Neuropsychological features of severe hospitalized coronavirus disease 2019 patients at clinical stability and clues for postacute rehabilitation. *Archives of Physical Medicine and Rehabilitation*, 102(1), 155–158.

Ntaios, G., Michel, P., Georgiopoulos, G., Guo, Y., Li, W., Xiong, J., et al. (2020). Characteristics and outcomes in patients with covid-19 and acute ischemic stroke: The global COVID-19 stroke registry. *Stroke*, 51(9), e254–e258. https://doi.org/10.1161/STROKEAHA.120.031208.

Ortelli, P., Ferrazzoli, D., Sebastianelli, L., Engl, M., Romanello, R., Nardone, R., et al. (2021). Neuropsychological and neurophysiological correlates of fatigue in post-acute patients with neurological manifestations of COVID-19: Insights into a challenging symptom. *Journal of the Neurological Sciences*, 420, 117271. https://doi.org/10.1016/j.jns.2020.117271.

Paterson, R. W., Brown, R. L., Benjamin, L., Nortley, R., Wiethoff, S., Bharucha, T., et al. (2020). The emerging spectrum of COVID-19 neurology: Clinical, radiological and laboratory findings. *Brain*, 143(10), 3104–3120.

Pensato, U., Muccioli, L., Pasini, E., Tappatà, M., Ferri, L., Volpi, L., et al. (2020). Encephalopathy in COVID-19 presenting with acute aphasia mimicking stroke. *Frontiers in Neurology*, 11, 587226. https://doi.org/10.3389/fneur.2020.587226.

Perrin, P., Collongues, N., Baloglu, S., Bedo, D., Bassand, X., Lavaux, T., et al. (2020). Cytokine release syndrome-associated encephalopathy in patients with COVID-19. *European Journal of Neurology*, 28(1), 248–258.

Priftis, K., Algeri, L., Villella, S., & Spada, M. S. (2020). COVID-19 presenting with agraphia and conduction aphasia in a patient with left-hemisphere ischemic stroke. *Neurological Sciences*, 41(12), 3381–3384.

Priftis, K., Prior, M., Meneghetti, L., Mercogliano, T., & Bendini, M. (2021). Alexia without agraphia in a post COVID-19 patient with left-hemisphere ischemic stroke. *Neurological Sciences*, 42(6), 2179–2181.

Raman, B., Cassar, M. P., Tunnicliffe, E. M., Filippini, N., Griffanti, L., Alfaro-Almagro, F., et al. (2021). Medium-term effects of SARS-CoV-2 infection on multiple vital organs, exercise capacity, cognition, quality of life and mental health, post-hospital discharge. *EClinicalMedicine*, 31, 100683. https://doi.org/10.1016/j.eclinm.2020.100683.

Rettenmaier, L. A., Abdel-Wahed, L., Abdelmotilib, H., Conway, K. S., Narayanan, N., & Groth, C. L. (2021). COVID-19-associated necrotizing encephalopathy presenting without active respiratory symptoms: A case report with histopathology. *Journal of NeuroVirology*. https://doi.org/10.1007/s13365-021-01042 3.

Scharpf, W., Katsafanas, C., & Ng, K. (2021). COVID-19 – associated ischemic stroke in a patient on therapeutic anticoagulation. *The Neurologist*, 26(3), 108–111.

Sharifi-Razavi, A., Karimi, N., Zarvani, A., Cheraghmakani, H., & Baghbanian, S. M. (2021). Ischemic stroke associated with novel coronavirus 2019: A report of three cases. *International Journal of Neuroscience*, 131(12), 1243–1247.

Teasdale, G., & Jennett, B. (1974). Assessment of coma and impaired consciousness. A practical scale. *Lancet*, 2(7872), 81–84.

Valencia Sanchez, C., Theel, E., Binnicker, M., Toledano, M., & McKeon, A. (2021). Autoimmune encephalitis after SARS-CoV-2 infection: Case frequency, findings, and outcomes. *Neurology*, 97(23), e2262–e2268. https://doi.org/10.1212/WNL.0000000000012931.

Varatharaj, A., Thomas, N., Ellul, M. A., Davies, N. W. S., Pollak, T. A., Tenorio, E. L., et al. and the CoroNerve Study Group (2020). Neurological and neuropsychiatric complications of COVID-19 in 153 patients: A UK-wide surveillance study. *The Lancet. Psychiatry*, 7(10), 875–882.

Woo, M. S., Malsy, J., Pöttgen, J., Seddiq Zai, S., Ufer, F., Hadjilaou, A., et al. (2020). Frequent neurocognitive deficits after recovery from mild COVID-19. *Brain Communications*, 2(2), fcaa205. https://doi.org/10.1093/braincomms/fcaa205.

World Health Organization (n.d.). WHO Coronavirus (COVID-19) dashboard. https://covid19.who.int/. Accessed 20 February 2022.

Zhou, H., Lu, S., Chen, J., Wei, N., Wang, D., Lyu, H., et al. (2020). The landscape of cognitive function in recovered COVID-19 patients. *Journal of Psychiatric Research*, 129, 98–102.

# 5

# COGNITIVE-LINGUISTIC DIFFICULTIES IN ADULTS WITH LONG COVID

*Louise Cummings*

## 5.1 Introduction

At the time of writing, the health and economic consequences of the COVID-19 pandemic are continuing to unfold. However, it is becoming increasingly clear that the true legacy of this crisis in global health may be the very large number of people who do not make a good recovery from COVID-19 infection. The prevalence of so-called Long COVID is beginning to be quantified. The Office of National Statistics (2022) stated that an estimated 2 million people living in private households in the UK (3.1% of the population) reported experiencing Long COVID as of 1 May 2022. Many of these individuals are adults of working age who are no longer able to work or have had to reduce their working hours because of debilitating physical and mental symptoms. The rehabilitation of these individuals will not only be costly in economic terms but will also require a significant evidence base to support medical interventions and therapies. Work on developing this evidence base is already underway. An area that has so far not received much attention is language and cognition. It will be argued in this chapter that subjective reports of cognitive-linguistic difficulties as part of the Long COVID syndrome are supported by findings from an experimental study of adults with Long COVID. Amongst other things, these adults present with a marked reduction in the informativeness of their spoken discourse that is related to the cognitive demands of different discourse production tasks. The implications of these findings for the role of speech-language pathology in the rehabilitation of these individuals are discussed.

## 5.2 Long COVID: some background

The COVID-19 pandemic has demonstrated the devastating consequences that a novel virus can have on susceptible human populations around the world.

DOI: 10.4324/9781003257318-5

By 12 March 2022, the World Health Organization reported 6,029,852 deaths from SARS-CoV-2, the novel coronavirus that causes COVID-19 disease. Whilst mortality rates vary with different countries and regions, there is widespread consensus that SARS-CoV-2 has a case fatality rate (mortality in individuals with the disease) of 1% compared to 9.7% in severe acute respiratory syndrome (SARS) and 34% in Middle East respiratory syndrome (MERS) (Petersen et al. 2020). Even in those who survive infection with the SARS-CoV-2 virus, there is a considerable burden of illness, often lasting many months. In a study of 143 Italian patients discharged from COVID-19 hospitalisation, only 18 patients (12.6%) were completely free of any COVID-19 symptoms when assessed a mean of 60.3 days after onset of the first symptom. A further 32% of patients had one or two symptoms, and 55% had three or more symptoms (Carfi et al. 2020). The term "Long COVID" has been coined by people with persistent COVID symptoms to describe the lingering illness that they are experiencing. The World Health Organization (2021) has developed a clinical case definition of what it calls "post COVID-19 condition":

> Post COVID-19 condition occurs in individuals with a history of probable or confirmed SARS CoV-2 infection, usually 3 months from the onset of COVID-19 with symptoms and that last for at least 2 months and cannot be explained by an alternative diagnosis. Common symptoms include fatigue, shortness of breath, cognitive dysfunction but also others and generally have an impact on everyday functioning. Symptoms may be new onset following initial recovery from an acute COVID 19 episode or persist from the initial illness. Symptoms may also fluctuate or relapse over time.

This definition recognises that alongside physical symptoms such as fatigue and breathlessness, adults with Long COVID also frequently report an array of cognitive-linguistic difficulties described as "brain fog." This expression captures problems with memory, a lack of attention and concentration, word-finding difficulty in conversation, and struggles with reading and writing. In my work with adults who have Long COVID, many participants have described in detail the nature of these cognitive-linguistic disturbances and the impact of these problems on work and other daily activities. It will be noted from the following testimonies of some of these adults that these symptoms extend well beyond the 12-week period described previously by the World Health Organization:

### *31-year-old woman; 8 months post-onset (reading):*

My reading was impacted severely around July–August 2020. I simply couldn't read one page. My head was spinning, I did not understand what I was reading. At the moment it's still hard to read and understand everything 100%. It takes me much more time than before. Prior to COVID

I would spend hours reading (at work + minimum 1h for my pleasure at home). This is impacted now. I also find it hard to follow scientific articles or books.

### 33-year-old woman; 6 months post-onset (topic of conversation):

I often forget what the question was midway through answering and if we tangent during the conversation I will have no idea where we started.

### 61-year-old man; 7 months post-onset (memory):

Seems to be worse. I write more lists. Often struggle to find words and names. When I get into a good phase I find things and projects I've "dropped" and/or forgotten about. I started filling this in a week or so ago, and have just remembered I didn't finish it.

### 52-year-old woman; 10 months post-onset (language comprehension):

Sometimes I feel like I didn't hear it right, and I don't have hearing issues. I think I'm really not understanding what I'm hearing.

### 31-year-old woman; 8 months post-onset (word-finding difficulty):

I lose track of my thought process and struggle to find the right word, or I use the wrong one without realising.

### 53-year-old woman; 10 months post-onset (attention and concentration):

I notice I often "zone out" and miss what is being said. I sometimes struggle to pay attention for long periods.

### 60-year-old woman; 5 months post-onset (language problems):

Family and friends understand my word blindness, word substitution and losing my way during a sentence etc. It can be highly embarrassing with strangers or those who don't know me well especially with medical matters so I minimise those.

That cognitive-linguistic difficulties should be reported as part of the Long COVID syndrome is not entirely unexpected. It was apparent to Chinese doctors who treated early cases of COVID-19 infection in Wuhan that the SARS-CoV-2 virus affects many organs and systems in the body other than the lungs and respiration (Li et al. 2020). This includes the nervous system. Neurological symptoms (e.g., headache) and complications (e.g., cerebral hemorrhage) are recognised clinical features of patients with COVID-19 infection (Collantes et al. 2021). Also, the SARS-CoV-2 virus has been detected in neural tissue on postmortem examination (Paniz-Mondolfi et al. 2020), although central nervous system (CNS) involvement caused by direct neuroinvasion is believed to be rare relative to CNS sequelae related to systemic hyper-inflammation (Najjar et al. 2020). Neurological findings from seriously ill and deceased patients with COVID-19 infection may not relate directly to non-hospitalised adults with moderate COVID illness. But they do provide a tentative basis for investigating if cognitive-linguistic difficulties in Long COVID might have a neurological basis or are a consequence of factors like fatigue in the Long COVID syndrome.

## 5.3  An experimental study

In October 2020, I was motivated by increasing media reports and personal accounts of cognitive-linguistic issues in Long COVID to start collecting data from adults who were not making a good recovery from their COVID infections. I contacted several people who were active on online Long COVID support groups in the UK. It was clear to me that reports of brain fog by users of these groups were too numerous and consistent for these difficulties to be a rare feature of Long COVID and that some investigation of these difficulties was warranted. On 15 October 2020, I conducted my first online interview of an adult with Long COVID. The participant was a 61-year-old genetic pathologist who contracted SARS-CoV-2 in March 2020 at the beginning of the first wave of the COVID pandemic in the UK. He was still experiencing significant symptoms some seven months after his acute illness. That case is published elsewhere (Cummings 2021a). It prompted me to embark on an experimental study to establish if there were identifiable cognitive-linguistic deficits in these adults and if such impairments that did exist were neurological consequences of COVID-19 infection or were related to the debilitating fatigue that is reported by people with Long COVID.

## *Method*

### *Participants*

Recruitment to the study was conducted by means of posts on Long COVID and myalgic encephalomyelitis/chronic fatigue syndrome (ME/CFS) support groups on Facebook and other forms of social media. The participants were adults who resided in the UK, Ireland, Canada, USA, Australia, Brazil, and Belgium. They emailed me directly after reading posts about the study. All healthy (non-COVID) participants were recruited from amongst academic colleagues, former students, and personal contacts in Hong Kong, mainland China, Belgium, Ireland, and the UK. Each participant signed a consent form and received an information sheet about the study. COVID participants were asked to complete a 38-item questionnaire about their lifestyle and general health prior to COVID infection and the onset and development of their COVID illness. A similar questionnaire was completed by ME/CFS participants. The study was approved by the Human Subjects Ethics Sub-Committee of The Hong Kong Polytechnic University.

Subjects were recruited to one of six groups in the study (see Table 5.1 in Appendix). Adults with Long COVID who reported cognitive-linguistic difficulties ("brain fog") were assigned to a COVID experimental group. Adults with COVID who did not report cognitive-linguistic difficulties were assigned to a COVID control group. Because several COVID participants spoke English as a second language, it was necessary to form a separate group of these subjects and to have a control group of L2 English speakers without COVID. There was also a control group of healthy participants who had not had COVID. A further control group of participants with ME/CFS was included in the study.

The chief reason COVID and ME/CFS control groups were used in the study was that the debilitating fatigue that is a feature of Long COVID is a potential performance limitation on language and cognition. Fatigue adversely impacts cognitive-linguistic performance in healthy individuals and in individuals with conditions like ME/CFS. It is noteworthy that language and cognitive problems are also documented in adults with ME/CFS (Moss 1995; Daly et al. 2001; Park et al. 2001). In the absence of COVID and ME/CFS control participants, the reduced performance of COVID experimental participants on the tasks in the study may simply reflect the fatigue of these participants rather than any COVID-related neurological dysfunction.

With one exception, COVID participants in the study remained at home during their illness. Most received medical advice by telephone, and several had the assistance of paramedics for breathing difficulties and other symptoms (see Figures 5.1 and 5.2 in Appendix for symptoms at onset and overall symptoms, respectively). A few COVID participants attended accident and emergency departments at their local hospitals or had short one- or two-day admissions to hospital for treatment of symptoms. The lack of extended periods of hospitalisation was more a sign of the parlous condition of many medical facilities and health systems at the start of the pandemic than an indication that the symptoms of participants were mild in nature and did not require intensive medical support. The age, gender, and educational background of all participants in the study are displayed in Table 5.1. The occupational status and pre-COVID lifestyles of the 92 COVID participants in the study are displayed in Table 5.2. None of the participants had a pre-existing language disorder or any condition (e.g., traumatic brain injury) that would place them at risk of such a disorder.

Amongst the 92 adults with COVID in the study, 52 received a clinical diagnosis of COVID infection by a physician, 16 had a positive PCR test, 20 had a positive antibody test, and 4 had a positive PCR *and* antibody test (see Table 5.3 in Appendix).

## Interviews

All interviews were conducted online because of COVID restrictions and the geographical distance between the author and participants. Skype or Zoom was used in accordance with the preference of participants. Each participant was interviewed on a date and at a time of their choice. Interviews lasted approximately one hour. One participant became upset at her performance on the tasks and was interviewed in two sessions conducted over consecutive days. All other participants were fully tested in a single session. Adults with COVID were interviewed on average 351.7 days (11.7 months) after the onset of their COVID symptoms. The time between symptom onset and interviews ranged from 102 to 572 days (3.4 to 19.1 months). It should be noted that the timing of interviews of all COVID participants exceeded the 12-week period stipulated in the clinical case definition of the post COVID-19 condition adopted by the World Health Organization.

## Tasks and materials

A series of 12 tasks was conducted during each interview. All tasks were administered by the author, who used a standard set of prompts and presented tasks in the same order. Test sessions were recorded using two digital voice recorders (Sony ICD-UX560F) and the record function on either Skype or Zoom. The tasks had previously been used in a study of language in adults with neurodegeneration (Cummings 2020) and had been found to be effective in eliciting high-quality data for linguistic analysis. Each task and its associated instructions are shown as follows:

(1) *Immediate recall*: A 100-word story titled "Sam and Fred" was read aloud to each participant, who was then asked to recall it immediately. Instruction: "I'm going to tell you a short story. I want you to listen to it carefully. I will then ask you to tell it back to me."

(2) *Cookie Theft picture description*: This is the picture description task from the Boston Diagnostic Aphasia Examination (Goodglass et al. 2001). Participants were asked to describe a black-and-white line drawing of a domestic scene whilst viewing the image. Instruction: "Here is a picture I would like you to look at. Tell me everything you see going on in this picture."

(3) *Sentence generation*: Participants are auditorily presented with two, three, and four words and are asked to generate a brief sentence. Instruction: "I'm going to give you words and I want you to put them in a brief sentence. Don't worry about the order of the words. You can use the words in any order."

(4) *Flowerpot Incident narration*: Participants are shown six black-and-white line drawings in sequence and are asked to tell a story based on the pictures. Instruction: "Here are six pictures. Please take a couple of minutes to look at each of them. I am then going to ask you to tell a story based on the pictures."

(5) *Phonemic (letter) fluency*: Participants are asked to generate words beginning with the letters "F," "A," and "S" in 60 seconds. Instruction: "Tell me as many words as possible that begin with the letter 'F.' Do not use names like *Fred* and multiple words with the same stem but different endings like *friend, friends, friendly*. You have 60 seconds. I will start the stopwatch as soon as you give me the first word with 'F.'"

(6) *Semantic (category) fluency 1*: Participants are asked to generate the names of animals in 60 seconds. Instruction: "Tell me as many names of animals as possible. They can be the names of domestic animals, wild animals, or exotic animals. You have 60 seconds. I will start the stopwatch as soon as you give me the first name of an animal."

(7) *Semantic (category) fluency 2*: Participants are asked to generate the names of vegetables in 60 seconds. Instruction: "Tell me as many names of vegetables as possible. They can be the names of vegetables from all over the world. You have 60 seconds. I will start the stopwatch as soon as you give me the first name of a vegetable."

(8) *Cinderella story*: Participants are shown a wordless picture book of the Cinderella story. The book is then closed, and participants are asked to narrate the story. Instruction: "I'm sure you are familiar with the story of Cinderella. I am going to use these pictures to refresh your memory of the story. I will scroll down the pictures and stop at each one. If you are happy with a picture, just say "okay." If you need me to explain how the picture relates to the story, please let me know. When we get to the end of the pictures, I am going to ask you to tell me the full Cinderella story."

(9) *Procedural discourse 1*: Participants are asked to describe the steps that someone would go through to make a cheese and ham sandwich. Instruction: "Can you talk me through all the steps or stages needed to make a cheese and ham sandwich?"

(10) *Procedural discourse 2*: Participants are asked to describe the steps that someone would go through to write a letter to someone. Instruction: "Can you talk me through all the steps or stages needed to write a letter to someone?"

(11) *Confrontation naming*: Participants are shown 20 black-and-white line drawings of objects and animals and are asked to name them. Instruction: "I'm

going to give you a number and I would like you to give me the name of the thing next to it."

(12) *Delayed recall:* Participants are asked to recall the 100-word story (Sam and Fred story) that was read aloud to them at the beginning of the session. Instruction: "I told you a short story at the start of the session. Can you tell me that story back again now?"

## Results

The number of essential propositions, correct words, and other responses to each of the 12 tasks was counted. Generalised linear models (GLM) with Poisson distribution were then fitted separately, with the count from each task as the outcome variable and COVID status (i.e., +/- COVID) as the (categorical) predictor variable. The more common independent-samples t-test is inappropriate in this case because count data do not meet the assumption of normal distribution.

The mean and standard deviation for all 12 tests across the six groups in the study are displayed in Table 5.4 in the Appendix. The effect of age, gender, and education on test performance was analysed separately using GLM with Poisson distribution with the count from each task as the outcome variable and age, gender, and education as the predictor variables. There were significant positive effects of age (increasing age resulting in better performance) in 5 of 12 tasks: flowerpot-incident narration ($z=2.439$, $p<0.05$); letter fluency ($z=2.750$, $p<0.05$); category fluency for vegetables ($z=2.126$, $p<0.05$); sandwich-making procedural discourse ($z=2.631$, $p<0.05$); and confrontation naming ($z=2.654$, $p<0.05$). Male subjects performed significantly better than female subjects on letter fluency ($z=2.351$, $p<0.05$) but performed significantly worse than female subjects on category fluency for vegetables ($z=-2.085$, $p<0.05$). There was an effect of education on performance in only one test. Participants with under 17 years of education performed significantly worse on Cinderella narration ($z=-3.655$, $p<0.001$) than participants with 17 or more years of education.

The performance of COVID experimental participants in the study was significantly weaker than that of healthy participants, COVID control participants, and ME/CFS participants in several tests (see Tables 5.5–5.7 in Appendix). The most marked reduction in performance was observed relative to healthy participants, with COVID participants achieving significantly lower scores than healthy participants on 7 of 12 tests: immediate recall ($z=-4.18$, $p<0.001$); delayed recall ($z=-6.47$, $p<0.001$); Cookie Theft picture description ($z=-2.03$, $p<0.05$); flowerpot-incident narration ($z=-2.65$, $p<0.05$); Cinderella narration ($z=-5.98$, $p<0.001$); letter fluency ($z=-7.49$, $p<0.001$); and category fluency for animals ($z=-3.69$, $p<0.001$). However, COVID experimental participants also performed significantly less well than COVID control participants with no self-reported cognitive-linguistic difficulties on 4 of 12 tests: immediate recall ($z=-4.09$, $p<0.001$); delayed recall ($z=-5.33$, $p<0.001$); letter fluency ($z=-7.96$, p<0.001); and Cinderella narration (z=−4.06, p<0.001). COVID experimental participants performed significantly less well than ME/CFS participants, with whom they share debilitating levels of fatigue, on 3 of 12 tasks: immediate recall (z=−1.97, p=0.05); delayed recall (z=−3.89, p<0.001); and Cinderella narration (z=−3.06, p<0.001).

Other between-group comparisons were also revealing. There were only two significant differences between L2 English speakers with COVID and L2 English healthy participants (compared to significant differences on seven tests in native English speakers). L2 English speakers with COVID had significantly poorer performance than L2 English healthy participants on letter fluency (z=−2.45, p<0.05) and category fluency for vegetables (z=2.64, p<0.05) (Table 5.8). The performance of ME/CFS participants and COVID control participants was significantly poorer than the performance of healthy participants on letter fluency only (z=5.66, p<0.001 and z=2.04, p<0.05, respectively). Finally, there was only one significant difference between COVID control participants and ME/CFS participants. The letter fluency performance of ME/CFS participants was significantly poorer than the letter fluency performance of COVID control participants (z=−6.61, p<0.001).

To establish if there is a relationship between cognitive functions measured by means of immediate and delayed verbal recall (tests 1 and 12) and letter fluency (test 5) on the one hand and informativeness during discourse production (tests 2, 4 and 8) on the other hand, Spearman's rank correlation coefficients were calculated. For healthy participants, there was a small to moderate correlation between immediate recall and flowerpot narration (r=0.46) and between delayed recall and flowerpot narration (r=0.38). For COVID experimental participants, there was a small correlation between letter fluency and flowerpot narration (r=0.33). For COVID control participants, there was a moderate to large correlation between immediate recall and flowerpot narration (r=0.70) and between delayed recall and flowerpot narration (r=0.67). There was a moderate correlation between delayed recall and flowerpot narration (r=0.58) in L2 English COVID participants. There was a small to moderate correlation between letter fluency and Cookie Theft picture description (r=0.40) and a moderate correlation between letter fluency and flowerpot narration (r=0.60) in L2 English healthy participants.

## 5.4 Discussion

Speech, language, swallowing, and cognitive problems are well-recognised sequelae of infectious disease in children and adults (Cummings 2019). It is therefore not surprising that dysarthria, dysphagia, and cognitive and language disorders are reported in adults with severe COVID disease requiring hospitalisation (Dawson et al. 2020; Ellul et al. 2020; Priftis et al. 2020, 2021). What is remarkable, however, is that the adults in this study, who were not hospitalised and had milder forms of infection, also present with marked cognitive-linguistic difficulties.

Moreover, these difficulties were evident many months after the onset of COVID illness when one might expect any cognitive-linguistic disturbance related to acute infection to have resolved. Whilst there has been some evidence to date of cognitive deficits in people who have recovered from COVID infection (Hampshire et al. 2021) and in people with Long COVID (Graham et al. 2021), this is the first study to find evidence of specific language deficits in individuals with Long COVID (see also Cummings 2021b).

A clear finding of this study is that adults with Long COVID have reduced discourse informativeness. The informativeness of spoken discourse in participants with Long COVID was significantly reduced relative to healthy participants in the study, COVID participants who did not report cognitive deficits ("brain fog"), and participants with ME/CFS. This latter finding suggests that reduced informativeness is not a consequence of the performance limitation that extreme fatigue in Long COVID can place on cognitive processing. Although reduced informativeness was evident in COVID participants who are native speakers of English, it was not a feature of COVID participants in the study who speak English as a second language. This latter finding may simply be a consequence of the small number of participants in the two L2 English groups or the heterogeneity in the linguistic backgrounds of the L2 English participants in the study. It would be interesting to repeat this investigation with much larger groups of L2 English participants of similar language backgrounds to establish if this result still obtains.

The reduction in informativeness increased incrementally with the cognitive challenge of the discourse production tasks used in the study. The smallest decrement in informativeness was found in the Cookie Theft picture-description task, a task in which participants were required to generate an informative description based on a single scene whilst in receipt of pictorial support. Informativeness was more compromised during the Flowerpot Incident narration, a task during which participants had to integrate information across a sequence of six pictures, also whilst in receipt of pictorial support. This integration could only be achieved if participants were able to draw inferences that linked events and characters in the story. The need to undertake temporal and causal inferences, present events in the correct order or sequence, and relate characters' actions to their motivations and mental states placed greater cognitive demands on the narrator than those required to generate a description based on a single scene. Finally, informativeness was most compromised during Cinderella narration. Where Cookie Theft picture description and Flowerpot Incident narration made few demands on memory – participants viewed pictures throughout these tasks – the narration of the Cinderella story in the absence of pictures placed considerable demands on memory. Also, the number of events and characters in this task well exceeds those in the other discourse production tasks. This greater informational load and high demand on memory surpassed the cognitive capacities of most COVID participants in the study, with a significant decrease in their informativeness during this task as a result. Moreover, this decrease appeared not to be mitigated by the inevitable priming that is achieved when the mental script of a well-known fictional narrative like the Cinderella story is activated.

A question of some interest is why this reduced informativeness is occurring during discourse production by the COVID participants in the study. It is not on account of any structural language deficits on the part of these participants. Individuals with Long COVID were able to produce well-formed and meaningful language. This was indicated not only by their performance during spontaneous conversation but also by their sentence-generation and confrontation-naming scores, which were the same as those of healthy participants in the study. COVID participants had access to the grammatical structures and lexical repertoire that was required to produce informative discourse. Instead, the difficulties with informativeness of these participants lie squarely within the underlying cognitive skills that are required to generate informative discourse. Speakers draw on these cognitive skills to foreground some information and leave other information implicit in the background of a story, to sequence information so that the hearer can construct a coherent mental representation of the events in a story, and to explain the actions of characters through causal, temporal, and mental state inferences. The demands of this high-level information processing on memory and other cognitive abilities such as executive functioning are considerable. It is decreased efficiency of the cognitive skills that permit these high-level discourse processes to come about that is responsible for the reduced informativeness of people with Long COVID in the study. This point warrants further examination.

The production of informative discourse involves a complex array of cognitive-linguistic processes. To produce an informative story, a speaker must establish what a hearer does not know and must be told explicitly (equally, what a hearer already knows and does not need to be told). The attribution of knowledge (and ignorance) to the mind of a hearer involves *theory of mind* skills. During spoken discourse, speakers also strive to present information in a manner that can be readily assimilated by the hearer. Hearers can achieve better comprehension of discourse when they are told events in the order in which they occurred. If John crashed his car and then phoned the police, it is not facilitative of comprehension for a hearer to be told first that John phoned the police and only much later that he crashed his car. The ordering or sequencing of information occurs during our planning of discourse and uses *executive function* skills. A skilled narrator must also know how to introduce characters into a story and make subsequent reference to them through use of pronouns. If this introduction is performed poorly (e.g., the narrator says *"The king wants a wife for his son"* when there is no prior mention of the king) or if pronominal reference is used inadequately (e.g., the pronoun "she" is used when it is not clear if the intended referent is *Cinderella*, the *wicked stepmother*, or the *fairy godmother*), a hearer cannot track characters over consecutive utterances. Certain linguistic selections must occur alongside cognitive skills like mental state reasoning for a speaker to introduce characters into a story and for a hearer to succeed in tracking them.

When these different cognitive-linguistic skills come together smoothly, a speaker can achieve a high level of discourse informativeness. When they break down, discourse informativeness is compromised to a greater or lesser extent. To illustrate the reduced informativeness of the COVID participants in the study, consider the following Cinderella narrative produced by a male participant aged 36.9 years. He was 7.7 months post onset of symptoms:

### Cinderella narrative:

Cinderella (.) is walking with her horse to a well she meets a man (0.2) she then goes only cos I know the story goes home er and the (.) wicked mother and ugly sisters are there she has to work (.) doing the menial jobs such as the sweeping (.) she's friends with the animals (.) uhm (.) they're mean to her and they (.) tear apart her (.) clothing (.) er she goes (.) to the ball (.) meets the fairy godmother (.) who (.) gives her glass slippers and uses magic to turn her into a (.) to enable her to wear a beautiful dress she meets prince charming she has to leave her slipper falls off her foot on the stair (.) she (0.2) meets him again (.) and they get married.

This participant produced 13 of 50 essential propositions and obtained an informativeness score of 26%. His performance on this narrative-production task fell between 3 and 4 standard deviations below the mean score of healthy participants in the study. This speaker's reduced informativeness can be explained as follows. He omits considerable information. There is no mention of the circumstances that led to Cinderella living with her stepmother and stepsisters, why the ball was organised, and where it was held. We are not told why or when Cinderella must leave the ball – she must leave because the spell will be broken at midnight – or that a search was launched to find the owner of the glass slipper. As well as omitting information, the speaker with COVID relates events in the wrong order. He states that Cinderella meets the fairy godmother *after* she goes to the ball when, in fact, she meets her *before* she attends the ball. The fairy godmother and her magic spell must be presented first in the story for Cinderella to have the clothing and transport that she needs to attend the ball.

This participant also displays some anomalies in his use of pronominal reference. A hearer will identify the noun phrase *the animals* as the intended referent of the pronoun *they* in line 4. This noun phrase is, after all, proximal to the pronoun. However, the *actual* referent is the distal noun phrase *the wicked mother and ugly sisters* in lines 2 and 3. This potential misunderstanding on the part of the hearer will likely be resolved as more information is presented by the speaker – it becomes increasingly apparent from context that the pronoun refers to the stepmother and stepsisters and not to the animals. However, the speaker should avoid the need for the hearer to revise his assignment of a referent to the pronoun by using a construction that contains an explicit noun phrase:

> the (.) wicked mother and ugly sisters are there she has to work (.) doing the menial jobs such as the sweeping (.) she's friends with the animals (.) uhm (.) **the stepmother and stepsisters** are mean to her and they (.) tear apart her (.) clothing [. . .]

It is contended that the reduced informativeness of speakers with Long COVID in this study has its basis in cognitive dysfunction and is not a primary language impairment. In this connection, it is interesting to note that letter fluency (a measure of executive function) and immediate and delayed verbal recall were also areas of marked difficulty in the performance of participants with Long COVID in the study. The performance of COVID experimental participants in letter fluency and verbal recall was significantly poorer than these same cognitive areas in healthy participants, COVID control participants, and participants with ME/CFS (immediate and delayed recall only). Moreover, whilst there was a small to moderate correlation between immediate recall and flowerpot narration ($r$=0.46) and between delayed recall and flowerpot narration ($r$=0.38) in healthy participants, and a moderate to large correlation between immediate recall and flowerpot narration ($r$=0.70) and between delayed recall and flowerpot narration ($r$=0.67) in COVID control participants, the opposite pattern was evident for COVID experimental participants: there was no correlation between immediate and delayed recall and flowerpot narration and a small correlation between letter fluency and informativeness during flowerpot narration ($r$=0.33). It is possible that in COVID participants with cognitive-linguistic difficulties, cognitive and language functions that were highly integrated pre-COVID were operating less efficiently following COVID-19 infection. Cognitive performance in areas like executive function has been found to be associated with measures of discourse informativeness in earlier studies (Coelho et al. 1995; Mozeiko et al. 2011). The findings of the current study are consistent with this earlier work and point to a cognitive basis of this discourse difficulty in people with Long COVID.

Fatigue was consistently reported amongst the participants with Long COVID in this study (see Figure 5.2 in Appendix). It is well known that fatigue can serve as a performance limitation on language and cognition. To determine if this factor was contributing to the cognitive-linguistic difficulties of adults with Long COVID, a group of participants with ME/CFS was included in the study. ME/CFS is another clinical condition in which sufferers experience debilitating fatigue. Except for letter fluency, the performance of the ME/CFS participants on the tasks in the study did not differ significantly from that of healthy participants. Meanwhile, the ME/CFS participants performed significantly better than COVID experimental participants on tests of immediate and delayed recall and informativeness during Cinderella narration. Although the ME/CFS control group was comparatively small, these findings suggest that fatigue may not be playing a significant role in the cognitive-linguistic difficulties of adults with Long COVID in this study.

## 5.5 Implications

This study found evidence of cognitive-linguistic difficulties in adults with Long COVID. These adults initially experienced mild-to-moderate COVID infection that did not require hospitalisation. Despite this fact, they had significant cognitive-linguistic difficulties in three areas: immediate and delayed verbal recall; verbal fluency (letter and category); and discourse informativeness. Moreover, these difficulties were evident on average 351 days, or 11 months, after the onset of their COVID symptoms. This time span far exceeds the 12 weeks that is used to diagnose the Long COVID syndrome and suggests that the symptom referred to as "brain fog" is a particularly persistent feature of the post-COVID 19 condition.

It is important to acknowledge that people with Long COVID who participated in the study probably presented with milder cognitive-linguistic difficulties than those found in the wider population of Long COVID sufferers. Many COVID participants had wanted to take part earlier in the study but were too unwell to do so. By the time they came forward to participate, they had already experienced considerable improvement of their cognitive-linguistic difficulties. If these same participants had been assessed several months earlier, it is likely that their cognitive-linguistic problems would have been more severe still. These same remarks apply with equal relevance to the ME/CFS participants in the study. Many people with ME/CFS are too debilitated by their condition to participate in research studies. Consequently, the ME/CFS participants who participated in the study are also likely to have milder difficulties than the ME/CFS population in general (but even then, their letter fluency performance was significantly weaker than that of healthy participants). It is likely that both groups of participants occupy the milder end of a spectrum of cognitive-linguistic difficulties which also has more severe manifestations.

Participants with Long COVID in this study had significant problems with discourse informativeness even as their structural language skills were intact. They could generate well-formed sentences and name pictures with the same degree of accuracy as healthy participants in the study. They had intact auditory verbal comprehension as evidenced by their ability to follow complex task instructions and engage in spontaneous conversation with the author. They could also convey the steps needed to perform simple, everyday tasks as well as healthy participants without COVID. These linguistic areas are problematic for speakers with aphasia where an impairment of language structure is a *primary* language disorder.

Notwithstanding their strong grammatical and lexical-semantic abilities, the adults with Long COVID in this study struggled to harness these expressive language skills to produce informative discourse. Because their discourse problems are related to cognitive difficulties, the language difficulties of adults with Long COVID are most appropriately characterised as a type of cognitive-communication disorder. Speech-language pathologists are familiar with the assessment and treatment of cognitive-communication disorders from their work with adults who have traumatic brain injury (TBI), right-hemisphere damage (RHD), and neurodegenerative conditions like Alzheimer's dementia. It is noteworthy that the production of informative discourse is also a documented difficulty in adults with these conditions (see Power et al. [2020] for TBI; Ash et al. [2017] for neurodegeneration; Marini [2012] for RHD). The results of this study suggest that we must now add Long COVID to the group of cognitive-communication disorders within a wider nosology of language disorder.

This study has several implications for the clinical management of people with Long COVID. First, the cognitive-linguistic difficulties of the adults with Long COVID in this study were sufficiently limiting to affect the ability of 93.48% of them to undertake work duties. These difficulties often persisted long after physical symptoms such as breathlessness and heart palpitations had improved. Occupational health assessments must address cognitive-linguistic issues, and Long COVID clinics must support individuals who have these difficulties. Positive steps in this direction include the recommendation to undertake neurocognitive assessment in people with Long COVID based on a recent Delphi study conducted amongst primary and secondary care doctors (Nurek et al. 2021). Second, the presence of cognitive-linguistic difficulties in adults with Long COVID suggests a need for the inclusion of speech-language pathologists and neuropsychologists in the multidisciplinary teams that are involved in the rehabilitation of these clients. These teams will lack the necessary expertise to manage individuals with Long COVID if they limit their membership to medical professionals in fields like respiratory medicine and neurology.

Third, the language difficulties of adults with Long COVID in this study were revealed through discourse production tasks such as Cinderella narration. They would not have come to light if these adults had been assessed using standardised language batteries such as the Boston Diagnostic Aphasia Examination (Goodglass et al. 2001). Many participants in the study expressed frustration that they had undergone cognitive assessments by neurologists and others, only to be told that their cognitive skills were in the normal range. This was not consistent with the difficulties that they were experiencing, with many participants reporting that their cognitive-linguistic problems had an adverse impact on all aspects of their lives. It appears likely that clinicians will need to adopt more sensitive tools of assessment if they are to succeed in identifying cognitive-linguistic difficulties of adults with Long COVID and "brain fog."

## 5.6 Summary

This study has found that adults with Long COVID who report "brain fog" have significant cognitive-linguistic difficulties. The performance of adults with Long COVID in this study on several language tasks was significantly weaker than the performance of healthy participants, participants with COVID who do not report brain fog, and participants with ME/CFS. These difficulties were present many months after the onset of COVID symptoms and occurred in people who initially had mild to moderate illness. The adults with Long COVID in this study exhibited reduced informativeness in discourse alongside problems with verbal fluency (letter and category) and immediate and delayed verbal recall. Their structural language skills remained largely intact. These difficulties do not appear to be related to fatigue in Long COVID but are a consequence of cognitive problems. Reduced discourse informativeness is a well-recognised linguistic feature of adults with cognitive dysfunction related to TBI, RHD, and neurodegeneration. Consistent with the diagnostic terminology used of these adults, the cognitive-linguistic difficulties of adults with Long COVID are most appropriately classified as a cognitive-communication disorder.

## Acknowledgements

The author would like to acknowledge Dr Phoebe Lin, Department of English and Communication, The Hong Kong Polytechnic University, for her statistical work on this chapter. Her contribution is very gratefully acknowledged.

## Bibliography

Ash, S., Jester, C., York, C., Kofman, O. L., Langey, R., Halpin, A., Firn, K., Dominguez Perez, S., Chahine, L., Spindler, M., Dahodwala, N., Irwin, D. J., McMillan, C., Weintraub, D., & Grossman, M. (2017). Longitudinal decline in speech production in Parkinson's disease spectrum disorders. *Brain and Language*, 171, 42–51.

Carfì, A., Bernabei, R., Landi, F., & Gemelli Against COVID-19 Post-Acute Care Study Group (2020). Persistent symptoms in patients after acute COVID-19. *JAMA*, 324(6), 603–605. https://doi.org/10.1001/jama.2020.12603.

Coelho, C. A., Liles, B. Z., & Duffy, R. J. (1995). Impairments of discourse abilities and executive functions in traumatically brain-injured adults. *Brain Injury*, 9(5), 471–477.

Collantes, M. E. V., Espiritu, A. I., Sy, M. C. C., Anlacan, V. M. M., & Jamora, R. D. G. (2021). Neurological manifestations in COVID-19 infection: A systematic review and meta-analysis. *Canadian Journal of Neurological Sciences*, 48(1), 66–76.

Cummings, L. (2019). Infectious diseases and communication disorders. In J. S. Damico & M. J. Ball (Eds.), *The SAGE encyclopedia of human communication sciences and disorders* (pp. 905–908). Thousand Oaks, CA: SAGE.

Cummings, L. (2020). *Language in dementia*. Cambridge: Cambridge University Press.

Cummings, L. (2021a). COVID-19 and language: A case study. *International Journal of Language Studies*, 15(3), 1–24.

Cummings, L. (2021b). Cognitive-linguistic difficulties in COVID-19: A longitudinal case study. *International Journal of Speech & Language Pathology and Audiology*, 9, 8–19.

Daly, E., Komaroff, A. L., Bloomingdale, K., Wilson, S., & Albert, M. S. (2001). Neuropsychological function in patients with chronic fatigue syndrome, multiple sclerosis, and depression. *Applied Neuropsychology*, 8(1), 12–22.

Dawson, C., Capewell, R., Ellis, S., Matthews, S., Adamson, S., Wood, M., Fitch, L., Reid, K., Shaw, M., Wheeler, J., Pracy, P., Nankivell, P., & Sharma, N. (2020). Dysphagia presentation and management following COVID-19: An acute care tertiary Centre experience. *The Journal of Laryngology & Otology*, https://doi.org/10.1017/S0022215120002443.

Ellul, M. A., Benjamin, L., Singh, B., Lant, S., Michael, B. D., Easton, A., Kneen, R., Defres, S., Sejvar, J., & Solomon, T. (2020). Neurological associations of COVID-19. *Lancet Neurology*, 19, 767–783.

Goodglass, H., Kaplan, E., & Barresi, B. (2001). *Boston diagnostic aphasia examination* (3rd ed.). Baltimore, MD: Lippincott Williams & Wilkins.

Graham, E. L., Clark, J. R., Orban, Z. S., Lim, P. H., Szymanski, A. L., Taylor, C., DiBiase, R. M., Jia, D. T., Balabanov, R., Ho, S. U., Batra, A., Liotta, E. M., & Koralnik, I. J. (2021). Persistent neurologic symptoms and cognitive dysfunction in non-hospitalized Covid-19 "long haulers." *Annals of Clinical and Translational Neurology*, 8(5), 1073–1085.

Hampshire, A., Trender, W., Chamberlain, S. R., Jolly, A. E., Grant, J. E., Patrick, F., Mazibuko, N., Williams, S. C., Barnby, J. M., Hellyer, P., & Mehta, M. A. (2021). Cognitive deficits in people who have recovered from COVID-19. *EClinicalMedicine*, 39, 101044. doi:10.1016/j.eclinm.2021.101044.

Li, X., Wang, L., Yan, S., Yang, F., Xiang, L., Zhu, J., Shen, B., & Gong, Z. (2020). Clinical characteristics of 25 death cases with COVID-19: A retrospective review of medical records in a single medical center, Wuhan, China. *International Journal of Infectious Diseases*, 94, 128–132.

Marini, A. (2012). Characteristics of narrative discourse processing after damage to the right hemisphere. *Seminars in Speech and Language*, 33(1), 68–78.

Moss, S. E. (1995). Cognitive/linguistic deficits associated with chronic fatigue syndrome. *Journal of Chronic Fatigue Syndrome*, 1(3–4), 95–100.

Mozeiko, J., Le, K., Coelho, C., Krueger, F., & Grafman, J. (2011). The relationship of story grammar and executive function following TBI. *Aphasiology*, 25(6–7), 826–835.

Najjar, S., Najjar, A., Chong, D. J., Pramanik, B. K., Kirsch, C., Kuzniecky, R. I., Pacia, S. V., & Azhar, S. (2020). Central nervous system complications associated with SARS-CoV-2 infection: Integrative concepts of pathophysiology and case reports. *Journal of Neuroinflammation*, 17(1), 231. doi:10.1186/s12974-020-01896-0.

Nurek, M., Rayner, C., Freyer, A., Taylor, S., Järte, L., MacDermott, N., & Delaney, B. C. (2021). Recommendations for the recognition, diagnosis, and management of long COVID: A Delphi study. *British Journal of General Practice*, 71(712), e815–e825. https://doi.org/10.3399/BJGP.2021.0265.

Office of National Statistics (2022). Prevalence of ongoing symptoms following coronavirus (COVID-19) infection in the UK: 1 March 2022. www.ons.gov.uk/peoplepopulationandcommunity/healthandsocialcare/conditionsanddiseases/bulletins/prevalenceofongoingsymptomsfollowingcoronaviruscovid19infectionintheuk/1june2022. Accessed 14 July 2022.

Paniz-Mondolfi, A., Bryce, C., Grimes, Z., Gordon, R. E., Reidy, J., Lednicky, J., Sordillo, E. M., & Fowkes, M. (2020). Central nervous system involvement by severe acute respiratory syndrome coronavirus-2 (SARS-CoV-2). *Journal of Medical Virology*, 92(7), 699–702. doi:10.1002/jmv.25915.

Park, P., Youngman, P., & Moss, S. E. (2001). Chronic fatigue syndrome: The role of the speech-language pathologist. *ASHA Leader*, 6(7), 4–5,11.

Petersen, E., Koopmans, M., Go, U., Hamer, D. H., Petrosillo, N., Castelli, F., Storgaard, M., Al Khalili, S., & Simonsen, L. (2020). Comparing SARS-CoV-2 with SARS-CoV and influenza pandemics. *Lancet Infectious Disease*, 20, e238–e244. https://doi.org/10.1016/S1473.3099(20)30484.9.

Power, E., Weir, S., Richardson, J., Fromm, D., Forbes, M., MacWhinney, B., & Togher, L. (2020). Patterns of narrative discourse in early recovery following severe traumatic brain injury. *Brain Injury*, 34(1), 98–109.

Priftis, K., Algeri, L., Villella, S., & Spada, M. S. (2020). COVID-19 presenting with agraphia and conduction aphasia in a patient with left-hemisphere ischemic stroke. *Neurological Sciences*, 41(12), 3381–3384.

Priftis, K., Prior, M., Meneghetti, L., Mercogliano, T., & Bendini, M. (2021). Alexia without agraphia in a post COVID-19 patient with left-hemisphere ischemic stroke. *Neurological Sciences*, 42, 2179–2181.

World Health Organization (2021). A clinical case definition of post COVID-19 condition by a Delphi consensus, 6 October 2021. www.who.int/publications/i/item/WHO-2019-nCoV-Post_COVID-19_condition-Clinical_case_definition-2021.1. Accessed 29 November 2021.

# APPENDIX

**TABLE 5.1** Characteristics of study participants

| Study group | N | Age (mean) | Age (range) | Gender (M/F) | Education (years) |
|---|---|---|---|---|---|
| **COVID experimental participants** | 69 | 49.1 years | 24.0–64.3 years | 5 M/64 F | 29 under 17 years 40 over 17 years |
| **COVID control participants** | 11 | 46.5 years | 30.9–60.6 years | 3 M/8 F | 4 under 17 years 7 over 17 years |
| **ME/CFS participants** | 11 | 49.2 years | 29.3–64.8 years | 1 M/10 F | 5 under 17 years 6 over 17 years |
| **Healthy participants** | 26 | 48.2 years | 18.1–64.6 years | 10 M/16 F | 7 under 17 years 19 over 17 years |
| **L2 English COVID participants**[1] | 12 | 43.2 years | 31.2–62.8 years | 0 M/12 F | 2 under 17 years 10 over 17 years |
| **L2 English control participants**[2] | 13 | 38.3 years | 18.3–60.8 years | 3 M/10 F | 1 under 17 years 12 over 17 years |
| **TOTAL** | 142 | 47.3 years | 18.1–64.8 years | 22 M/120 F | 48 under 17 years 94 over 17 years |

[1] First languages of participants: Mandarin Chinese; Dutch; Romanian; Polish; Portuguese; Italian; Shona (Zimbabwe)

[2] First languages of participants: Mandarin Chinese; Cantonese Chinese; French; Spanish; Dutch

**TABLE 5.2** Occupational status and pre-COVID lifestyle of COVID participants

| Occupational status | | Pre-COVID lifestyle | | |
|---|---|---|---|---|
| Role | % | Lifestyle question | YES | NO |
| Administration | 5.4% | Did you have chronic health problems before COVID-19? | 53.3% | 46.7% |
| Business | 6.5% | | | |
| Creative industries | 3.3% | Did you have a normal body weight for your age, gender, and height before COVID-19? | 53.3% | 46.7% |
| Education | 21.7% | | | |
| Emergency workers | 4.4% | Pre-COVID, did you consume alcoholic beverages? | 67.4% | 32.6% |
| Finance | 5.4% | | | |
| Health, social care, and medicine | 33.7% | Pre-COVID, did you smoke or vape? | 5.4% | 94.6% |
| Retail | 1.1% | | | |
| Research | 2.2% | Pre-COVID, did you take exercise? | 79.4% | 20.6% |
| Retired | 2.2% | | | |
| Unemployed | 7.6% | Pre-COVID, did you eat a well-balanced diet? | 85.9% | 14.1% |
| Wellness and coaching | 5.4% | | | |
| Other | 1.1% | | | |

**TABLE 5.3** The test and diagnostic status of COVID participants

| | Antibody | PCR test | Antibody & PCR test | Clinical diagnosis |
|---|---|---|---|---|
| **COVID experimental Participants** | 14 | 13 | 3 | 39 |
| **COVID control Participants** | 1 | 2 | 1 | 7 |
| **L2 English COVID Participants** | 5 | 1 | 0 | 6 |
| **TOTAL** | 20 | 16 | 4 | 52 |

**TABLE 5.4** Mean and standard deviation (SD) for all tasks and participants

| | Healthy | COVID control | COVID exp | L2 COVID | L2 healthy | ME/CFS |
|---|---|---|---|---|---|---|
| **Test 1** | 9.73 | 10.45 | 7.77 | 7.96 | 8.62 | 9.05 |
| Immediate recall | (1.97) | (1.59) | (2.01) | (2.45) | (1.99) | (1.37) |
| **Test 2** | 7.79 | 7.77 | 6.9 | 5.96 | 6.69 | 7.14 |
| Cookie Theft picture | (1.27) | (0.9) | (1.43) | (1.99) | (1.15) | (1.42) |
| **Test 3** | 5.23 | 5.45 | 5 | 3.75 | 4.69 | 4.82 |
| Sentence generation | (0.86) | (0.82) | (1.03) | (1.42) | (1.11) | (0.6) |
| **Test 4** | 13.85 | 12.82 | 12.3 | 11.29 | 12.42 | 13.23 |
| Flowerpot narration | (2.94) | (2.94) | (2.73) | (2.38) | (1.79) | (3.39) |

*(Continued)*

**TABLE 5.4** (Continued)

| | Healthy | COVID control | COVID exp | L2 COVID | L2 healthy | ME/CFS |
|---|---|---|---|---|---|---|
| **Test 5** | 48.08 | 53.27 | 37 | 31.25 | 37 | 34.45 |
| Letter fluency | (10.85) | (14.45) | (11.51) | (9.49) | (10.32) | (11.17) |
| **Test 6** | 25.81 | 23.45 | 21.74 | 18.17 | 18.69 | 23.82 |
| Animal fluency | (4.72) | (6.68) | (6.68) | (3.81) | (4.7) | (6.37) |
| **Test 7** | 15.31 | 17.18 | 15.16 | 14.17 | 10.46 | 16.18 |
| Vegetable fluency | (3.73) | (3.46) | (4.42) | (4.26) | (3.26) | (2.99) |
| **Test 8** | 32.1 | 31.82 | 26.91 | 32 | 34.23 | 30.59 |
| Cinderella narration | (5.77) | (5.15) | (7.03) | (7.98) | (5.93) | (7.91) |
| **Test 9** | 6.69 | 6.82 | 6.46 | 5.04 | 4.65 | 6.68 |
| Sandwich making | (0.98) | (0.98) | (0.99) | (0.92) | (0.94) | (1.31) |
| **Test 10** | 6.58 | 7.27 | 6.29 | 6.21 | 6.12 | 6.82 |
| Letter writing | (1.42) | (1.42) | (1.32) | (1.03) | (1.42) | (1.23) |
| **Test 11** | 17.62 | 18.27 | 17.71 | 13.75 | 13.15 | 18.73 |
| Confrontation naming | (2.08) | (1.35) | (1.84) | (3.33) | (4.1) | (1.1) |
| **Test 12** | 9.38 | 9.77 | 6.51 | 7.25 | 8.42 | 8.86 |
| Delayed recall | (2.08) | (1.98) | (2.21) | (3.14) | (1.88) | (1.91) |

**TABLE 5.5** Test performance of COVID experimental participants vs. healthy participants

| Test | coefficient | standard error | z value | p-value |
|---|---|---|---|---|
| **Test 1** Immediate recall | −0.23 | 0.05 | −4.18 | **0.00** |
| **Test 2** Cookie theft picture | −0.12 | 0.06 | −2.03 | **0.04** |
| **Test 3** Sentence generation | −0.05 | 0.10 | −0.45 | 0.66 |
| **Test 4** Flowerpot narration | −0.12 | 0.04 | −2.65 | **0.01** |
| **Test 5** Letter fluency | −0.26 | 0.03 | −7.49 | **0.00** |
| **Test 6** Animal fluency | −0.17 | 0.05 | −3.69 | **0.00** |
| **Test 7** Vegetable fluency | −0.01 | 0.06 | −0.16 | 0.87 |
| **Test 8** Cinderella narration | −0.18 | 0.03 | −5.98 | **0.00** |
| **Test 9** Sandwich making | −0.03 | 0.06 | −0.55 | 0.58 |
| **Test 10** Letter writing | −0.04 | 0.06 | −0.70 | 0.48 |
| **Test 11** Confrontation naming | 0.01 | 0.05 | 0.10 | 0.92 |
| **Test 12** Delayed recall | −0.37 | 0.06 | −6.47 | **0.00** |

**TABLE 5.6** Test performance of COVID experimental participants vs. COVID control participants

| Test | coefficient | standard error | z value | p-value |
|---|---|---|---|---|
| **Test 1** Immediate recall | −0.30 | 0.07 | −4.09 | **0.00** |
| **Test 2** Cookie theft picture | −0.12 | 0.08 | −1.43 | 0.15 |
| **Test 3** Sentence generation | −0.09 | 0.14 | −0.62 | 0.53 |
| **Test 4** Flowerpot narration | −0.04 | 0.06 | −0.64 | 0.52 |

| Test | coefficient | standard error | z value | p-value |
|---|---|---|---|---|
| **Test 5** Letter fluency | −0.36 | 0.05 | −7.96 | **0.00** |
| **Test 6** Animal fluency | −0.08 | 0.07 | −1.13 | 0.26 |
| **Test 7** Vegetable fluency | −0.13 | 0.08 | −1.58 | 0.11 |
| **Test 8** Cinderella narration | −0.17 | 0.04 | −4.06 | **0.00** |
| **Test 9** Sandwich making | −0.05 | 0.09 | −0.60 | 0.55 |
| **Test 10** Letter writing | −0.15 | 0.09 | −1.69 | 0.09 |
| **Test 11** Confrontation naming | −0.03 | 0.08 | −0.41 | 0.68 |
| **Test 12** Delayed recall | −0.41 | 0.08 | −5.33 | **0.00** |

**TABLE 5.7** Test performance of COVID experimental participants vs. ME/CFS participants

| Test | coefficient | standard error | z value | p-value |
|---|---|---|---|---|
| **Test 1** Immediate recall | −0.15 | 0.08 | −1.97 | **0.05** |
| **Test 2** Cookie theft picture | −0.03 | 0.09 | −0.39 | 0.70 |
| **Test 3** Sentence generation | 0.04 | 0.15 | 0.25 | 0.80 |
| **Test 4** Flowerpot narration | −0.07 | 0.06 | −1.14 | 0.25 |
| **Test 5** Letter fluency | 0.07 | 0.06 | 1.29 | 0.20 |
| **Test 6** Animal fluency | −0.09 | 0.07 | −1.36 | 0.17 |
| **Test 7** Vegetable fluency | −0.07 | 0.08 | −0.80 | 0.42 |
| **Test 8** Cinderella narration | −0.13 | 0.04 | −3.06 | **0.00** |
| **Test 9** Sandwich making | −0.03 | 0.09 | −0.37 | 0.71 |
| **Test 10** Letter writing | −0.08 | 0.09 | −0.91 | 0.36 |
| **Test 11** Confrontation naming | −0.06 | 0.08 | −0.74 | 0.46 |
| **Test 12** Delayed recall | −0.31 | 0.08 | −3.89 | **0.00** |

**TABLE 5.8** Test performance of L2 English COVID participants vs. L2 English healthy participants

| Test | coefficient | standard error | z value | p-value |
|---|---|---|---|---|
| **Test 1** Immediate recall | −0.08 | 0.10 | −0.81 | 0.42 |
| **Test 2** Cookie theft picture | −0.12 | 0.11 | −1.03 | 0.30 |
| **Test 3** Sentence generation | −0.22 | 0.20 | −1.14 | 0.25 |
| **Test 4** Flowerpot narration | −0.10 | 0.08 | −1.16 | 0.25 |
| **Test 5** Letter fluency | −0.17 | 0.07 | −2.45 | **0.01** |
| **Test 6** Animal fluency | −0.03 | 0.09 | −0.31 | 0.76 |
| **Test 7** Vegetable fluency | 0.30 | 0.12 | 2.64 | **0.01** |
| **Test 8** Cinderella narration | −0.07 | 0.05 | −1.37 | 0.17 |
| **Test 9** Sandwich making | 0.08 | 0.13 | 0.62 | 0.53 |
| **Test 10** Letter writing | 0.02 | 0.11 | 0.13 | 0.89 |
| **Test 11** Confrontation naming | 0.04 | 0.11 | 0.41 | 0.68 |
| **Test 12** Delayed recall | −0.15 | 0.10 | −1.48 | 0.14 |

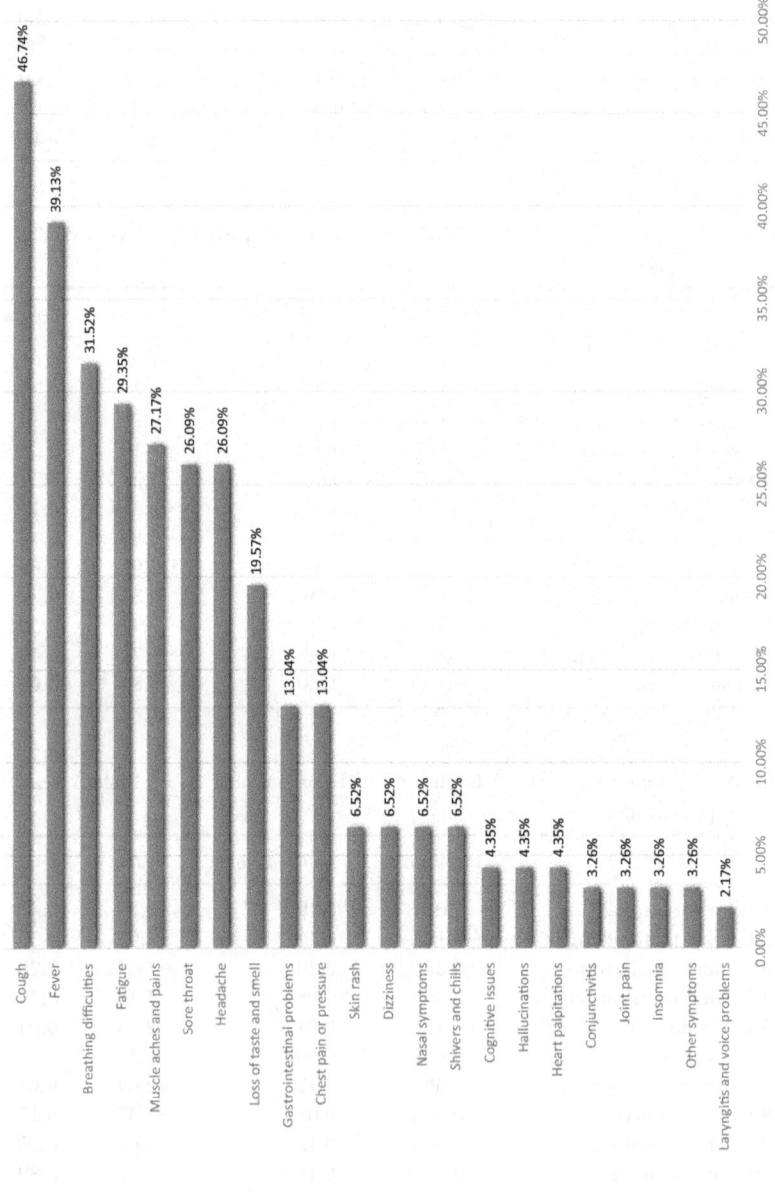

**FIGURE 5.1** Symptoms at COVID onset for the 92 participants with COVID in the study

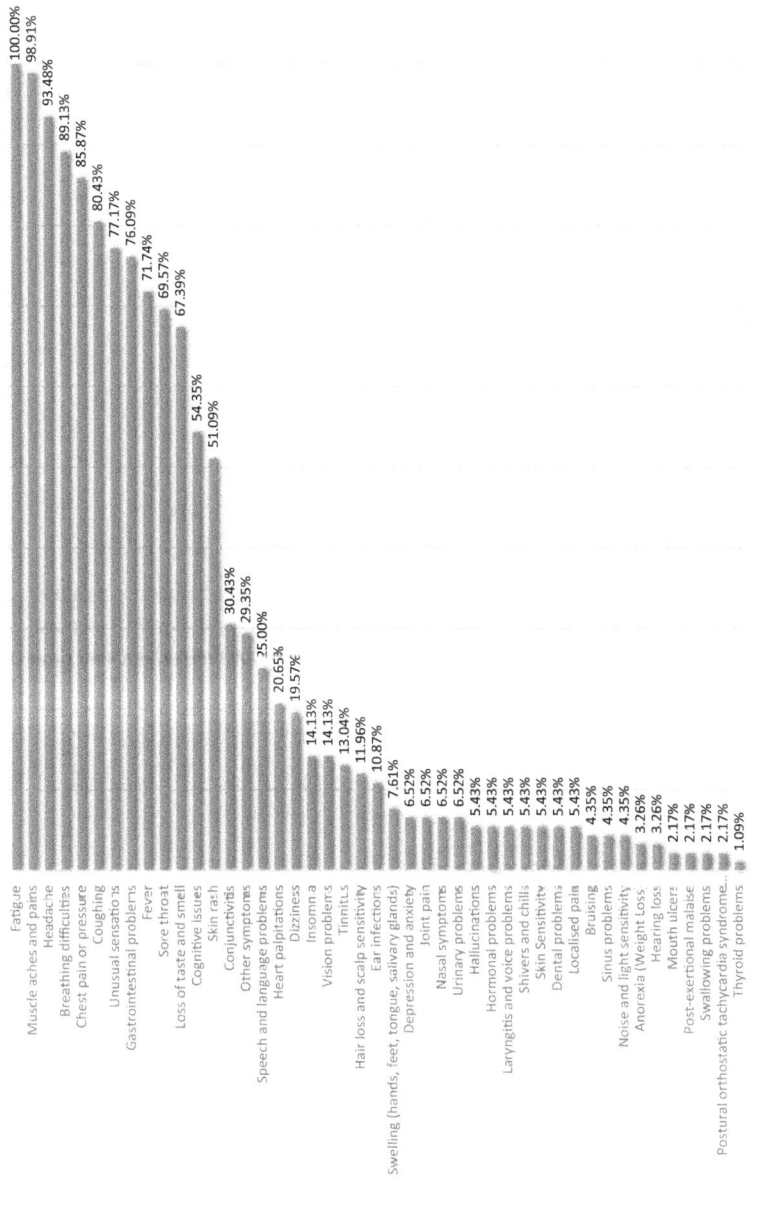

**FIGURE 5.2** Overall COVID symptoms for the 92 participants with COVID in the study

# 6

# COMMUNICATION-RELATED QUALITY OF LIFE IN ADULTS WITH LONG COVID

*Louise Cummings*

---

**43-year-old woman with Long COVID; 8.6 months post onset:**

> "I am unable to do a tiny fraction of a life. Unable to care for myself or my children. Unable to work and generate income. Unable to read, write, speak. Long COVID is crippling physically and mentally. The pain and impairment are just too vast to put across."

---

## 6.1 Introduction

The COVID-19 pandemic continues to pose health and economic challenges for populations around the world. But behind the large and growing deaths from COVID-19 lies a more insidious threat to human well-being and economic stability. This is the threat posed by Long COVID. It is now known that as many as one in seven people who contract SARS-CoV-2 still have symptoms 12 weeks after the onset of their illness (Office for National Statistics 2021). These children and adults have been variously referred to as having Long COVID, the post-COVID syndrome, or more informally as COVID long haulers. People with Long COVID can suffer debilitating physical and cognitive symptoms, with many unable to return to work and resume their social roles due to these difficulties. A set of cognitive-linguistic problems (so-called "brain fog") has proved to be particularly challenging for individuals with Long COVID (Callan et al. 2022). This group of problems is still rather poorly defined and includes behaviours such

DOI: 10.4324/9781003257318-6

as word-finding difficulties, poor memory, and lack of concentration. The consistent reporting of language and communicative problems by people with Long COVID has prompted the author to investigate the nature of these difficulties (Cummings 2021a, 2021b; see Chapter 5 this volume). This chapter extends this investigation by considering the impact of these problems on the quality of life of adults with Long COVID.

The chapter unfolds as follows. Definitions of Long COVID are continually revised as more becomes known about the onset, clinical presentation, and progression of the condition. In section 6.2, Long COVID is defined using the most recent definition adopted by the World Health Organization. This section will also consider risk factors for the development of Long COVID, the prevalence of the condition, and the types of physical and cognitive symptoms that constitute the post-COVID syndrome. Cognitive-linguistic difficulties in people with Long COVID can persist after physical symptoms have resolved and are often the difficulties that most compromise occupational and social functioning. In section 6.3, the nature of these difficulties is considered by examining extracts from the personal narratives of adults with Long COVID who report symptoms of "brain fog." These qualitative reflections are then supplemented in section 6.5 by the findings of a survey of 973 adults with Long COVID. This survey aimed to quantify the effect of Long COVID on spoken and written communication skills and to investigate the impact of post-COVID communication difficulties on an individual's quality of life. The chapter concludes in section 6.7 with an assessment of the implications of these findings for the management of adults with Long COVID. It is argued that speech-language pathologists should play a significant role in the rehabilitation of people with Long COVID.

## 6.2 Long COVID: some background

On 6 October 2021, the World Health Organization published a clinical case definition of post-COVID-19 condition arrived at by a Delphi consensus. Whilst WHO acknowledges that this definition will need to be revised as new evidence emerges about COVID-19, it is nonetheless a valuable starting point for our discussion of Long COVID:

> Post COVID-19 condition occurs in individuals with a history of probable or confirmed SARS CoV-2 infection, usually 3 months from the onset of COVID-19 with symptoms and that last for at least 2 months and cannot be explained by an alternative diagnosis. Common symptoms include fatigue, shortness of breath, cognitive dysfunction but also others and generally have an impact on everyday functioning. Symptoms may be new onset following initial recovery from an acute COVID-19 episode or persist from the initial illness. Symptoms may also fluctuate or relapse over time. (World Health Organization 2021)

The noteworthy features of this definition include the persistence of symptoms **3 months** after COVID onset with a duration of at least **2 months**. There must be **no alternative diagnosis** of the symptoms, which can include **physical problems** (e.g., fatigue) and **cognitive dysfunction**. Symptoms have an impact on everyday functioning. They may **persist** from the acute COVID illness or may be **new onset**. They may also **fluctuate or relapse** over time.

When examined as part of a definition, these features somehow fail to reflect the true magnitude of the post COVID-19 condition. This condition is a lived reality for millions of people worldwide and will be with us for years to come in the form of a large burden of illness and economic inactivity. It is for these reasons that there is now considerable research effort directed towards understanding Long COVID and its impact on people's lives. In this section, we throw light on this largely hidden part of the COVID-19 pandemic by examining the prevalence, symptoms, and risk factors for this chronic condition.

The prevalence of Long COVID varies considerably across studies, ranging from 4.7% to 80% according to a recent review of 25 observational studies (Carbrera Martimbianco et al. 2021). In a systematic review and meta-analysis of 15 studies examining 47,910 patients, Lopez-Leon et al. (2022) estimated that 80% of patients infected with SARS-CoV-2 developed one or more long-term symptoms. Jacobson et al. (2021) found that at 3–4 months post-COVID-19 diagnosis, 81.8% of hospitalised patients and 64.2% of non-hospitalised patients had any COVID symptoms, suggesting a significant burden of long-term illness even in patients with milder COVID illness in the acute stage. The prevalence of Long COVID in children has also been investigated. In a review of 14 studies, Zimmermann et al. (2021) reported that the prevalence of persistent COVID symptoms in children varied considerably from 4% to 66%. Similarly high Long COVID prevalence figures are reported in other countries and territories. The prevalence of Long COVID symptoms at 12 weeks in 2,198 participants in Bangladesh was 16.1% (Hossain et al. 2021). Osikomaiya et al. (2021) examined 274 patients attending the COVID-19 outpatient clinic in Lagos State, Nigeria. More than one-third (40.9%) had persistent COVID-19 symptoms after discharge.

Symptoms in Long COVID have been investigated in several large-scale studies. Over 60 physical and psychological symptoms were reported in a review of studies that examined 10,951 people with Long COVID (Michelen et al. 2021). In a study of 273,618 patients diagnosed with Long COVID, one in three patients had one or more features of Long COVID between three and six months after diagnosis of COVID-19. From most to least common, these features included anxiety/depression (15.49%); abdominal symptoms (8.29%); abnormal breathing (7.94%); "other" pain (7.19%); fatigue/malaise (5.87%); chest/throat pain (5.71%); headache (4.63%); cognitive symptoms (3.95%); and myalgia (1.54%). For two in five of these patients, they had no record of these features in the previous three months (i.e., they were new-onset features) (Taquet et al. 2021). The five most common long-term symptoms reported by Lopez-Leon et al. (2022)

were fatigue (58%); headache (44%); attention disorder (27%); hair loss (25%); and dyspnea (24%).

To control for background symptom prevalence, Wanga et al. (2021) compared symptom persistence (> 4 weeks) in people who received positive SARS-CoV-2 test results (n=698) and people with negative test results (n=2,437) in the United States between January 2020 and April 2021. More persons with positive test results (76.2%) reported persistence of at least one initially occurring symptom at four weeks compared with those with negative test results (69.6%). This higher prevalence was found in fatigue (22.5% versus 12.0%); change in sense of smell or taste (17.3% versus 1.7%); shortness of breath (15.5% versus 5.2%); cough (14.5% versus 4.9%); and headache (13.8% versus 9.9%).

A question of some interest is whether certain population groups are more at risk of Long COVID than others. Taquet et al. (2021) examined the electronic health records of 273,618 patients diagnosed with COVID-19 and reported a higher risk of Long COVID features in patients who had more severe COVID-19 illness and a slightly higher risk in women and in young adults. There was no difference in Long COVID risk between White and non-White patients. Female sex and increasing age and body mass index were associated with Long COVID in a study of 4,182 incident cases of COVID-19 in which individuals self-reported their symptoms prospectively in an app (Sudre et al. 2021). Younger age, female gender, rural residence, prior functional limitation, and smoking have been found to predict the length of Long COVID in a patient cohort in Bangladesh (Hossain et al. 2021). Old age, female sex, severe clinical status, a high number of comorbidities, hospital admission, and oxygen supplementation at the acute phase were risk factors for Long COVID in Carbrera Martimbianco's systematic review of 25 observational studies. The only factor that is consistently reported to increase the risk of Long COVID is female gender.

## 6.3 Brain fog in Long COVID

The term "brain fog" has been coined to characterise cognitive symptoms that are commonly reported by people with Long COVID. Davis et al. (2021) recorded cognitive symptoms, including problems with memory, in approximately 88% of adults of all ages in a study of 3,762 people with COVID illness lasting over 28 days. Many cognitive symptoms are present at the acute illness stage and then persist for weeks and months. Orrù et al. (2021) found cognitive impairment (brain fog, loss of concentration) in 40% of study participants who were currently positive for COVID-19. Cognitive symptoms were also reported in 47.06% of participants who had had COVID-19 but had not been positive for less than a month, 59.46% who had not been positive for at least a month, 47.40% who had not been positive for at least two months, and 48.68% who had not been positive for at least three months. Other cognitive symptoms appear to arise for the first time after the acute phase of illness. It is possible, however, that these symptoms are present during the acute phase of COVID-19 and are masked by physical symptoms and extended periods of rest. Cognitive problems may then become apparent for the first time as some physical symptoms improve and people with COVID start to resume work and social functions.

> ### 45-year-old woman; 21.1 months post onset:
>
> "Cognitively it felt like my brain was 'full' – I couldn't follow instructions, hold conversations, follow storylines or anything where I had to hold information in my head."

The symptom of brain fog is a constellation of wide-ranging cognitive and linguistic problems. These problems include issues with memory and concentration but also difficulties with speaking, reading, writing, and comprehension. Language is the vehicle through which we communicate with others, and its disruption has been one of the most distressing symptoms experienced by people with Long COVID. The author recorded the responses of 92 people with test-confirmed or clinically diagnosed COVID-19 as they characterised the impact of their illness on language across the four areas of speech and writing (expressive language) and comprehension and reading (receptive language) (see Chapter 5). Some understanding of the impact of COVID-19 on each of these areas can be gleaned from examining the comments of several study participants as they reflect on the effect of their illness on language skills (see Table 6.1).

Language difficulties have left previously articulate, skilled communicators unable to participate in conversation with family members and friends, enjoy hobbies such as reading, and struggling to complete tasks required of them in their occupational roles. Once mundane activities like writing a birthday card require rehearsal and additional time; considerable editing is needed to write a text. The frustration resulting from these difficulties is palpable in at least one of these participants. Another reported feeling embarrassed by his language and communication skills, even attempting to "cover" for his difficulties in conversation with others. It is unsurprising that these difficulties have left adults with Long COVID wanting to avoid communication with others, change the way in which they communicate with others, and reduce the frequency of communication with family members, friends, and colleagues. There is also a marked negative impact on the desire to communicate, with many adults with Long COVID no longer feeling motivated to communicate or confident enough to communicate with people other than family members (see Table 6.2).

**TABLE 6.1** Participant reports of impact of COVID-19 on language

*Receptive language*

| Comprehension | Reading |
|---|---|
| **Woman: 38.3 years; 18.3 months post onset:** "It's mostly when fatigued that I have difficulty following a conversation. It's not so much that I forget what they said – most of the time I don't even register what they're saying." | **Woman: 51.4 years; 10.6 months post onset:** "Reading has been a challenge – I was an avid reader, and it's like I can't digest the info – I can see the words, read the words, but it doesn't go in." |
| **Woman: 40.6 years; 18.6 months post onset:** "Someone says something to me and I have to sit and think for a minute to try to process what they've said and how I need to respond. If I'm asked a question with more than one part to it, I find I can only remember one part of the question." | **Woman: 45.6 years; 7.6 months post onset:** "I can't read. AAAAAARRRGGGHHH. One of my two jobs is to read large volumes of evidence for General Medical Council fitness to practise case examiner work. Brain fog descends after a couple of minutes, and I can't concentrate. I used to be in a book club and read a book every two to four weeks but have read nothing for pleasure." |

*Expressive language*

| Speech | Writing |
|---|---|
| **Man: 55.5 years; 17.9 months post onset:** "I can keep things going but I can start rambling and introduce things to cover for not knowing something. I sometimes get into a complete mess as I can't keep talking and think about what comes next at the same time." | **Woman: 61 years; 15.4 months post onset:** "The first birthday card I wrote after becoming ill was a disaster – my hand would not do what I wanted it to. I ruined it and had to find another one. I now practise what I'm going to write in a card and take lots of time over it. Rushing is impossible." |
| **Woman: 44.1 years; 10.8 months post onset:** "General easy chit-chat at home now easier, but it wasn't always easy as I couldn't string a sentence together for four months [. . .] I can now manage conversation on phone for longer, but I know when it's about to go [. . .] all of a sudden speech will become slurred." | **Woman: 51.3 years; 8.9 months post onset:** "I was wrong in saying the effects hadn't affected my written communication. Predictive text and auto correct mask the mistakes, but when I investigated, I was slower and made many more mistakes in writing too. I just go back and edit all the time." |

These responses provide sufficient evidence of a significant burden of communication disability and related impact on quality of life in adults with Long COVID to warrant further investigation. To this end, an online survey of 973 adults with Long COVID was conducted. The aim of the survey was twofold: to capture the type of communicative difficulties that occur in adults with Long

**TABLE 6.2** Participant reports of impact of COVID-19 on communication motivation, frequency, and mode

---

*Motivation to communicate*

---

**Woman: 53.6 years; 9 months post onset:**
"Sometimes I find I do not want to engage in conversation (I am usually very chatty) and will give one-word answers to people."

**Woman: 45.3 years; 15.2 months post onset:**
"To be honest, it [conversation] feels like a lot of hard work, and I'm not sure it's worth the effort at the moment."

**Woman: 42.3 years; 15.2 months post onset:**
"I tend to shy away from conversations with strangers as I come across as stupid, and that makes me feel vulnerable. Family make allowances for me, but out and about I withdraw."

**Woman: 61.6 years; 7.5 months post onset:**
"I do want to be connected with people still, but a lot of the time, I don't bother talking because I know the words will come out wrong, or I have too little energy to have a conversation."

**Woman: 50.9 years; 8 months post onset:**
"I will not participate in conversations as sometimes I just can't be bothered."

**Woman: 53.3 years; 22.2 months post onset:**
"Lost all confidence in joining in any academic conversation or with people that didn't know me before I had COVID, as I feel I come across as stupid and ill-informed."

---

*Frequency of communication*

---

**Woman: 43.8 years; 8.6 months post onset:**
"Decreased as embarrassed. Couldn't trust myself to say the right thing or behave normally. It was like I was very drunk or drugged."

**Man: 61.6 years; 7.4 months post onset:**
"Probably less than usual. I think on reflection I don't initiate so many calls as before."

**Woman: 61 years; 15.4 months post onset:**
"Family and friends understand my word blindness, word substitution, and losing my way during a sentence, etc. It can be highly embarrassing with strangers or those who don't know me well especially with medical matters, so I minimise those."

**Woman: 58.4 years; 16.3 months post onset:**
"I would have spoken to my daughter once a week, and now it's once a fortnight at most."

---

*Mode of communication*

---

**Woman: 53.6 years; 9 months post onset:**
"I have noticed I am reluctant to chat to family members via the phone and sometimes will ignore the phone."

**Woman: 42.3 years; 15.2 months post onset:**
"I'd rather communicate with others via text as I am in control of the speed of reading and replying."

**Woman: 64.3 years; 7.5 months post onset:**
"Because of the difficulties and the embarrassment I feel, I have reduced the communication I have with others face to face or on the phone and resort to messaging more."

**Woman: 51.4 years; 10.7 months post onset:**
"I find I'm texting to keep up with friends – it's easier and less tiring."

---

COVID and to examine the impact of these difficulties on a person's interpersonal relations, work and leisure experiences, and quality of life. The results of this survey are presented in section 6.4. But first, the contribution of communication to quality of life in people with Long COVID is examined.

## 6.4 Communication and quality of life in Long COVID

It has been documented in several studies to date that Long COVID has a significant adverse impact on a person's quality of life. In a review of studies examining 10,951 people with Long COVID, Michelen et al. (2021) found that 37% of patients reported reduced quality of life. Long COVID has been found to compromise quality of life across several domains, including social relationships, occupational functioning, and psychological well-being. Jacobs et al. (2020) examined 183 hospital-discharged patients who reported persistent COVID symptoms at 35 days. These patients gave poor to fair ratings on each of the following domains: quality of life (23.2%); mental health (16.9%); social relationships (60.4%); and active participation in social roles (31.5%). In their study of 3,762 people with COVID illness lasting over 28 days, Davis et al. (2021) found that 1,700 respondents (45.2%) required a reduced work schedule compared to pre-illness, and an additional 839 respondents (22.3%) were not working at the time of the survey due to illness.

These studies provide strong evidence that Long COVID compromises quality of life across a range of domains. But what is less clear is the *specific* contribution that communication problems make to quality of life and daily functioning in people with Long COVID. This is because the instruments used to measure quality of life in people with Long COVID do not assess communication as a unique domain. This can be illustrated by considering how Jacobs et al. (2020) and Davis et al. (2021) examine quality of life and functioning in their respective studies. Jacobs et al. used PROMIS® survey questions to assess general health, quality of life, physical health, mental health, social relationships, social active role, physical activity, emotional problems, and fatigue (Choi et al. 2011; PROMIS Health Organization 2018). The daily living activities examined in their study included dressing, walking, climbing stairs, meal preparation, washing dishes, sweeping, making the bed, lifting, lifting and carrying, and walking fast. Communication is not examined or even mentioned in this investigation.

In their study, Davis et al. consider the impact of memory and cognitive dysfunction on three aspects of language and communication: (1) the ability to communicate thoughts; (2) the ability to have conversations with others; and (3) the ability to follow simple instructions. Whilst this study at least acknowledges communication, it also omits any examination of the contribution that communication difficulties make to quality of life and daily functioning. Communication impairment is assessed as an *outcome* of cognitive dysfunction rather than as a *cause* of reduced functioning in areas such as work and social relationships. Clearly, a shift of focus is required to give greater prominence to communication problems in an explanation of poor quality of life and reduced functioning in people with Long COVID.

To address the omission of communication in instruments used to measure quality of life, speech-language pathologists have increasingly focused on communication-related quality of life (CRQoL) in their development of clinical scales and assessments. CRQoL is now assessed in clients with voice disorders, stuttering, and aphasia through dedicated instruments (Yaruss 2010; Zraick and Risner 2008; Hilari et al. 2003). One such instrument is the Quality of Communication Life (QCL) Scale. Devised by Paul et al. (2004) for the American Speech-Language-Hearing Association (ASHA), the QCL is designed to assess the impact of a communication disorder on an adult's relationships; communication interactions; participation in social, leisure, work, and education activities; and overall quality of life (2004, p. 1). The scale is designed to supplement measures of impairment and functional communication and is validated for use with adults who have communication disorders resulting from various neurological conditions (e.g., aphasia and dysarthria). The items used in the scale are displayed in Box 6.1 in the Appendix.

Whilst the QCL was not developed for use with adults with Long COVID, it can contribute to our understanding of the impact of impaired communication on quality of life and daily functioning in people with this condition. The scale assesses in a simple, transparent way the areas that are impacted by poor communication skills in adults with Long COVID. The QCL is normally administered in person, with the clinician assisting the client with marking up his or her responses to test items on a visual analogue scale (when necessary) and ensuring comprehension of task instructions and test items. In-person administration is not possible for adults with Long COVID, all of whom are geographically remote from the author and are unable to meet the author face to face in any event due to COVID restrictions. Also, in-person administration is not needed for adults with Long COVID who have no physical disability that requires the author's assistance in marking the visual analogue scale and who have adequate language comprehension skills to comply with task instructions. Along with adaptations to the scale that permit it to be administered online – to be outlined in the next section – these considerations were judged not to limit the utility of the QCL in understanding the impact of COVID-related communication difficulties on quality of life.

## 6.5 Exploring communication-related quality of life in Long COVID

To establish the impact of communication difficulties on quality of life and daily functioning in adults with Long COVID, an online survey was conducted in

February and March 2022. The survey link was posted on Twitter and on Long COVID Facebook groups in the UK and Europe. It was shared widely amongst the Long COVID community. The survey was eventually completed by 973 people in 32 countries (see Table 6.3). It was part of a wider study of cognitive-linguistic difficulties in adults with COVID-19 which was approved by the Human Subjects Ethics Sub-Committee of The Hong Kong Polytechnic University. Some respondents to the survey also participated in other parts of the study, whilst most respondents had no prior contact with the author and her work.

The survey was conducted in five parts (see Box 6.2 in Appendix). In part one, participants were required to read information about the study and the eligibility criteria that were required for participation. They were then asked to indicate that they satisfied the criteria for participation and that they consented to participate in the study. In part two, participants were asked to provide their date of birth, gender, ethnicity, educational background, employment status before their COVID illness, and their status as an English speaker. In part three, participants were asked to rate their physical health, mental health, and spoken and written communication skills before their COVID illness. They were also asked to indicate their preferred method of communication before becoming unwell with COVID-19. In part four, participants were asked about their COVID illness, including when their symptoms first developed and their test and diagnostic status. They were also asked to rate their physical and mental health and spoken and written communication skills since developing COVID. Part four also asked respondents about their employment status and preferred method of communication following COVID. There were several questions about Long COVID, including its severity and whether respondents were under medical supervision for their condition. Respondents were then asked to select statements that described their experience of brain fog. In part five, participants were presented with the items used in the Quality of Communication Life Scale. These items were appropriately modified for use in an online survey format, with respondents rating statements on a five-item scale from "strongly disagree" to "strongly agree" rather than on a visual analogue scale. The entire survey could be completed in under 15 minutes. The results of this survey are presented as follows:

*Participant characteristics:* There was a total of 973 respondents to the survey. They ranged in age from 18 to 80 years, with a mean age of 47.4 years. Most respondents were female (89.6%), had White British ethnicity (62.8%), and lived in the United Kingdom (69.4%). English was a first language for 83.6% of respondents. High levels of education were reported, with 40% of respondents having an undergraduate degree and 38.4% having a higher degree (see Table 6.3).

*Health before and after COVID-19:* Most respondents reported good to excellent physical health (96.6%) and mental health (94.8%) prior to COVID-19. This decreased significantly following COVID infection, with only 5.6% and 35.2%

**TABLE 6.3** Characteristics of 973 survey respondents

| Age | | | Gender | | |
|---|---|---|---|---|---|
| Age (mean): 47.4 years | | | Male: 101 (10.4%) | | |
| Age (range): 18–80 years | | | Female: 872 (89.6%) | | |

| Ethnicity | | | | | |
|---|---|---|---|---|---|
| White British: | 611 | 62.8% | Asian Other: | 8 | 0.8% |
| White Other: | 250 | 25.7% | Asian Pakistani: | 6 | 0.6% |
| White Irish: | 48 | 4.9% | Black British: | 6 | 0.6% |
| Mixed or Multiple Ethnicities: | 19 | 2.0% | Black Other: | 4 | 0.4% |
| Other Ethnic Group: | 9 | 0.9% | Asian Chinese: | 3 | 0.3% |
| Asian Indian: | 8 | 0.8% | Asian Bangladeshi: | 1 | 0.1% |

| Country | | | | | |
|---|---|---|---|---|---|
| United Kingdom | 675 | 69.4% | Jersey | 2 | 0.2% |
| United States of America | 99 | 10.2% | Portugal | 2 | 0.2% |
| Belgium | 61 | 6.3% | Switzerland | 2 | 0.2% |
| Netherlands | 37 | 3.8% | Austria | 1 | 0.1% |
| Ireland | 28 | 2.9% | Bahrain | 1 | 0.1% |
| Canada | 13 | 1.3% | Barbados | 1 | 0.1% |
| Spain | 10 | 1.0% | Bermuda | 1 | 0.1% |
| France | 8 | 0.8% | Brazil | 1 | 0.1% |
| Germany | 4 | 0.4% | Czech Republic | 1 | 0.1% |
| South Africa | 4 | 0.4% | Lebanon | 1 | 0.1% |
| Australia | 3 | 0.3% | Mexico | 1 | 0.1% |
| Norway | 3 | 0.3% | Saudi Arabia | 1 | 0.1% |
| Philippines | 3 | 0.3% | Singapore | 1 | 0.1% |
| Denmark | 2 | 0.2% | Slovakia | 1 | 0.1% |
| Finland | 2 | 0.2% | Sweden | 1 | 0.1% |
| Isle of Man | 2 | 0.2% | Thailand | 1 | 0.1% |

| Education | English language |
|---|---|
| Primary and secondary education only: 210 (21.6%) | English as a first language: 813 (83.6%) |
| University undergraduate degree: 389 (40%) | English as a second language: 109 (11.2%) |
| University higher degree: 374 (38.4%) | English as a third language: 51 (5.2%) |

reporting good to excellent physical health and mental health, respectively (see Table 6.4).

*Communication before and after COVID-19:* An equally marked decrease occurred in respondents' self-rated spoken and written communication skills following COVID infection. Prior to COVID-19, 99.8% of respondents rated their spoken communication skills good to excellent. This dropped to 41.6% following their COVID illness. A similar decrease was observed in written communication

**TABLE 6.4** Physical and mental health in respondents before and after COVID-19

| | Physical health | |
| | Before COVID | After COVID |
|---|---|---|
| **Excellent** | 467 (48.0%) | 8 (0.8%) |
| **Good** | 473 (48.6%) | 47 (4.8%) |
| **Poor** | 33 (3.4%) | 918 (94.4%) |
| | Mental health | |
| | Before COVID | After COVID |
| **Excellent** | 475 (48.8%) | 17 (1.7%) |
| **Good** | 448 (46.0%) | 326 (33.5%) |
| **Poor** | 50 (5.2%) | 630 (64.8%) |

skills, with 99.7% reporting good to excellent skills before COVID and 54.1% reporting good to excellent skills after COVID (see Table 6.5). Consistent with the perceived deterioration in communication skills, there was a marked change in how respondents chose to communicate with people after COVID-19. Prior to their illness, most respondents (61%) opted for face-to-face communication. Reflecting the communicative challenges caused by COVID-19, face-to-face communication was the preferred means of communication for just 12.6% respondents after their illness. Whilst there was a significant move away from face-to-face communication, with its high cognitive processing demands in real time, there was an equally marked shift towards the use of texts and emails. These written forms of communication afford the user more time for planning and editing of messages. Text use increased from 14.6% before COVID to 50.2% after COVID. Social media use also increased, from 3.5% before COVID to 6.8% after

**TABLE 6.5** Spoken and written communication in respondents before and after COVID-19

| | Spoken communication | |
| | Before COVID | After COVID |
|---|---|---|
| **Excellent** | 856 (88.0%) | 15 (1.5%) |
| **Good** | 115 (11.8%) | 390 (40.1%) |
| **Poor** | 2 (0.2%) | 568 (58.4%) |
| | Written communication | |
| | Before COVID | After COVID |
| **Excellent** | 847 (87.1%) | 43 (4.4%) |
| **Good** | 123 (12.6%) | 484 (49.7%) |
| **Poor** | 3 (0.3%) | 446 (45.9%) |

**TABLE 6.6** Preferred method of communication in respondents before and after COVID-19

*Preferred method of communication*

| Category | Before COVID | After COVID |
|---|---|---|
| **Phone calls** | 94 (9.7%) | 79 (8.1%) |
| **Texts** | 142 (14.6%) | 488 (50.2%) |
| **Emails** | 96 (9.9%) | 183 (18.8%) |
| **Video calls** | 13 (1.3%) | 34 (3.5%) |
| **Social media** | 34 (3.5%) | 66 (6.8%) |
| **Face-to-face communication** | 594 (61.0%) | 123 (12.6%) |

COVID. This increased use of social media most likely reflects the psychosocial support that many respondents received from participation in Facebook and other online groups for people with Long COVID (see Table 6.6).

*Employment before and after COVID-19:* For respondents, who are largely adults of working age, one of the most profound impacts of Long COVID has been on employment. Most respondents (67.9%) were employed full-time before developing COVID-19. Full-time employment for these respondents dropped to just 24.6% following their illness. There was a corresponding increase in all "no employment" categories after COVID-19, with the biggest increase registered for the category "not working due to disability." This increased from just 2.4% before COVID to 32.5% after COVID, an increase that reflected the high level of debilitation that people with Long COVID experienced and the work incapacity that this condition had caused (see Table 6.7).

*COVID-19 illness:* The onset, diagnosis, and testing of COVID-19 was also explored in the survey. Most respondents (33.4%) developed COVID-19 in the

**TABLE 6.7** Employment of respondents before and after COVID-19

*Employment*

| Category | Before COVID | After COVID |
|---|---|---|
| **Employed full-time** | 661 (67.9%) | 239 (24.6%) |
| **Employed part-time** | 206 (21.2%) | 187 (19.2%) |
| **Unemployed** | 10 (1.0%) | 42 (4.3%) |
| **Not working due to retirement** | 26 (2.7%) | 35 (3.6%) |
| **Not working due to disability** | 23 (2.4%) | 316 (32.5%) |
| **Student** | 10 (1.0%) | 8 (0.8%) |
| **Other** | 37 (3.8%) | 146 (15.0%) |

first quarter of 2020. This was when the pandemic first reached the UK. Onset of illness was also high in the fourth quarter of 2020 (16.9%) and the first quarter of 2021 (11.1%), when the UK experienced a second, severe wave of infection. Reflecting the lack of testing that was available at the start of the pandemic, most respondents (35%) had received a clinical diagnosis of COVID-19 only. Amongst respondents, 98.7% reported having Long COVID currently, and 81.2% are under medical supervision for the condition (see Table 6.8).

Turning to brain fog, at its worst, this was rated to be severe by 60.3% of respondents. Over time the severity of brain fog decreased. However, there was

**TABLE 6.8** COVID illness and brain fog in survey respondents

| *COVID illness* | | | | | | |
|---|---|---|---|---|---|---|
| **Onset** | First quarter 2020 | 325 | 33.4% | First quarter 2021 | 108 | 11.1% |
| | Second quarter 2020 | 130 | 13.4% | Second quarter 2021 | 18 | 1.8% |
| | Third quarter 2020 | 34 | 3.5% | Third quarter 2021 | 70 | 7.2% |
| | Fourth quarter 2020 | 164 | 16.9% | Fourth quarter 2021 | 97 | 9.9% |
| | Date omitted or incorrect | | | | 27 | 2.8% |
| **Diagnosis & testing** | Clinical diagnosis only | | | | 341 | 35.0% |
| | Positive PCR test only | | | | 301 | 31.0% |
| | Positive antibody test only | | | | 59 | 6.1% |
| | Clinical diagnosis and positive PCR test | | | | 123 | 12.6% |
| | Clinical diagnosis and positive antibody test | | | | 37 | 3.8% |
| | Positive PCR test and positive antibody test | | | | 34 | 3.5% |
| | Clinical diagnosis and positive PCR test and positive antibody test | | | | 78 | 8.0% |
| **Long COVID** | Long COVID currently | YES 98.7% | NO 1.3% | Currently under medical supervision for Long COVID | YES 81.2% | NO 18.8% |
| *Brain fog* | | | | | | |
| **Severity of brain fog at worst** | Severe | 587 | 60.3% | | | |
| | Moderate | 354 | 36.4% | | | |
| | Mild | 32 | 3.3% | | | |
| **Severity of brain fog currently** | Severe | 94 | 9.7% | | | |
| | Moderate | 598 | 61.4% | | | |
| | Mild | 281 | 28.9% | | | |

still a significant burden of impairment related to brain fog at the time of survey completion, with 61.4% rating their current brain fog as moderate in severity (see Table 6.8). A constellation of language difficulties occurred in brain fog. The most marked language problem was word-finding difficulty. This was reported by 93.1% of respondents (see Figure 6.1). Amongst 11 language difficulties explored in the survey, all but two were reported to occur in over 50% of respondents. This reflects the high burden of language and communication problems in this population of adults. These difficulties caused frustration and embarrassment for 83.2% and 54.9% of respondents, respectively. Long COVID also resulted in reduced frequency of communication with others and less desire to communicate with others in 71.3% and 65.8% of respondents, respectively (see Figure 6.1).

*Quality of Communication Life Scale:* The items in the QCL Scale were administered to respondents of the survey. Despite their communication difficulties, adults with Long COVID reported a high degree of autonomy, responsibility, and independence, with 79.9% reporting that they make their own decisions, 66.8% stating that they had household responsibilities, and 83.5% agreeing with the statement "I speak for myself." Respondents also indicated for the most part that they liked to talk to people (64%) and felt included in conversations by others (55.3%). However, this positive stance towards communication with others was not always realised in terms of actual communication, with fewer than half of respondents (48.1%) agreeing that they stayed in touch with family members and friends. This may simply have reflected pre-morbid patterns of communication between adults with Long COVID and friends and family. However, combined with the finding that 71.3% of respondents reported that they communicated less frequently with others since their COVID illness, it is likely that communication difficulties and communication-related fatigue were significant factors in limiting contact with family members and friends. Other positively rated items were "people understand me when I talk" (72.6%); "I keep trying when people don't understand me" (74.3%); "I use the telephone" (61.1%); "I follow news, sports, and stories on TV/ movies" (55.5%); and "I see the funny things in life" (66.2%). Clearly, adults with post-COVID communication difficulties were still able to engage in meaningful communicative interactions with others, sought out ways to undertake those interactions (e.g., use the telephone), enjoyed certain leisure activities (e.g., watching TV), and appreciated humorous moments in their daily lives.

Notwithstanding these positively rated items, there was considerable disagreement expressed by respondents towards several items on the scale. Most respondents (55.9%) did not agree that it was easy for them to communicate, whilst just under half of respondents (49.1%) were confident that they can communicate. These findings confirm the many narrative comments describing communicative difficulties and reduced confidence in communication produced by adults with Long COVID (see Tables 6.1 and 6.2). There was a significant impact of these communicative difficulties on survey participants' self-esteem and occupational and familial roles. Only 34.7% of respondents agreed with the statement "I like

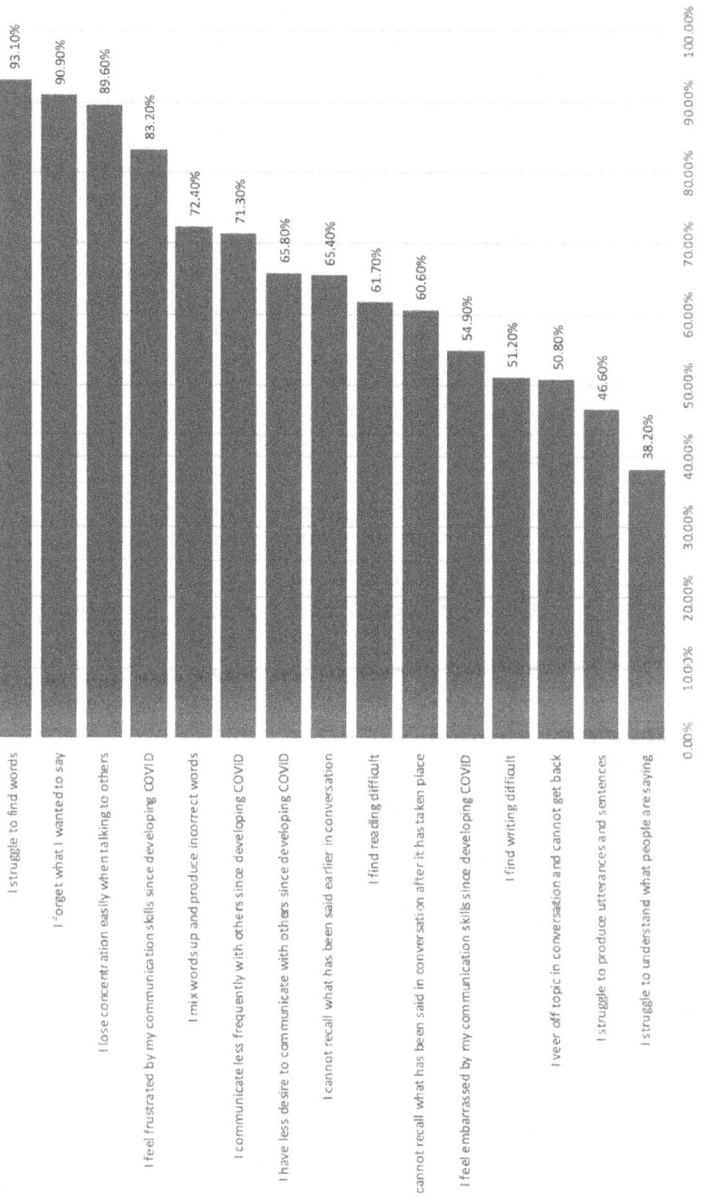

**FIGURE 6.1**   Language and communication in Long COVID brain fog

myself." Some 69.3% of respondents did not agree with the statement "I meet the communication needs of my job or college," and 62.9% disagreed with the statement "My role in the family is the same." Also, 74.8% of respondents disagreed with the statement "I get out of the house and do things." Communication problems almost certainly contributed to this reduced participation in activities outside the home – adults with Long COVID are unlikely to participate in activities outside the home, especially social activities, if communication skills are compromised. Fatigue and general debilitation are also features of Long COVID and are likely to be equally significant factors in preventing adults from participating in a range of activities outside the home. Most worryingly of all is that some 68.3% of respondents did not agree with the statement "In general, my quality of life is good." The impact of communication difficulties on self-esteem and on functioning in occupational, familial, and social domains resulted in reduced life quality for most survey respondents.

**TABLE 6.9** Respondent ratings of items in the modified QCL scale

*Quality of communication life scale*

|  | Strongly disagree | Somewhat disagree | Neither agree nor disagree | Somewhat agree | Strongly agree |
|---|---|---|---|---|---|
| I like to talk with people | 7.1% | 19.3% | 9.6% | 37.8% | 26.2% |
| It's easy for me to communicate | 14.5% | 41.4% | 14.4% | 23.3% | 6.4% |
| My role in the family is the same | 30.3% | 32.6% | 7.5% | 16.5% | 13.1% |
| I like myself | 17.1% | 29.3% | 18.9% | 22.6% | 12.1% |
| I meet the communication needs of my job or college | 44.0% | 25.3% | 7.9% | 18.6% | 4.2% |
| I stay in touch with family and friends | 9.7% | 31.3% | 10.9% | 35.5% | 12.6% |
| People include me in conversations | 3.4% | 18.1% | 23.2% | 37.6% | 17.7% |
| I follow news, sports, and stories on TV/movies | 10.0% | 22.3% | 12.2% | 40.3% | 15.2% |
| I use the telephone | 7.1% | 21.5% | 10.3% | 41.2% | 19.9% |
| I see the funny things in life | 4.7% | 14.4% | 14.7% | 44.5% | 21.7% |
| People understand me when I talk | 1.7% | 13.2% | 12.5% | 49.2% | 23.4% |
| I keep trying when people don't understand me | 2.9% | 11.2% | 11.6% | 47.8% | 26.5% |
| I make my own decisions | 0.9% | 9.4% | 9.8% | 38.6% | 41.3% |
| I am confident that I can communicate | 7.1% | 28.7% | 15.1% | 34.9% | 14.2% |
| I get out of the house and do things | 48.8% | 26.0% | 7.1% | 12.9% | 5.2% |
| I have household responsibilities | 11.2% | 13.6% | 8.4% | 31.5% | 35.3% |
| I speak for myself | 0.4% | 6.2% | 9.9% | 38.4% | 45.1% |
| In general, my quality of life is good | 33.7% | 34.6% | 11.7% | 15.6% | 4.4% |

## 6.6 Discussion

The results of the survey combined with an examination of the personal narratives of adults with Long COVID reveal a high burden of communication disability amongst this population. The impact of this disability on functioning and quality of life is considerable. In this section, that impact is explored further by examining how adults with Long COVID perceive the consequences of their illness on communication and the implications of their communicative difficulties for their ability to work, maintain social relationships, pursue leisure activities, and fulfil family responsibilities. The sudden onset and persistent nature of communication problems led many participants to express concern about the medical causes of these problems and to voice anxiety about the likelihood of recovery. These understandable worries about their communication problems and what they may signal about future health are also explored.

A striking feature of adults with Long COVID is how perceptive these adults are about their language and communication difficulties. Many of these adults can give detailed accounts of specific language problems, such as word-finding difficulties, substitution and reversal of sounds, syllables, letters and words, sentence-processing problems, and written language difficulties (see Table 6.10). These accounts often state the exact contexts in which language and communication difficulties arise. Respondents were adept at describing the communicative partners who were present; compensations that were adopted (e.g., the use of mime); consequences of poor communication (e.g., not getting a job); and feelings that are triggered when communication is problematic (e.g., shame). Metaphorical descriptions were often used to capture the experience of poor communication, such as when a word-finding difficulty was described in the following terms: "It was as if the word was behind a wall." Linguistic features relating to meaning and grammar are skilfully captured, such as when a respondent expressed that she could not distinguish between the different (homonymous) senses of the word *bank*. The author's overall impression is that adults with Long COVID are not only keenly aware of their communication difficulties but that they are also able to characterise them in a range of sophisticated ways:

**TABLE 6.10** Self-reported language and communication problems in Long COVID

| *Word-finding difficulties* |
| --- |

| **Woman: 54.8 years; 11.2 months post-onset:** | **Woman: 45.3 years; 15.2 months post-onset:** |
| --- | --- |
| "My close friends and family are aware and are able to fill in the gaps or help me find the word that's just out of reach . . . When they say it, I recognise it immediately. My husband reminded | "I struggle to find the right words quite a lot. Yesterday, after I'd discovered I had missed last month's credit card payment, I said to my wife, 'What's the word for if you hope someone might choose to not |

*(Continued)*

---
*Word-finding difficulties*

---

me that I mimed holding a phone to my ear two nights ago when I could not remember the word 'telephone.' I sometimes give a long-winded explanation of something in an attempt to remember the correct word."

**Woman: 61.6 years; 7.5 months post-onset:**

"At its worst, I couldn't even think of the word 'cat' to tell my husband what our cat was doing (he went blind through COVID). It was as if the word was behind a wall. That was very upsetting."

charge the default payment fee . . . What's the word for someone to say I won't have to pay it . . . The only word I can think of is 'sway' . . . Could they sway the payment . . . but I don't think that's the right word . . . or is it 'sway'? She very patiently said it's 'waive.' Of course it is! Not a difficult word!"

**Woman: 64.3 years; 7.5 months post-onset:**

"I have had to pause and allow other people to suggest the word I am so obviously looking for."

---
*Substitution and reversal of sounds, syllables, letters, words*

---

**Woman: 61.6 years; 7.5 months post-onset:**

"I remember distinctly typing a complete 7 letter word in reverse order without even thinking about it. I couldn't even do that normally (I'm a proficient touch typist)."

**Woman: 45.6 years; 17.8 months post onset:**

"I bought a new dishwasher, and when I was talking to my mum to tell her I was buying a silver one, I kept visualising silver but saying the word 'gold' to her."

**Woman: 49.5 years; 11.2 months post onset:**

"Sometimes I use words which are not words but vaguely sound like the word that I am trying to say. Sometimes I will say a word that rhymes with the word that I am trying to say."

**Woman: 52.9 years; 7.4 months post-onset:**

"I found after the first three to four months, I had almost forgotten how to speak. Didn't know until I started speaking – would stop, badly swap words around. Could not pronounce certain words at all. Swapping syllables."

**Woman: 51.4 years; 8.9 months post-onset:**

"Often type incorrect letter or words. Sometimes like dyslexia, sometimes completedly (sic) the wrong word."

---
*Sentence-processing problems*

---

**Woman: 43.8 years; 8.6 months post-onset:**

"It made me not be able to converse. I found it so difficult to understand what was being said to me. I couldn't begin to respond."

**Woman: 58.3 years; 17.8 months post-onset:**

"I had a job interview. Halfway through answering a question, I not only forgot what I was saying and the question. Needless to say, I didn't get the job."

*(Continued)*

*Sentence-processing problems*

**Woman: 49.5 years; 11.2 months post-onset:**

"I sometimes start a sentence somewhere in the middle and don't know how I'm going to finish it."

**Woman: 59.8 years; 7.5 months post-onset:**

"One example was when I had to call my works Pensions Dept regarding an early retirement application. I found it impossible to take in the information and had to ask them to slow down and even wait while I tried to process what they were telling me. I found I was unable to write down the information so in the end I had to make three separate calls asking just one or two questions at a time."

**Woman: 45.6 years; 7.6 months post-onset:**

"I frequently mix up words at the end of sentences or if I have moved on to think about something else while completing the sentence."

**Woman: 47.3 years; 17.1 months post-onset:**

"I often mix up words or struggle to understand the correct meaning of a word in a conversation (e.g., when someone talks about a 'bank,' I am confused if it's a riverbank or an actual bank)."

*Written-language difficulties*

**Woman: 38 years; 6.8 months post-onset:**

"Writing is difficult. I make much more mistakes than usual, grammatical ones, but also just writing words I didn't want to write. Once I wrote to a friend I would come to her 'after eating my child' instead of 'giving him his dinner.'"

**Woman: 48.4 years; 12.1 months post-onset:**

"Writing can have interesting consequences. It often seems completely lucid, sensible, and well-written. When looking back, it can be quite incredible what I have written. Sometimes a sentence doesn't make sense, but mostly it will be a case of missing out information and spelling, grammar, or punctuation mistakes. As an English teacher, this fills me with shame."

There is also a high level of awareness amongst adults with Long COVID that they are no longer able to cope with the communicative demands of their occupational roles, social relationships, leisure activities, and family responsibilities. Participants expressed this change in communicative performance in a wide range of ways, with statements often comparing language and communication skills in each of these domains *now* to how these skills were used *before* their COVID illness. The loss of language and communication skills required for employment was an area of particular concern for adults with Long COVID. Most of these adults are of working age. Many had demanding professional roles prior to their COVID illness, and the impact of their illness on their professional identity was keenly felt. Respondents expressed feelings of fear that their communication skills may never return. The communicative loss was characterised by one respondent as going from being "at the top of my game" to being "second or third division at best" (see Table 6.11).

The loss of social relationships and networks was a dominant theme, with many participants reporting that friends and family members no longer make contact or have reduced contact, possibly because the adult with Long COVID and communication difficulties is no longer fulfilling the needs of others. Consistent with the finding on the QCL Scale that 62.9% of respondents reported a change in their family role, participants reported an inability to fulfil normal parental duties like assisting children with homework and participating in parent-teacher evenings at their children's school. One participant reported how her husband "now has a different wife." Leisure activities such as sociable meals with

**TABLE 6.11** Self-reported impact of communication difficulties on work, leisure, social relationships, and family responsibilities

---

*Occupational roles*

---

**Woman: 31.5 years; 8.5 months post-onset:**
"I used to read for a living. Now I struggle if text is more than a paragraph. Typing is a struggle, and I misspell more."
**Woman: 41.1 years; 16.2 months post-onset:**
"As a clinical lead in psychiatry, my job is all about talking, listening, reflecting, and evaluating – synthesising really pertinent information and making complex risk assessments. I'm terrified I will never get back to feeling fit enough to do this."
**Man: 55.5 years; 18 months post-onset:**
"I'm used to working with plays from 16th/17th centuries, so am adept at 'difficult' language. I haven't tested this, but as with much else, I get the impression that I have gone from being right at the top of my game, as would be needed in my role as a teacher in a number of top schools (and with results to match), to being second or third division at best."
**Woman: 45.3 years; 15.2 months post-onset:**
"With coaching clients, I am fully present and listen incredibly carefully – that's a key part of the job. I'm usually very good at then being able to go back to things they mentioned earlier (earlier that session or indeed a session many months earlier) and make connections, etc. But quite often at the moment, I'm not so able to do that."

---

*Social relationships*

---

**Woman: 43.8 years; 8.6 months post-onset:**
"[Conversation is] too hard and confusing to do but craved social inclusion as felt so isolated."
**Woman: 44.1 years; 10.8 months post-onset:**
"People do not have the same contact with me. I rarely hear from many of my friends or certain members of the family. Maybe it's because with my communication problems I no longer fulfil their needs."

---

*(Continued)*

---

*Social relationships*

---

**Woman: 42.3 years; 15.2 months post-onset:**
"I struggle to communicate with strangers and am more withdrawn than I was before."
**Woman: 49.6 years; 7 months post-onset:**
"From an extrovert, garrulous teacher who craved company and an audience to a reticent, hermetic recluse with a vow of silence, seeking peace, who has lost their exuberant confidence and now feels a sense of vulnerability in social settings."

---

*Leisure activities*

---

**Woman: 55.5 years; 22.3 months post-onset:**
"I also used to be an avid reader, reading at least a book a week, but no longer read at all."
**Woman: 44.1 years; 10.8 months post-onset:**
"This is something I miss, a sociable meal with my husband and children and with our friends/family and their children."
**Woman: 37.2 years; 9.3 months post-onset:**
"I find myself zoning in and out of films. I tend to miss things these days and have to rewind and rewatch as I've missed key points. I have also noticed that if I can't lip-read the person speaking, I struggle to keep up and follow the conversation."
**Woman: 40.9 years; 18.4 months post-onset:**
"I don't watch difficult films or series for the moment, making it easy for myself to follow. If it's too difficult, I find myself scrolling back several minutes to see it again to understand. Worst case it has been that I had to do that three to four times."

---

*Family responsibilities*

---

**Woman: 45.6 years; 7.6 months post-onset:**
"[I] find I have 'tuned out' of conversations, e.g., in the car when child telling me about the day at school."
**Woman: 44.1 years; 10.8 months post-onset:**
"My family have been affected the most, my kids have a different mum, my husband now has a different wife."
"I've struggled to even attend a parents evening on Zoom. I can't focus on the screen, process the words being said, or respond appropriately."
"Of all the things Long COVID has taken away from me, it's the ability to speak properly after an evening meal. An evening meal has always been a family time for us to share what's happened in the day. The energy involved in digestion affects my cognitive ability and language. Therefore, I am unable to speak after we've eaten food."
"Homeschooling was horrendous. I couldn't even read words. I was blending words like a child. Long COVID has affected my ability to read. I can no longer help my children with their homework."

---

other families, reading for relaxation, and watching films with complex plot lines were also reported to be compromised by communication difficulties in Long COVID (see Table 6.11).

Many adults with Long COVID expressed anxieties about the medical causes of their communication problems. The onset of language and communication

**TABLE 6.12** Self-reported medical concerns relating to communication problems

| *Stroke* | *Dementia* |
|---|---|
| **Woman: 49.6 years; 15.5 months post-onset:** | **Woman: 41.1 years; 16.2 months post-onset:** |
| "In October [2020] I had some type of extreme event, but a stroke was ruled out. This is where all the language problems started to happen. I lost the ability to communicate for around 18 hours. This just wasn't finding words – I had no language or comprehension of language at all." | "It feels like some sort of dementia, like bits of my brain that used to/should work just don't anymore." |
| | **Woman: 56.4 years; 8.3 months post-onset:** |
| | "I sometimes felt that I had dementia as could not remember what I was trying to say." |
| **Woman: 49.6 years; 7 months post-onset:** | **Woman: 43.8 years; 8.6 months post-onset:** |
| "Is this what dementia or a stroke feels like? Is this the lived experience of someone with autism?" | "The neurological symptoms which mimic dementia, autism, MS, and others are very worrying." |

difficulties was sudden for some of these adults. This led to a concern that they had sustained a stroke. For other adults, the loss of language and communication skills created an anxiety that they were developing dementia or another neurological disorder. Most adults with Long COVID had received an extensive range of medical investigations, including MRI and CT scans, ECGs, blood tests, and X-rays. With few exceptions, these investigations produced normal results. The lack of medical explanation of the language difficulties that these adults experienced gave rise to concerns that their communication problems may be permanent in nature and may indicate a poor long-term prognosis for their health (see Table 6.12).

The significant impact of communication problems in Long COVID on the four domains of employment, social relationships, leisure, and family responsibilities culminated in a marked reduction in quality of life. Participants expressed this reduction through their responses to the survey and in their personal narratives. Only 20% of those who responded to the items in the QCL Scale reported that their quality of life was good. The personal narratives of adults with Long COVID vividly captured this reduced quality of life. There was a profound sense of loss of the once-fulfilling lives that had been taken away by Long COVID and its accompanying communication problems. The core of one's being, expressed in terms of "purpose and identity" and "soul," had been torn apart. No part of one's existence was untouched by Long COVID and the impairments of language and communication that affected many of those with the condition. Long COVID had truly destroyed people's lives, with many individuals fearing that they might never make a full recovery (see Table 6.13).

**TABLE 6.13** Self-reported quality of life in adults with Long COVID

---

*Quality of life*

---

**Woman: 49.6 years; 7 months post-onset:**
"To have your son with autism with whom you'd done intensive interaction, PECS, and Makaton gaze at you perplexed as you struggle to sign "I can't talk" whilst bedridden tore my soul in two. To then experience slurring and stuttering, word loss, to feel as if your IQ dropped."
**Woman: 44.1 years; 10.8 months post-onset:**
"Long COVID and my communication problems have affected every part of my life. They have taken away everything I had [. . .] This has had a massive impact on my life, taken away my purpose and identity."
**Man: 55.5 years; 18 months post-onset:**
"I am certainly not what I was prior to early 2020, and the nature of my hearing and communication issues have affected my quality of life substantially."

---

## 6.7 Implications

This chapter has presented evidence of a significant burden of communication difficulties in adults with Long COVID. These difficulties have impacted employment, social relationships, leisure activities, and family responsibilities and have served to reduce quality of life in these adults. Long COVID presents unique challenges for agencies that must address the ongoing health and economic needs of people with this condition. This section briefly considers ways in which health service providers and employers can support adults with Long COVID who experience communication difficulties as part of their condition.

*Long COVID clinics:* Health systems around the world are increasingly recognising the complex medical needs of clients with Long COVID. Many have established dedicated Long COVID clinics.[1] In the UK, there are 90 post-COVID assessment clinics under the auspices of the NHS (National Health Service 2022). Similar Long COVID clinics are also operating in several countries across the European Union (Baraniuk 2022). These clinics are typically staffed by specialists in respiratory medicine, infectious diseases, and paediatrics. However, speech and language therapists have not to date been consistently part of the multidisciplinary teams that assess and treat people with Long COVID (Royal College of Speech and Language Therapists 2021). The inclusion of speech and language therapy (SLT) in multidisciplinary teams that manage the health needs of people with Long COVID is one of eleven recommendations in a report published by the Royal College of Speech and Language Therapists in the UK in 2021. Other recommendations include the need to upskill the SLT workforce to address the communication and swallowing problems of this new group of clients and to conduct research into the presentation of COVID-19 and Long COVID in the community (non-hospitalised patients). The combined aim of these recommendations is to ensure that any person with communication and swallowing needs after COVID-19 receive "timely, person-centred rehabilitation" that will "support and maximize their mental health and wellbeing, participation in society, and ability to return to work" (RCSLT 2021, p. 19). The extent to which this aim can be achieved depends ultimately on funding, both of Long COVID recovery services but also regular SLT services that have experienced significant backlogs due to the pandemic.

*Return to work:* The non-linear recovery of people with Long COVID presents unique challenges for occupational health and human resource professionals who must manage return to work for people with this chronic condition. People with Long COVID may return to work for days or weeks in some cases, only to experience a significant relapse in their condition that requires them to take a further period of sickness absence. Phased returns that facilitate work re-entry for people with other health conditions are often of an intensity and duration that exceed the physical and cognitive capacities of people with Long COVID. These issues are not lost on the Royal College of Speech and Language Therapists in the UK. It calls on speech and language therapists to make the wider public and other health and care professionals aware of the communication and swallowing problems experienced by people with Long COVID and of the implications of these problems for work re-entry. The College's eleventh recommendation in its 2021 report states that "[m]ore information needs to be provided specifically on the impact of Long COVID and implications for people returning to work" (RCSLT 2021, p. 20).

There is clearly a job of work to be done to encourage better understanding amongst occupational health and human resource professionals of how communication problems affect return to work for people with Long COVID. One 44-year-old woman with significant communication difficulties studied by the author (Cummings 2021b) received excellent support from her occupational health consultant, remarking, "I continue to be really well supported by Dr XXX. I genuinely would not be getting through this without him." Her experience is far from universal, however. The author studied a 49-year-old woman who had marked communication difficulties following COVID-19. She described her treatment by her human resources department in the following terms:

> I expected support and empathy at a raw, vulnerable moment. Their belittling tone, aggressive agenda, and patronisation when I couldn't express myself without word loss was highly insensitive and haunting. Tears of frustration at speech loss were perceived as a histrionic expression of stress. I felt invisible, humiliated, unheard, and alone.

To ensure a high standard of support for people with Long COVID, the Chartered Institute of Personnel and Development (CIPD) recently published a report in which it made several recommendations to assist employees with Long COVID in returning to work (CIPD 2022). These recommendations can be implemented by *i*ndividual employees, *g*roups, *l*ine managers, *o*rganisations, and *o*utside resources (the IGLOO framework). By avoiding barriers and encouraging facilitators at each of these levels, the CIPD argues that a successful return to work can be navigated by people with Long COVID. A communication-related facilitator at the group level, for example, is to take conversations at an employee's pace.

## 6.8 Summary

This chapter has examined the impact of Long COVID on language and communication skills and the effect of impairment of these skills on daily functioning and quality of life in people with this chronic condition. Drawing on evidence from an online survey and personal narratives of adults who have not made a good recovery from their COVID illnesses, the chapter has demonstrated that there is a significant burden of communication disability in adults with Long COVID. Moreover, this disability compromises functioning in a range of areas, including work, social relationships, leisure activities, and family responsibilities. The combined effect of reduced participation in these areas of functioning is a marked reduction in the quality of life of people with Long COVID. The chapter concludes by recommending a prominent role for speech-language pathology in the rehabilitation of people with Long COVID and for increased awareness amongst occupational health and human resource professionals of how communication difficulties can affect return to work for adults with this condition.

## Note

1. It is worth remarking that access to these clinics, even when they do exist, has been patchy at best. As one 55-year-old man from the UK remarked in my study, "I have given up on my Long COVID referral ever leading to anything."

## Acknowledgements

The author would like to acknowledge Dr Phoebe Lin, Department of English and Communication, The Hong Kong Polytechnic University, for her excellent assistance with the online survey in this study. I am also hugely indebted to Samantha Berry and Kerry Davies, who tirelessly promoted the survey to members of the Long COVID community. The large number of responses is entirely due to their efforts.

## References

Baraniuk, C. (2022). Covid-19: How Europe is approaching long covid. *British Medical Journal*, 376. https://doi.org/10.1136/bmj.o158.

Cabrera Martimbianco, A. L., Pacheco, R. L., Bagattini, Â. M., & Riera, R. (2021). Frequency, signs and symptoms, and criteria adopted for long COVID-19: A systematic review. *International Journal of Clinical Practice*, 75(10), e14357. doi:10.1111/ijcp.14357.

Callan, C., Ladds, E., Husain, L., Pattinson, K., & Greenhalgh, T. (2022). "I can't cope with multiple inputs": A qualitative study of the lived experience of "brain fog" after COVID-19. *BMJ Open*, 12(2), e056366. doi:10.1136/bmjopen-2021-056366.

Chartered Institute of Personnel and Development (2022). Working with long COVID: Research evidence to inform support. www.cipd.co.uk/knowledge/fundamentals/relations/absence/long-covid-report#gref. Accessed 27 February 2022.

Choi, S. W., Victorson, D. E., Yount, S., Anton, S., & Cella, D. (2011). PROMIS Short-Form v1.0 – Dyspnea – Functional Limitations 5. https://eprovide.mapi-trust.org/instruments/patient-reported-outcomes-measurement-information-system-short-form-v1.0-dyspnea-functional-limitations-5b. Accessed 14 February 2022.

Cummings, L. (2021a). COVID-19 and language: A case study. *International Journal of Language Studies*, 15(3), 1–24.

Cummings, L. (2021b). Cognitive-linguistic difficulties in COVID-19: A longitudinal case study. *International Journal of Speech & Language Pathology and Audiology*, 9, 8–19.

Davis, H. E., Assaf, G. S., McCorkell, L., Wei, H., Low, R. J., Re'em, Y., et al. (2021). Characterizing long COVID in an international cohort: 7 months of symptoms and their impact. *EClinicalMedicine*, 38, 101019. doi:10.1016/j.eclinm.2021.101019.

Hilari, K., Byng, S., Lamping, D. L., & Smith, S. C. (2003). Stroke and aphasia quality of life scale-39 (SAQOL-39): Evaluation of acceptability, reliability, and validity. *Stroke*, 34(8), 1944–1950.

Hossain, M. A., Hossain, K. M. A., Saunders, K., Uddin, Z., Walton, L. M., Raigangar, V., et al. (2021). Prevalence of Long COVID symptoms in Bangladesh: A prospective inception cohort study of COVID-19 survivors. *BMJ Global Health*, 6, e006838.

Jacobs, L. G., Gourna Paleoudis, E., Lesky-Di Bari, D., Nyirenda, T., Friedman, T., Gupta, A., et al. (2020). Persistence of symptoms and quality of life at 35 days after hospitalization for COVID-19 infection. *PLoS One*, 15(12), e0243882. doi:10.1371/journal.pone.0243882.

Jacobson, K. B., Rao, M., Bonilla, H., Subramanian, A., Hack, I., Madrigal, M., et al. (2021). Patients with uncomplicated coronavirus disease 2019 (COVID-19) have long-term persistent symptoms and functional impairment similar to patients with severe COVID-19: A cautionary tale during a global pandemic. *Clinical Infectious Diseases*, 73(3), e826–e829. doi:10.1093/cid/ciab103.

Lopez-Leon, S., Wegman-Ostrosky, T., Perelman, C., Sepulveda, R., Rebolledo, P. A., Cuapio, A., & Villapol, S. (2022). More than 50 long-term effects of COVID-19: A systematic review and meta-analysis. *MedRxiv*, 11(1), 16144. doi:10.1101/2021.01.27.21250617.

Michelen, M., Manoharan, L., Elkheir, N., Cheng, V., Dagens, A., Hastie, C., et al. (2021). Characterising long COVID: A living systematic review. *BMJ Global Health*, 6(9), e005427. doi:10.1136/bmjgh-2021-005427.

National Health Service (2022). Guidelines for supporting our NHS people affected by Long COVID. www.england.nhs.uk/publication/guidelines-for-supporting-our-nhs-people-affected-by-long-covid/. Accessed 25 February 2022.

Office for National Statistics (2021). Prevalence of ongoing symptoms following coronavirus (COVID-19) infection in the UK: 1 April 2021. www.ons.gov.uk/peoplepopulationandcommunity/healthandsocialcare/conditionsanddiseases/bulletins/prevalenceofongoingsymptomsfollowingcoronaviruscovid19infectionintheuk/1april2021. Accessed 7 February 2022.

Orrù, G., Bertelloni, D., Diolaiuti, F., Mucci, F., Di Giuseppe, M., Biella, M., et al. (2021). Long-COVID syndrome? A study on the persistence of neurological, psychological and physiological symptoms. *Healthcare (Basel)*, 9(5), 575. doi:10.3390/healthcare9050575.

Osikomaiya, B., Erinoso, O., Wright, K. O., Odusola, A. O., Thomas, B., Adeyemi, O., et al. (2021). "Long COVID": Persistent COVID-19 symptoms in survivors managed in Lagos State, Nigeria. *BMC Infectious Diseases*, 21(1), 304. doi:10.1186/s12879-020-05716-x.

Paul, D. R., Frattali, C. M., Holland, A. L., Thompson, C. K., Caperton, C. J., & Slater, S. C. (2004). *Quality of communication life scale*. Rockville, MD: American Speech-Language-Hearing Association.

PROMIS Health Organization (2018). PROMIS scale v1.2 – Global health. www.healthmeasures.net/index.php?option=com_instruments&view=measure&id=778. Accessed 14 February 2022.

Royal College of Speech and Language Therapists (2021). Long COVID and speech and language therapy: Understanding the mid- to long-term speech and language therapy needs and the impact on services. www.rcslt.org/news/new-rcslt-report-on-long-covid-and-speech-and-language-therapy/. Accessed 26 February 2022.

Sudre, C. H., Murray, B., Varsavsky, T., Graham, M. S., Penfold, R. S., Bowyer, R. C., et al. (2021). Attributes and predictors of long COVID. *Nature Medicine*, 27(4), 626–631.

Taquet, M., Dercon, Q., Luciano, S., Geddes, J. R., Husain, M., & Harrison, P. J. (2021). Incidence, co-occurrence, and evolution of long-COVID features: A 6-month retrospective cohort study of 273,618 survivors of COVID-19. *PLoS Medicine*, https://doi.org/10.1371/journal.pmed.1003773.

Wanga, V., Chevinsky, J. R., Dimitrov, L. V., Gerdes, M. E., Whitfield, G. P., Bonacci, R. A., et al. (2021). Long-term symptoms among adults tested for SARS-CoV-2 – United States, January 2020-April 2021. *Morbidity and Mortality Weekly Report*, 70(36), 1235–1241.

World Health Organization (2021). A clinical case definition of post COVID-19 condition by a Delphi consensus, 6 October 2021. www.who.int/publications/i/item/WHO-2019-nCoV-Post_COVID-19_condition-Clinical_case_definition-2021.1. Accessed 8 February 2022.

Yaruss, J. S. (2010). Assessing quality of life in stuttering treatment outcomes research. *Journal of Fluency Disorders*, 35(3), 190–202.

Zimmermann, P., Pittet, L. F., & Curtis, N. (2021). How common is Long COVID in children and adolescents? *Pediatric Infectious Disease Journal*, 40(12), e482–e487. doi:10.1097/INF.0000000000003328.

Zraick, R. I., & Risner, B. Y. (2008). Assessment of quality of life in persons with voice disorders. *Current Opinion in Otolaryngology & Head and Neck Surgery*, 16(3), 188–193.

# APPENDIX

## BOX 6.1: TEST ITEMS USED IN THE QUALITY OF COMMUNICATION LIFE SCALE

| Item # | Item | Score |
|--------|------|-------|
| 1. | I like to talk with people. | _____ |
| 2. | It's easy for me to communicate. | _____ |
| 3. | My role in the family is the same. | _____ |
| 4. | I like myself. | _____ |
| 5. | I meet the communication needs of my job or school. | _____ |
| 6. | I stay in touch with family and friends. | _____ |
| 7. | People include me in conversations. | _____ |
| 8. | I follow news, sports, and stories on TV/movies. | _____ |
| 9. | I use the telephone. | _____ |
| 10. | I see the funny things in life. | _____ |
| 11. | People understand me when I talk. | _____ |
| 12. | I keep trying when people don't understand me. | _____ |
| 13. | I make my own decisions. | _____ |
| 14. | I am confident that I can communicate. | _____ |
| 15. | I get out of the house and do things. | _____ |
| 16. | I have household responsibilities. | _____ |
| 17. | I speak for myself. | _____ |
| 18. | In general, my quality of life is good. | _____ |

## BOX 6.2: ONLINE SURVEY ADMINISTERED TO ADULTS WITH LONG COVID

### *Cognitive-linguistic difficulties in adults with COVID-19*

You are invited to participate in a study conducted by Professor Louise Cummings who is a staff member of the Department of English and Communication in The Hong Kong Polytechnic University. The project has been approved by the Human Subjects Ethics Sub-Committee (HSESC) (or its Delegate) of The Hong Kong Polytechnic University (HSESC Reference Number: HSEARS20210712001).

The aim of this study is to understand the impact of the SARS-CoV-2 virus on language and communication in adults with COVID-19 infection. In the following questionnaire, you will be asked to provide some personal information such as your date of birth and educational background. You will also be asked questions about your COVID illness and its impact on your communication skills. The responses require you to tick boxes and enter numbers to grade statements. The entire questionnaire can be completed in under 15 minutes and will not cause you any discomfort or psychological stress. All information related to you will remain confidential and will be identifiable by codes only known to the researcher.

To participate in this study, you must satisfy the following criteria:

- You must be 18 years of age or older.
- You must have had COVID-19 confirmed through testing (PCR test or antibody test) *or* have received a clinical diagnosis of COVID-19.
- You must have experienced Long COVID, defined as the persistence of COVID symptoms beyond 3 months from the onset of illness.
- You must have experienced cognitive-linguistic difficulties (so-called "brain fog") as part of your Long COVID.

To give your consent to participate in the study, please tick the boxes next to each of the following statements:

- I satisfy the criteria required for participation in this study ☐
- I give my consent to participate in this study ☐

If you would like to obtain more information about this study, please contact me at any time by email (louise.cummings@polyu.edu.hk) or telephone on (852) 2766 7978.

If you have any complaints about the conduct of this research study, please do not hesitate to contact Miss Cherrie Mok, Secretary of the Human Subjects Ethics Sub-Committee of The Hong Kong Polytechnic University in writing (c/o Research Office of the University), stating clearly the responsible person and department of this study as well as the HSESC Reference Number.

Thank you for your interest in participating in this study.

Professor Louise Cummings

Principal Investigator

---

Date of birth: ☐

Gender: ☐ male   ☐ female

Ethnicity: ☐ White: British   ☐ White: Irish   ☐ White: Other
☐ Black: British   ☐ Black: Other
☐ Asian: Indian   ☐ Asian: Pakistani   ☐ Asian: Bangladeshi
☐ Asian: Chinese   ☐ Asian: Other
☐ Mixed or Multiple Ethnicities   ☐ Other Ethnic Group

Education:
☐ Primary and secondary education only
☐ University undergraduate degree
☐ University higher degree

Employment before COVID-19 illness:
☐ Employed full-time   ☐ Employed part-time   ☐ Unemployed
☐ Not working due to retirement   ☐ Not working due to disability
☐ Student   ☐ Other

Which of the following best describes your use of English?
☐ I speak English as a native or first language
☐ I speak English as a second language
☐ I speak English as a third language

Which of the following describes your physical health **before** COVID-19?
☐ Excellent   ☐ Good   ☐ Poor

Which of the following describes your mental health **before** COVID-19?
☐ Excellent   ☐ Good   ☐ Poor

Which of the following describes your spoken communication skills **before** COVID-19?

☐ Excellent ☐ Good ☐ Poor

Which of the following describes your written communication skills **before** COVID-19?

☐ Excellent ☐ Good ☐ Poor

**Before** developing COVID, my preferred method of communication with others was:

☐ phone calls ☐ texts ☐ emails
☐ video calls ☐ social media ☐ face-to-face communication

When did you first develop symptoms of COVID-19? Please try to give a specific date. ☐

Which of the following categories applies to you? Please tick as many boxes as necessary:

☐ Clinical diagnosis of COVID-19

☐ Positive PCR test

☐ Positive antibody test

Which of the following describes your physical health **following** COVID-19?

☐ Excellent ☐ Good ☐ Poor

Which of the following describes your mental health **following** COVID-19?

☐ Excellent ☐ Good ☐ Poor

Which of the following describes your spoken communication skills **following** COVID-19?

☐ Excellent ☐ Good ☐ Poor

Which of the following describes your written communication skills **following** COVID-19?

☐ Excellent ☐ Good ☐ Poor

Which of the following categories applies to you currently?

☐ Employed full-time ☐ Employed part-time ☐ Unemployed
☐ Not working due to retirement ☐ Not working due to disability
☐ Student ☐ Other

Are you currently experiencing Long COVID? ☐ Yes ☐ No

Are you currently under medical supervision for Long COVID?

☐ Yes ☐ No

Have you had brain fog as part of Long COVID?   ☐ Yes   ☐ No

Which of the following describes your brain fog **at its worst**?

☐ Severe      ☐ Moderate      ☐ Mild

Which of the following describes your brain fog **currently**?

☐ Severe      ☐ Moderate      ☐ Mild

Which of the following statements applies to your brain fog? Please tick as many boxes as necessary:

☐ I struggle to find words

☐ I struggle to produce utterances and sentences

☐ I mix words up and produce incorrect words

☐ I find reading difficult

☐ I find writing difficult

☐ I struggle to understand what people are saying

☐ I lose concentration easily when talking to others

☐ I veer off topic in conversation and cannot get back

☐ I forget what I wanted to say

☐ I cannot recall what has been said earlier in conversation

☐ I cannot recall what has been said in conversation after it has taken place

☐ I communicate less frequently with others since developing COVID

☐ I have less desire to communicate with others since developing COVID

☐ I feel embarrassed by my communication skills since developing COVID

☐ I feel frustrated by my communication skills since developing COVID

**Since** developing COVID, my preferred method of communication with others is:

☐ phone calls   ☐ texts        ☐ emails

☐ video calls   ☐ social media ☐ face-to-face communication

**Quality of Communication Life Scale★**

Is today an especially good, average, or especially bad day for you?

☐ Especially good   ☐ Average   ☐ Especially bad

Before reading each of the following statements, ask yourself "Even though I have difficulty communicating after COVID. . . . " Then rank each statement from 1 (strongly disagree) to 5 (strongly agree) or indicate "does not apply":

☐ I like to talk with people

☐ It's easy for me to communicate

☐ My role in the family is the same

☐ I like myself

☐ I meet the communication needs of my job or college (such as typing, giving and following directions, reading)

☐ I stay in touch with family and friends

☐ People include me in conversations

☐ I follow news, sports, and stories on TV/movies

☐ I use the telephone

☐ I see the funny things in life

☐ People understand me when I talk

☐ I keep trying when people don't understand me

☐ I make my own decisions

☐ I am confident that I can communicate

☐ I get out of the house and do things (such as sports, dinner, shows, parties)

☐ I have household responsibilities (such as shopping, cooking, home repairs)

☐ I speak for myself

☐ In general, my quality of life is good

* Items in this section are adapted from the following: Paul, D. R., Frattali, C. M., Holland, A. L., Thompson, C. K., Caperton, C. J., & Slater, S. C. (2004) *Quality of Communication Life Scale*. Rockville, MD: American Speech-Language-Hearing Association.

# 7

# MANAGEMENT OF VOICE DISORDERS IN COVID-19

*Emerald J. Doll*

## 7.1 Introduction

In March 2020 the novel respiratory syndrome coronavirus 2 (SARS-CoV-2) pandemic became widespread in the United States. Minimal information about the coronavirus was known except the severity of the contagion and the likelihood of imminent hospitalisations of people with COVID-19. Like all medical professionals, speech-language pathologists (SLPs) who treat voice and upper airway disorders had to quickly adjust their assessment and treatment practices. To maximise safety and minimise risk, personal protective equipment (PPE) was integrated into in-person care, and therapy modality changed from in-person to virtual delivery. Such practice guidelines were proposed by the Centers for Disease Control and Prevention (CDC), Occupational Safety and Health Association (OSHA), local infectious-disease and infection-control specialists, as well as various speech and language associations like the American-Speech-Language-Hearing Association. This chapter examines some of these guidelines as they relate to the management of voice disorders. The impacts of the COVID-19 pandemic on the voice and airways are just beginning to emerge. These impacts are examined based on current research and clinical practice. Finally, as the severity of the pandemic declines, the considerations and research discussed in this chapter may be applicable to facilitating safe and effective voice-care delivery in future public health emergencies and for COVID-related voice and upper airway concerns.

DOI: 10.4324/9781003257318-7

## 7.2 Telemedicine

### 7.2.1 Voice and upper airway evaluations

At the beginning of the COVID-19 pandemic, all non-essential in-person appointments were postponed, leaving 1 in 13 (7.6%) adults annually with a voice problem in the United States uncared for (Bhattacharyya 2014). Despite new restrictions of physical distancing and quarantine protocols, patient care remained the priority. Medical disciplines were forced to quickly adapt their practices when the Centers for Medicare and Medicaid Services advised maximum use of all telehealth modalities as a feasible and appropriate alternative to in-person services. An expedited literature review supported this recommendation by suggesting that telemedicine could reduce the spread of COVID-19 by decreasing in-person visits, reducing emergency visits, and preserving healthcare resources (Bokolo 2020).

Medicaid defines telemedicine as "an avenue to improve a patient's health by providing a synchronous platform for interactive two-way communication between the patient and a clinician, and a cost-effective alternative to traditional in-person way of providing medical care" (Centers for Medicare and Medicaid Services 2021). ASHA supported telemedicine as early as 2005 when it was deemed an appropriate service delivery for speech-language pathology and audiology services (Georgeadis and Krumm 2007). The efficacy of telemedicine in speech-language pathology services has been broadly supported (Duffy et al. 1997). This includes the assessment and treatment of specific voice and speech conditions including spasmodic dysphonia, vocal tremor, muscle tension dysphonia, and hypokinetic dysarthria in Parkinson's disease (Constantinescu et al. 2010). Virtual assessment for these and other voice and airway conditions was especially indicated when distance prohibited in-person evaluations (Duffy et al. 1997; Health Resources and Service Administration 2021). More recently, surveys have revealed 87% of patients were highly satisfied with their ENT telemedicine consultation (Fieux et al. 2020). In another study, 98% of patients surveyed were satisfied with their virtual voice assessment, 84% believed further face-to-face voice assessment follow-up would be beneficial, and 83% liked the option of virtual care in the future (Watters et al. 2021).

When in-person appointments were limited to conserve PPE and follow physical distancing recommendations (Murphy 2020), SLPs and laryngologists were tasked with reviewing voice and upper airway patients' medical charts for risk factors to determine the appropriate modality of care (Mattei et al. 2020). Patients appropriate for a telemedicine assessment were those without a high risk for cancer or airway compromise and that were elective and not time sensitive. Ideally, a comprehensive assessment of vocal function should consist of a thorough case history, patient-reported outcome measures, auditory-perceptual assessments, vocal function studies (i.e., acoustic and aerodynamic data), and stroboscopy (Roy et al. 2013; Patel et al. 2018). Unfortunately, aerodynamic testing (apart from s/z ratio and maximum phonation time [MPT]) and endoscopy currently cannot be completed remotely. Fortunately, other segments of the comprehensive evaluation can be completed virtually, with a growing literature providing insight into such virtual method's reliability and validity.

Auditory-perceptual judgments is one area of virtual assessment that has been examined. In one study, auditory-perceptual judgements of pre-recorded dysphonic voices were consistent when delivered via different web platforms to 10 experienced SLPs and 10 experienced laryngologists (Dahl et al. 2021). Further, post-treatment auditory-perceptual comparisons have been achieved by saving voice samples collected via voicemail recordings into the patient electronic medical record (Castillo-Allendes et al. 2021).

On the contrary, acoustic measures (smoothed cepstral peak prominence, low-to-high spectral energy ratio, and harmonic-to-noise ratio) of dysphonic voices are not consistent across web platforms (Weerathunge et al. 2021). Thus, one voice sample collected and measured acoustically across Zoom and the same one collected and measured through Cisco Webex is likely to generate different values. Nonetheless, remote acoustic assessment has its benefits. Specifically, the smartphone voice-assessment application VoiceEvalU8 (Grillo 2017) has been designated as a novel and low-cost way to collect acoustic data remotely for interpretation and clinical care (Schneider et al. 2021). Though VoiceEvalU8 does not have available normative data for comparison, it could be utilised for pre- and post-intervention comparisons (Schneider et al. 2021). Similarly, other literature suggests that low-tech MPT, voice range profile (VRP), and s/z ratio for pre- and post-evaluation and/or therapy comparisons (Castillo-Allendes et al. 2021; Doll et al. 2021) are typically warranted until the patient can be evaluated in person.

Stroboscopy is the gold standard for diagnosing dysphonia and assessing vocal fold biomechanics and physiology. Despite evidence supporting telemedicine assessments, voice professionals had concerns about proceeding without visualisation of the larynx as the pandemic surged. However, the alternative to postponing the evaluation until the unforeseen future when a laryngeal endoscopy could be completed was considered to be far worse. In August 2020, ASHA's Special Interest Group Coordinating Committee of Voice and Upper Airway Disorders provided a statement of support to proceed with therapy in lieu of stroboscopic evaluation, stipulating that the telemedicine assessment consist of a thorough case history, auditory-perceptual analysis, vocal-function testing if able and appropriate, and extensive stimulability tasks to assess appropriateness of telemedicine therapy versus in-person evaluation. If the SLP and the laryngologist agreed to proceed with therapy without an in-person evaluation, the risks and benefits associated with providing treatment in absence of a confirmed dysphonia etiology need to be explicitly communicated with the patient. Furthermore, it was strongly advised that the patient return for a comprehensive voice or upper airway evaluation, including laryngeal evaluation when appropriate (Castillo-Allendes et al. 2021; Doll et al. 2021).

During the pandemic, studies have continued to support these altered practices. Perceptual ratings of urgent versus non-urgent voice samples linked with medical histories were accurately rated 86% of the time for urgent voices and 77% for non-urgent voices (Fujiki et al. 2021). Another study found that patients who received a telemedicine laryngology evaluation had comparable diagnoses and care at their follow-up in-person laryngology appointment with laryngeal imaging (Choi et al. 2021). The authors further stated "that while laryngoscopy is still essential to confirm diagnosis and provide appropriate management, telemedicine may be a feasible alternative to provide suitable empiric therapy until laryngoscopy can be safely performed" (Choi et al. 2021, p. 1). As it stands, ASHA's support of deferred endoscopic evaluation is no longer recommended by any agency. A comprehensive voice evaluation must be completed in person following COVID-19 pre-screening, and CDC recommended PPE (American Speech-Language-Hearing Association 2020).

### 7.2.2  Voice and upper airway therapy

Voice and upper airway therapy with a facemask is not ideal. It potentially hinders and impedes both the patient's performance and the SLP's ability to model vocal tasks, e.g., semi-occluded vocal tract (SOVT) exercises of straw phonation, cup bubbles, lip trills, raspberries, external biofeedback from a Kleenex or hand for flow phonation, and tongue stretches. Though some tasks can be performed with the mask on, the patient's mouth cannot be monitored, and visual modeling cannot be provided by the SLP. Teletherapy has proven to be the ideal platform for therapy because patient and clinician can safely remain maskless.

Research comparing voice and upper airway therapy via telehealth versus in person prior to the COVID-19 pandemic showed comparable outcomes for those with a variety of voice disorders (Mashima et al. 2003; Mashima and Brown 2011; Kelchner 2013; Rangarathnam et al. 2016), including vocal fold nodules (Mashima et al. 2003; Fu et al. 2015); vocal fold oedema, unilateral vocal fold paralysis, and hyperfunction (Mashima et al. 2003); muscle tension dysphonia (Rangarathnam et al. 2015); Parkinson's disease (Howell et al. 2009); and the functional breathing disorder, paradoxical vocal fold motion (PVFM) (Towey 2012). Additionally, intensive voice therapy comprised of one in-person appointment, followed by three telemedicine appointments a week for three weeks resulted in significant improvements in perceptual ratings, voice-handicap index total and physical scores, mean fundamental frequency, mean airflow rate, and stroboscopy ratings, including mucosal wave, vocal fold edge, and glottic closure (Fu et al. 2015).

Other research has implicated reduced medical costs via telemedicine versus in-person PVFM treatment (Towey 2012). Further, telemedicine may improve access to voice and airway services in geographic areas where this sub-specialty is not typically available (Duffy et al. 1997; Mashima and Brown 2011; Becker and

Gillespie 2021); increase convenience for both the provider and patient whilst reducing travel burdens (Kelchner 2013); reduce time off work and childcare needs whilst allowing support persons to help the patient during virtual sessions (Macoir et al. 2021); and shorten appointment wait times whilst reducing COVID-19 exposure.

The frequency of telemedicine has increased as result of the pandemic, and SLPs plan to continue to utilise telemedicine in their practice (Macoir et al. 2021). Due to teletherapy's convenience and ease, it has become a standard modality for voice therapy, peri-operative therapy, cough suppression, and respiratory retraining. As it stands, the biggest teletherapy challenges for SLPs are lack of familiarity and confidence with the technology and process of remote service delivery (Cantarella et al. 2021; Becker and Gillespie 2021). Telemedicine decreases the visibility of a patient's face and body, eliminates opportunity for hands-on manipulation, and presents potential acoustic signal distortions and other technological issues. These barriers require the clinician's instruction during telemedicine to be flexible, innovative, and creative to successfully guide the patient's behavioural changes.

When visual monitoring of the patient's entire body is reduced, repositioning of the patient or the camera may be required. The clinician can zoom the camera out to allow full-body visualisation when working on breathing, body alignment, or stretching and zoom the camera in to improve visibility of facial and upper trunk nuances. To encourage appropriate posture, patients should position the camera at eye level to avoid craning their head forward, up, or down. Absence of hands-on manipulation of the larynx or body requires clear verbal instruction, description, modeling, and questioning to verify physical changes and self-administered pressure.

The nuances of auditory features of voicing (e.g., forward focus, flow, pressed phonation) during therapy tasks can be difficult to differentiate over a web platform. Some studies have provided recommendations to optimise acoustic signals from both the SLP and the patient for specific web platforms (Dahl et al. 2021; Weerathunge et al. 2021). However, these suggested settings may not improve acoustic distortions or be applicable to all programmes. The SLP should consider providing in-depth explanations, rationales, and goals of tasks, along with increased clinician prompting of kinesthetic and/or auditory check-ins to guide the patient's progress. In addition, the SLP should frequently calibrate his or her auditory-perceptual judgement with the acoustic output and the patient's responses.

The computer software programme may have enhancements that remove computer-perceived noise. Thus, sustained voiceless fricatives during respiratory retraining therapy or loud sustained phonation during Lee Silverman Voice Therapy (LSVT) or Speak OUT! may not be audible to the clinician. Without the signal, the task cannot be monitored for maladaptive behaviours such as increased effort, strain, reduced airflow, etc. Though visual monitoring is still applicable, it may not be enough to identify maladaptive behaviours. Questions for the patient can include "Did it feel the same throughout?" "Did you notice any pushing/effort?" "Did that feel easy?" If the patient answers something other than "yes," such as "pretty close," "no," "fairly close," deeper questioning may be required, along with explanations as to why pushing/effort/reduced airflow during tasks should be avoided. Alternative methods may include using a phone for the auditory signal feedback and muting the computer programme to maintain the video, since the phone will not exclude the patient's phonatory signal. Further guidance on how to implement telemedicine into SLP practice can be gleaned from other clinics and from those who have shared their own experiences and recommendations (Strohl et al. 2020).

Despite the accessibility and convenience of telehealth, it may not be appropriate for every individual. Foremost, the SLP must ensure that the patient has the cognitive, behavioural, and mental status to participate in telemedicine. They should also have suitable resources for accessing telemedicine, including internet access and appropriate technology (Duffy et al. 1997; Macoir et al. 2021). It is the provider's responsibility to ensure protection of the patient's privacy and all platforms are encrypted and compliant with the Health Insurance Portability and Accountability Act (HIPAA). The SLP should verify insurance coverage and/or payment, state laws and regulations, licensure policies, professional liability insurance, billing, and coding.

## 7.3 In-person medicine

### 7.3.1 Voice and upper airway evaluations

At the beginning of the pandemic, patients who were suspected of having a high-risk laryngeal pathology or airway compromise were more likely to be triaged for in-person voice and airway evaluations with visualisation (Gillespie and Gartner-Schmidt 2016). Other potential reasons patients were triaged for in-person evaluation included a lack of stimulability for vocal improvement during their telemedicine evaluation (Gillespie and Gartner-Schmidt 2016), lack of progression through or discharge from therapy, and when in-person appointments during the pandemic were considered safer (Castillo-Allendes et al. 2021; Doll et al. 2021). In-person voice and airway evaluations were re-initiated when PPE became more readily available and when many clinics began to require COVID-19 RT-PCR testing prior to aerosolising generating procedures (AGPs) like laryngeal endoscopy (Rameau et al. 2020).

Rigid and flexible endoscopy of the upper airways with or without stroboscopy is considered an AGP, which is defined as a procedure that could produce higher concentrations of respiratory particles as compared to coughing, sneezing, talking, and breathing. Current literature, however, neither supports nor negates this procedure as an AGP. The American Academy of Otolaryngology-Head and Neck Surgery (2020) stated that endoscopy itself is not an AGP. Rather, it may trigger aerosolising behaviours such as coughing, sneezing, and gagging and therefore, healthcare agencies continue to categorise it as an AGP (Mick and Murphy 2020). Since endoscopy may produce increased aerosols or cause aerosolising behaviours, an SLP or an ENT performing this procedure may be at a higher risk of contracting SARS-CoV-2 and therefore should maintain appropriate PPE during the procedure. If anesthetic is utilised for flexible endoscopy, spraying viscous anesthetic gel into patients' nostrils is also considered an AGP (Rameau et al. 2020; Tan et al. 2020). Additional precautions might involve placing a mask over the patient's mouth during flexible endoscopy in case the patient sneezes and/or coughs (Tan et al. 2020).

For all in-person appointments, safety precautions should be frequently evaluated, and modifications made depending on the rates of infection in the community; the severity of transmission; patients' COVID-19 status; the procedures, tests, and tasks typically completed during the appointment; and availability of COVID-19 testing. To ensure appropriate donning and doffing protocols, SLPs should confirm the minimum PPE recommended for AGPs by facility, local, state, and professional agencies (Doll et al. 2021). Additionally, patients should continue to wear a barrier mask to further reduce transmission risk depending on local infection rates and local or state guidelines.

During a comprehensive voice evaluation a thorough case history, patient-reported outcome measures, auditory-perceptual analysis, acoustics and aerodynamics measures, and stroboscopic evaluation should be completed (Roy et al. 2013; Patel et al. 2018). As of September 2021, CDC recommended that patients receive a COVID RT-PCR test prior to an AGP such as endoscopy within 24 to 72 hours of the AGP (Castillo-Allendes et al. 2021; Rameau et al. 2020; Reddy et al. 2020). Self-quarantine between testing and the clinic visit is also advised to the patient. Patients should also be screened upon clinic arrival for any COVID-19 symptoms. If patients are symptomatic, despite a negative test, clinicians should consider postponing their appointment. Asymptomatic patients who test negative may still be carriers of COVID-19; therefore, a barrier mask and protective eyewear worn by the provider performing an AGP is recommended at a minimum. Guidelines are constantly evolving based on newly learnt information (Doll et al. 2021). For example, the Omicron variant increased transmission of COVID-19, escalating use of an N95 or powered air purifying respirator (PAPR) in place of a barrier mask during AGPs. As the Omicron variant surged, public health officials endorsed wearing N95/PAPR and face shield/goggles during any in-person appointment with or without an AGP.

If a provider plans to perform an AGP on a patient who is unable to receive COVID-19 testing due to availability, providers must assume patients are COVID-19 positive and use appropriate PPE. ASHA recommends following CDC guidelines for PPE when an AGP is performed, including N95 or PAPR, protective eyewear such as face shield or goggles, gown, and gloves (Givi et al.

2020; Lammers et al. 2020; Namasivayam-MacDonald and Riquelme 2020; Rameau et al. 2020; Reddy et al. 2020). The clinician should perform the AGP in a negative pressure room if available (Givi et al. 2020; Lammers et al. 2020; Namasivayam-MacDonald and Riquelme 2020; Rameau et al. 2020; Reddy et al. 2020) or allow full-room ventilation between patients per Occupational Safety and Health Administration (OSHA) guidelines. It is recommended that an AGP should only be performed when patients are asymptomatic. If patients are symptomatic or test positive for COVID-19, the evaluation should be postponed for a given period (e.g., 21 days) unless deemed essential due to suspected high-risk laryngeal pathology or airway compromise. If clinicians are performing an AGP within 21 to 90 days after a patient tests positive for COVID-19, COVID-19 testing may not be indicated secondary to high false positive rates. If a patient does not receive a COVID-19 test due to a recent COVID-19 infection and continues to screen negative for COVID-19 symptoms, clinicians should presume the patient's COVID-19 status is unknown and use full PPE when performing the AGP with the patient and a standard room without need for room closure.

For essential visits with COVID-19 positive patients or symptomatic patients with unknown COVID-19 status, full PPE should be utilised (Givi et al. 2020; Rameau et al. 2020; Reddy et al. 2020). The AGP should be conducted in a negative pressure room if available (Givi et al. 2020; Lammers et al. 2020; Namasivayam-MacDonald and Riquelme 2020; Rameau et al. 2020; Reddy et al. 2020), or the examination room should be unoccupied for a period of time following the AGP.

Data concerning presence or absence of a face mask worn by a patient during acoustic measurements has been conflicting. A published review of this literature found that there were significant acoustic voice-characteristic changes with a face mask versus without a mask. However, the authors indicated that fundamental frequency and aerodynamic measures of MPT were comparable in both conditions (Gama et al. 2021). To achieve validity for comparison with normative data, clinicians should have the patient remove their face mask during acoustic testing. For collecting aerodynamic measures such as mean airflow rate, mean peak air pressure, aerodynamic resistance, and phonation threshold pressure, the patient's barrier face masks must be removed.

## 7.3.2 Equipment

All equipment utilised – such as acoustic, aerodynamic, and endoscopy instruments – should be cleaned per manufacture recommendations. In addition, on-site verification of high-level processing and disinfection control protocol within facilities is required. Aerodynamic tubing should be discarded between patients. Microphone covers should be considered with reservation as their effects on acoustic signals are unknown and pose risk to valid comparisons to existing normative data.

**TABLE 7.1** PPE for evaluation with aerosol-generating procedure

*PPE for Evaluation with AGP (endoscopy with or without stroboscopy)*

| Status | Day of COVID-19 Screening | Appointment | Mask | Eye Protection | Gown | Gloves | Room Requirement | Room Closure |
|---|---|---|---|---|---|---|---|---|
| COVID-19 negative★ | Asymptomatic | Proceed | Barrier | Yes | No | No | Standard room | No |
| COVID-19 negative★ | Symptomatic | Consider postponing | N95/PAPR | Yes | Yes | Yes | Negative pressure room if available | Yes if standard room |
| Unknown | Asymptomatic | Proceed | N95/PAPR | Yes | Yes | Yes | Negative pressure room if available | Yes if standard room |
| Unknown | Symptomatic | Consider postponing | N95/PAPR | Yes | Yes | Yes | Negative pressure room if available | Yes if standard room |
| COVID-19 positive | Symptomatic/asymptomatic | Consider postponing | N95/PAPR | Yes | Yes | Yes | Negative pressure room if available | Yes if standard room |
| Post COVID-19 positive | Symptomatic/asymptomatic | 21 days post COVID-19 positive | N95/PAPR | Yes | Yes | Yes | Standard room | No |

★COVID-19 negative test confirmed with COVID RT-PCR test

### 7.3.3  Voice and upper airway therapy

The voice community has expressed concern about the potentially aerosol-generating nature of voice and breathing exercises performed in voice therapy. A preliminary study measured visualised exhaled vapor from two e-cigarette users to determine the velocity and therefore droplet trajectory during voice exercises (Giovanni et al. 2022). Whispered voice and loud tasks, similar to LSVT exercises, had higher velocities than normal speech. SOVT exercises (i.e., sustained /v/ and /ʒ/ and straw phonation) also had higher air velocities when compared to vowels. Blowing through a straw and sustaining /f/ and /ʃ/, as a patient might do during a respiratory retraining maneuver, led to faster airflow velocities than loud speech. SOVT exercises with delayed onset of phonation had initial high-velocity flow that quickly decreased during phonation. Though some voiceless consonants during speech generated high velocities, the highest velocity occurred during deep inhalation followed by a long exhalation. These results revealed great variability in air velocities during these tasks, though the velocities generated were lower than reported velocities for coughing and sneezing. The authors concluded this preliminary data of voice and upper airway task velocities are not considered any riskier than standard speech (Giovanni et al. 2022).

A recent systematic review of speech pathology literature incorporating 39 studies similarly examined aerosol-generating behaviours (AGBs) such as coughing, speaking, breathing, singing, sustained phonation, and loud voicing (Chacon et al. 2021). They concluded that current speech pathology literature has low levels of evidence supporting these behaviours as aerosol-generating or that any of these behaviours were riskier than others. This review pointed out many limitations of these studies, including the parameters explored and outcomes measured. The methodological approaches applied between studies were highly variable and not comparable. Also, there is a paucity of research related to singing as an AGB. They further stated that all AGBs had a low risk of generating aerosols, except cough, which had a moderate risk and the highest number of studies for review. They concluded that the associated risks between behaviours needs to be examined and SLPs should treat all AGBs as though they are high risk. Since AGBs are present in everyday communication and speech (Chacon et al. 2021) and loud voicing and voice exercises are comparable to standard speech (Giovanni et al. 2022), then universal safety measures, including appropriate PPE, should be used during in-person therapy sessions.

## 7.4  Voice and upper airway patients

Not only has the COVID-19 pandemic altered voice and upper airway management, but it has also dramatically impacted how we communicate. Virtual platforms were quickly implemented, and face masks became the new normal, all of which were unfamiliar in our daily lives. Though COVID-19's direct and indirect relationship to dysphonia and upper airway disorders is yet to be fully understood, studies are emerging.

An online survey of 1,575 participants during the COVID-19 lockdown in Ireland found the prevalence of dysphonia to be 33% and the incidence was 28%. The incidence of those who developed dysphonia during the lockdown was 85%. The top four vocal tract discomfort (VTD) symptoms were dry throat, feeling of irritation, tickling sensation, and tightness. The prevalence of VTD symptoms was 68%, and the incidence was 50%. The incidence of those who developed VTD symptoms during lockdown was 73% (Kenny 2020). A published review found those with a face mask versus those without a face mask had a significant increase in self-rated vocal effort and fatigue. There was also an increase, though not significant, in voice handicap index (VHI) scores, a questionnaire measuring the psychosocial effects of voice disorders (Jacobson et al. 1997), and VTD symptoms of dryness, throat clearing, globus, and breathiness whilst speaking (Gama et al. 2021). In a different study, a quarter of patients who had mild-to-moderate COVID-19 developed dysphonia (Lechien et al. 2020), and those with milder COVID-19 infections had muscle tension dysphonia (MTD), globus, and chronic cough induced laryngeal hypersensitivity (Miles et al. 2022). Amongst those with COVID-19 and dysphonia, there was a higher prevalence of cough, chest pain, sticky sputum, arthralgia, diarrhea, headaches, fatigue, nausea, and vomiting, as well as increased severity of dyspnea, dysphagia, nasal obstruction, and throat, ear, and face pain compared to non-dysphonic patients (Lechien et al. 2020).

Given the nature of COVID-19, those with more severe COVID-19 illness often require hospitalisation and intubation or mechanical ventilation that likely increases their risk of laryngeal injury or airway compromise. Supporting this notion, a systematic review and meta-analysis of laryngeal injury and upper airway symptoms during surgery with short-term endotracheal intubation found laryngeal injuries to be common and mild (Brodsky et al. 2021). The authors reported 80% did not have any injuries; 9%–84% had vocal fold oedema; 4% had vocal fold hemorrhages; and less than 1% had vocal fold paralysis or arytenoid dislocation. The most common post-extubation symptoms were dysphagia, pain, cough, sore throat, and dysphonia (Brodsky et al. 2021). Following a 12+ hour prolonged mechanical ventilation, 57% of patients had a vocal fold ulceration or granulation tissue and significantly worse patient-reported breathing and vocal symptoms 10 weeks post-extubation than those patients without laryngeal injury (Shinn et al. 2019). Both studies support the impression that prolonged intubation and mechanical ventilation increase the risk of laryngeal injury.

A retrospective chart review of 20 of 24 COVID-19 patients presenting with laryngeal complaints who were hospitalised, 18 were intubated for an average of 14 days, 10 underwent a tracheostomy, 19 experienced dysphonia, 17 complained of dyspnea, and 6 suffered from dysphagia. For those patients who required intubation, laryngeal evaluation revealed 50% had vocal fold paralysis or paresis; 39% and laryngeal oedema, granulation, and/or ulcers; 22% had subglottic/tracheal stenosis; and 17% had posterior glottic stenosis (Neevel et al. 2021). It is concluded that prolonged intubation and tracheostomies are major contributors to dysphonia, airway compromise, and dysphagia in those with COVID-19 infection (Miles et al. 2022). MTD was common in patients who had milder COVID-19 infections (Miles et al. 2022) or those who suffered from COVID-19 but had not undergone intubation (Neevel et al. 2021).

Finally, whilst the implications of COVID-19 and its long-term effect on voice and upper airway are still not fully understood, post-COVID syndrome or "long COVID" may lead to long-term voice and upper airway symptoms, including cough, shortness of breath, and dysphonia (Lechien et al. 2020; Naunheim et al. 2020; Raveendran et al. 2021; Song et al. 2021; Miles et al. 2022). In particular, persistent cough is one of the most frequent symptoms of long COVID (Raveendran et al. 2021) and may be a hypersensitive cough from the COVID-19 infection causing a neuroinflammatory response and/or vagal nerve injury (Song et al. 2021). As our understanding of the pathophysiology of laryngeal sequelae of COVID-19 infections improves, the care of voice and upper airway disorders should continue to evolve.

## 7.5  Summary

In conclusion, throughout the COVID-19 pandemic the management of voice and upper airway disorders continues to evolve to maximise safety and effectiveness in patient care. When assessing safety associated with current practice, clinicians must consider the current rates and risks of COVID infection in the community and the urgency of the patient's referral to guide decision-making. Additional considerations include availability of COVID-19 testing, PPE, and the type of procedure and tasks performed at the appointment. Maintaining flexibility between in-person and telemedicine appointments helps ensure maximum safety for all and optimise continued patient care.

Voice and upper airway disorders during the COVID-19 pandemic have manifested in many ways, including increased difficulty with communication secondary to use of masks, increased telecommunication during the pandemic, laryngeal sequelae such as postintubation injuries, vocal fold impairments, and emerging data on post-COVID-19 viral laryngeal sensory neuropathy. Whether laryngeal complications are directly related to a COVID-19 infection or occurred secondary to the COVID-19 pandemic, SLP services should continue to play an important role in voice and upper airway management.

## References

American Academy of Otolaryngology-Head and Neck Surgery (2020). Guidance for return to practice for otolaryngology-head and neck surgery. Part one. www.entnet. org/wp-content/uploads/2021/04/guidance_for_return_to_practice_part_one_ update_070120.pdf. Accessed 8 March 2022.

American Speech-Language-Hearing Association (2020). SLP service delivery considerations in health care during coronavirus/COVID 19. www.asha.org/slp/healthcare/slp-service-delivery-considerations-in-health-care-during-coronavirus/. Accessed 8 March 2022.

Becker, D. R., & Gillespie, A. I. (2021). In the Zoom where it happened: Telepractice and the voice clinic in 2020. *Seminars in Speech and Language*, 42(1), 64–72.

Bhattacharyya, N. (2014). The prevalence of voice problems among adults in the United States. *Laryngoscope*, 124(10), 2359–2362.

Bokolo, A. J. (2020). Exploring the adoption of telemedicine and virtual software for care of outpatients during and after COVID-19 pandemic. *Irish Journal of Medical Science*, 190(1), 1–10.

Brodsky, M. B., Akst, L. M., Jedlanek, E., Pandian, V., Blackford, B., Price, C., et al. (2021). Laryngeal injury and upper airway symptoms after endotracheal intubation during surgery: A systematic review and meta-analysis. *Anesthesia and Analgesia*, 132(4), 1023–1032.

Cantarella, G., Barillari, M. R., Lechien, J. R., & Pignataro, L. (2021). The challenge of virtual voice therapy during the COVID-19 pandemic. *Journal of Voice*, 35(3), 336–337.

Castillo-Allendes, A., Contreras-Ruston, F., Cantor-Cutiva, L. C., Codino, J., Guzman, M., Malebran, C., et al. (2021). Voice therapy in the context of the COVID-19 pandemic: Guidelines for clinical practice. *Journal of Voice*, 35(5), 717–727.

Centers for Medicare and Medicaid Services (2021). Telemedicine. www.medicaid.gov/medicaid/benefits/telemedicine/index.html. Accessed 9 March 2022.

Chacon, A. M., Nguyen, D. D., McCabe, P., & Madill, C. (2021). Aerosol-generating behaviours in speech pathology clinical practice: A systematic literature review. *PLoS One*, 16(4), e0250308. https://doi.org/10.1371/journal.pone.0250308.

Choi, J. S., Yin, V., Wu, F., Bhatt, N. K., O'Dell, K., & Johns, M. 3rd (2021). Utility of telemedicine for diagnosis and management of laryngology-related complaints during COVID-19. *Laryngoscope*. doi:10.1002/lary.29838.

Constantinescu, G., Theodoros, D., Russell, T., Ward, E., Wilson, S., & Wootton, R. (2010). Assessing disordered speech and voice in Parkinson's disease: A telerehabilitation application. *International Journal of Language & Communication Disorders*, 45(6), 630–644.

Dahl, K. L., Weerathunge, H. R., Buckley, D. P., Dolling, A. S., Díaz-Cádiz, M., Tracy, L. F., et al. (2021). Reliability and accuracy of expert auditory-perceptual evaluation of voice via telepractice platforms. *American Journal of Speech-Language Pathology*, 30(6), 2446–2455.

Doll, E. J., Braden, M. N., & Thibeault, S. L. (2021). COVID-19 and speech-language pathology clinical practice of voice and upper airway disorders. *American Journal of Speech-Language Pathology*, 30(1), 63–74.

Duffy, J. R., Werven, G. W., & Aronson, A. E. (1997). Telemedicine and the diagnosis of speech and language disorders. *Mayo Clinic Proceedings*, 72(12), 1116–1122.

Fieux, M., Duret, S., Bawazeer, N., Denoix, L., Zaouche, S., & Tringali, S. (2020). Telemedicine for ENT: Effect on quality of care during Covid-19 pandemic. *European Annals of Otorhinolaryngology, Head and Neck Diseases*, 137(4), 257–261.

Fu, S., Theodoros, D. G., & Ward, E. C. (2015). Delivery of intensive voice therapy for vocal fold nodules via telepractice: A pilot feasibility and efficacy study. *Journal of Voice*, 29(6), 696–706.

Fujiki, R. B., Sanders, P. W., Sivasankar, M. P., & Halum, S. (2021). Determining medical urgency of voice disorders using auditory-perceptual voice assessments performed by speech-language pathologists. *Annals of Otology, Rhinology, and Laryngology*. doi:10.1177/00034894211032779.

Gama, R., Castro, M. E., van Lith-Bijl, J. T., & Desuter, G. (2021). Does the wearing of masks change voice and speech parameters? *European Archives of Oto-Rhino-Laryngology*. doi:10.1007/s00405-021-07086-9.

Georgeadis, A. C., & Krumm, M. (2007). Telehealth and telepractice. https://academy. pubs.asha.org/2007/12/telehealth-and-telepractice/. Accessed 8 March 2022.

Gillespie, A. I., & Gartner-Schmidt, J. (2016). Immediate effect of stimulability assessment on acoustic, aerodynamic, and patient-perceptual measures of voice. *Journal of Voice*, 30(4), 507.E9–507.E14. doi:10.1016/J.JVOICE.2015.06.004.

Giovanni, A., Radulesco, T., Bouchet, G., Mattei, A., Révis, J., Bogdanski, E., et al. (2022). Transmission of droplet-conveyed infectious agents such as SARS-CoV-2 by speech and vocal exercises during speech therapy: Preliminary experiment concerning airflow velocity. *European Archives of Oto-Rhino-Laryngology*, 278(5), 1687–1692.

Givi, B., Schiff, B. A., Chinn, S. B., Clayburgh, D., Iyer, N. G., Jalisi, S., et al. (2020). Safety recommendations for evaluation and surgery of the head and neck during the COVID-19 pandemic. *JAMA Otolaryngology – Head and Neck Surgery*, 146(6), 579–584.

Grillo, E. U. (2017). An online telepractice model for the prevention of voice disorders in vocally healthy student teachers evaluated by a smartphone application. *Perspectives of the ASHA Special Interest Groups*, 2(3), 63–78.

Health Resources and Service Administration (2021). What is telehealth? https://telehealth.hhs.gov/patients/understanding-telehealth/. Accessed 8 March 2022.

Howell, S., Tripoliti, E., & Pring, T. (2009). Delivering the Lee Silverman Voice Treatment (LSVT) by web camera: A feasibility study. *International Journal of Language and Communication Disorders*, 44(3), 287–300.

Jacobson, B. H., Johnson, A., Grywalski, C., Silbergleit, A., Jacobson, G., Benninger, M. S. (1997). The Voice Handicap Index (VHI): Development and validation. *American Journal of Speech-Language Pathology*, 6(3), 66–69.

Kelchner, L. (2013). Telehealth and the treatment of voice disorders: A discussion regarding evidence. *Perspectives on Voice and Voice Disorders*, 23(3), 88–94.

Kenny, C. (2020). Dysphonia and vocal tract discomfort while working from home during COVID-19. *Journal of Voice*. doi:10.1016/j.jvoice.2020.10.010.

Lammers, M. J. W., Lea, J., & Westerberg, B. D. (2020). Guidance for otolaryngology health care workers performing aerosol generating medical procedures during the COVID-19 pandemic. *Journal of Otolaryngology – Head and Neck Surgery*, 49, 36. https://doi.org/10.1186/s40463-020-00429-2.

Lechien, J. R., Chiesa-Estomba, C. M., Cabaraux, P., Mat, Q., Huet, K., Harmegnies, B., et al. (2020). Features of mild-to-moderate COVID-19 patients with dysphonia. *Journal of Voice*. doi:10.1016/j.jvoice.2020.05.012.

Macoir, J., Desmarais, C., Martel-Sauvageau, V., & Monetta, L. (2021). Proactive changes in clinical practice as a result of the COVID-19 pandemic: Survey on use of telepractice by Quebec speech-language pathologists. *International Journal of Language and Communication Disorders*, 56(5), 1086–1096.

Mashima, P. A., Birkmire-Peters, D. P., Syms, M. J., Holtel, M. R., Burgess, L. P., & Peters, L. J. (2003). Telehealth: Voice therapy using telecommunications technology. *American Journal of Speech-Language Pathology*, 12(4), 432–439.

Mashima, P. A., & Brown, J. E. (2011). Remote management of voice and swallowing disorders. *Otolaryngologic Clinics of North America*, 44(6), 1305–1316.

Mattei, A., Amy de la Bretèque, B., Crestani, S., Crevier-Buchman, L., Galant, C., Hans, S., et al. (2020). Guidelines of clinical practice for the management of swallowing disorders and recent dysphonia in the context of the COVID-19 pandemic. *European Annals of Otorhinolaryngology, Head and Neck Diseases*, 137(3), 173–175.

Mick, P., & Murphy, R. (2020). Aerosol-generating otolaryngology procedures and the need for enhanced PPE during the COVID-19 pandemic: A literature review. *Journal of Otolaryngology – Head and Neck Surgery*, 49(1), 29. doi:10.1186/s40463-020-00424-7.

Miles, A., McRae, J., Clunie, G., Gillivan-Murphy, P., Inamoto, Y., Kalf, H., et al. (2022). An international commentary on dysphagia and dysphonia during the COVID-19 pandemic. *Dysphagia*, 1–26. doi:10.1007/s00455-021-10396-z.

Murphy, J. (2020). Planning for reactivation of ambulatory care settings post – COVID-19 pandemic restrictions. *Journal of Ambulatory Care Management*, 43(4), 286–289.

Namasivayam-MacDonald, A. M., & Riquelme, L. F. (2020). Speech-language pathology management for adults with COVID-19 in the acute hospital setting: Initial recommendations to guide clinical practice. *American Journal of Speech-Language Pathology*, 29(4), 1850–1865.

Naunheim, M. R., Zhou, A. S., Puka, E., Franco, R. A. Jr, Carroll, T. L., Teng, S. E., et al. (2020). Laryngeal complications of COVID-19. *Laryngoscope. Investigative Otolaryngology*, 5(6), 1117–1124.

Neevel, A. J., Smith, J. D., Morrison, R. J., Hogikyan, N. D., Kupfer, R. A., & Stein, A. P. (2021). Postacute COVID-19 laryngeal injury and dysfunction. *OTO Open*, 5(3), 2473974X211041040. doi:10.1177/2473974X211041040.

Patel, R. R., Awan, S. N., Barkmeier-Kraemer, J., Courey, M., Deliyski, D., Eadie, T., et al. (2018). Recommended protocols for instrumental assessment of voice: American speech-language-hearing association expert panel to develop a protocol for instrumental assessment of vocal function. *American Journal of Speech-Language Pathology*, 27(3), 887–905.

Rameau, A., Young, V. N., Amin, M. R., & Sulica, L. (2020). Flexible laryngoscopy and COVID-19. *Otolaryngology-Head & Neck Surgery*, 162(6), 813–815.

Rangarathnam, B., Gilroy, H., & McCullough, G. H. (2016). Do patients treated for voice therapy with telepractice show similar changes in voice outcome measures as patients treated face-to-face? *EBP Briefs*, 11(5), 1–6.

Rangarathnam, B., McCullough, G. H., Pickett, H., Zraick, R. I., Tulunay-Ugur, O., & McCullough, K. C. (2015). Telepractice versus in-person delivery of voice therapy for primary muscle tension dysphonia. *American Journal of Speech-Language Pathology*, 24(3), 386–399.

Raveendran, A. V., Jayadevan, R., & Sashidharan, S. (2021). Long COVID: An overview. *Diabetes and Metabolic Syndrome: Clinical Research and Reviews*, 15(3), 869–875.

Reddy, P. D., Nguyen, S. A., & Deschler, D. (2020). Bronchoscopy, laryngoscopy, and esophagoscopy during the COVID-19 pandemic. *Head & Neck*, 42(7), 1634–1637.

Roy, N., Barkmeier-Kraemer, J., Eadie, T., Sivasankar, M. P., Mehta, D., Paul, D., et al. (2013). Evidence-based clinical voice assessment: A systematic review. *American Journal of Speech-Language Pathology*, 22(2), 212–226.

Schneider, S. L., Habich, L., Weston, Z. M., & Rosen, C. A. (2021). Observations and considerations for implementing remote acoustic voice recording and analysis in clinical practice. *Journal of Voice*. doi:10.1016/j.jvoice.2021.06.011.

Shinn, J. R., Kimura, K. S., Campbell, B. R., Sun Lowery, A., Wootten, C. T., Garrett, C. G., et al. (2019). Incidence and outcomes of acute laryngeal injury after prolonged mechanical ventilation. *Critical Care Medicine*, 47(12), 1699–1706. doi:10.1097/CCM.0000000000004015.

Song, W.-J., Hui, C. K. M., Hull, J. H., Birring, S. S., McGarvey, L., Mazzone, S. B., et al. (2021). Confronting COVID-19-associated cough and the post-COVID syndrome: Role of viral neurotropism, neuroinflammation, and neuroimmune responses. *The Lancet Respiratory Medicine*, 9(5), 533–544.

Strohl, M. P., Dwyer, C. D., Ma, Y., Rosen, C. A., Schneider, S. L., & Young, V. N. (2020). Implementation of telemedicine in a laryngology practice during the COVID-19 pandemic: Lessons learned, experiences shared. *Journal of Voice*. doi:10.1016/j.jvoice.2020.06.017.

Tan, V. Y. J., Zhang, E. Z. Y., Daniel, D., Sadovoy, A., Teo, N. W. Y., Kiong, K. L., et al. (2020). Respiratory droplet generation and dispersal during nasoendoscopy and upper respiratory swab testing. *Head & Neck*, 42(10), 2779–2781.

Towey, M. P. (2012). Speech therapy telepractice for vocal cord dysfunction (VCD): MaineCare (Medicaid) cost savings. *International Journal of Telerehabilitation*, 4(1), 37–40.

Watters, C., Miller, B., Kelly, M., Burnay, V., Karagama, Y., & Chevretton, E. (2021). Virtual voice clinics in the COVID-19 era: Have they been helpful? *European Archives of Otorhinolaryngology*, 278(10), 4113–4118.

Weerathunge, H. R., Segina, R. K., Tracy, L., & Stepp, C. E. (2021). Accuracy of acoustic measures of voice via telepractice videoconferencing platforms. *Journal of Speech, Language, and Hearing Research*, 64(7), 2586–2599.

# 8

# CLINICAL PRESENTATION OF PATIENTS WITH COVID-19 IN CRITICAL CARE FOLLOWING INTUBATION AND TRACHEOSTOMY

*Sarah Wallace*

## 8.1 Introduction

The COVID-19 pandemic has seen unprecedented numbers of patients globally develop life-threatening severe disease requiring hospitalisation and subsequent admission to intensive care. The need to provide this level of critical care has been and continues to be an enormous challenge for many countries across the world. The response led to unparalleled rapid clinical learning and logistical adaptations to practice affecting the whole multidisciplinary team (MDT) working in the intensive care unit (ICU). Dealing with a new disease resulted in simultaneous evolution of research and treatments, at pace and with global collaboration on a new scale. This was equally demonstrated by speech and language therapy (SLT) professionals involved in the frontline critical care response. Assimilating atypical observations and predicting ICU clinical and workforce needs whilst delivering patient care in stressful environments became the new norm.

Provision of SLT to UK ICUs pre-COVID-19 was geographically highly variable with shortages of funded posts and widespread inability to meet national staffing standards (Twose et al. 2021). A recent UK study found only 22% of ICUs directly funded SLT and the staffing ratio fell far short, with 1 SLT to 30 ICU beds compared to the recommended 1 to 10 beds (Faculty of Intensive Care Medicine and Intensive Care Society 2019) and 1 to 157 beds without ring-fenced SLT (Twose et al. 2022). The pandemic brought additional challenges for a stretched SLT critical care workforce. In April 2020, early in the first wave, whilst patients remained intubated, sedated, and inappropriate for SLT-specific intervention, many SLTs worked in support roles, such as proning teams. Meanwhile, rapid upskilling to meet the rising tide of extubated and/or tracheostomised critical care patients became a priority. The RCSLT facilitated SLT experts to deliver

DOI: 10.4324/9781003257318-8

educational webinars on clinical issues emerging in patients with SARS-CoV-2, with the first attracting over 1,000 global attendees. The profession was hungry for knowledge and providing medical updates and guidance on clinical adaptations whilst keeping staff safe from viral transmission was crucial. Calm reassurance and shared expertise reduced fears and empowered SLTs to work in COVID ICUs. Dissemination of knowledge and guidance has continued throughout the pandemic via webinars and collaborative research through the joint efforts of clinicians and international professional bodies. Consequently, the SLT critical care evidence base has been accelerated. Large numbers of patients with laryngeal dysfunction following intubation and tracheostomy increased awareness and elevated the value of SLT in ICU amongst MDT colleagues.

Globally, SLTs stepped up, delivering vital patient care and rehabilitation within ICUs and beyond. New opportunities to collaborate with ICU colleagues and professional bodies, such as the Intensive Care Society (ICS), were seized despite burgeoning SLT workloads. The UK ICS National Rehabilitation Collaborative formed in March 2020 and welcomed SLT to the top table, recognising early the potential large cohort of patients with laryngeal complications needing SLT (British Society of Rehabilitation Medicine and Intensive Care Society 2020; Intensive Care Society 2020). Collaborative research led to the development of the validated ICU rehabilitation screening tool (PICUPS), which crucially included identification of voice, swallowing, airway and communication needs (Turner-Stokes et al. 2021; Puthucheary et al. 2021). The ICS National Rehabilitation Collaborative with SLT continues to research and lobby for rehabilitation services. SLT experts also developed the SLT Pillar of the Professional Development Framework to support future SLT critical care workforce (Intensive Care Society 2021). Undoubtedly, the pandemic forged firm inter-professional links, to the benefit of all future critical care patients.

## 8.2 Challenges of working in the "COVID ICU"

The SLT role within the ICU MDT in swallowing, communication, and tracheostomy weaning is well evidenced (McGrath and Wallace 2014; McGrath 2014; Bonvento et al. 2017; McGrath, Ashby et al. 2020; McGrath, Wallace, Lynch et al. 2020; Wallace and McGrath 2021; Faculty of Intensive Care Medicine and Intensive Care Society 2019; National Confidential Enquiry into Patient Outcome and Death 2014). The virus presents unique challenges. This includes adapting practice to limit aerosols, wearing PPE, communicating wearing masks, lack of visitors, and working in crowded overspill ICUs with ventilators not designed for cuff-down "laryngeal" weaning with redeployed staff unfamiliar with tracheostomies. There has been insufficient recognition of viral exposure risk of SLT interventions (e.g., dysphagia assessment) by governments and restricted access to high-level PPE for many (Bolton et al. 2020). SLT experts and professional bodies urgently developed national and international consensus documents to protect staff and patients, support PPE access, and guide risk assessment (Vergara et al. 2020a, 2020b; Zaga et al. 2020; Freeman-Sanderson et al. 2021; McGrath, Brenner et al. 2020; Royal College of Speech and Language Therapists 2021a; Royal College of Nursing 2022).

All tracheostomy care procedures are acknowledged as potentially aerosol generating. This initially triggered caution, delaying cuff deflation, weaning, one-way valve, and oral trials. Increased knowledge and trust in PPE mean weaning has reverted to pre-COVID times. As new variants evolve, SLTs should continue to consider airbourne virus exposure risks carefully and use appropriate PPE protection (Vergara et al. 2020a, 2020b; Zaga et al. 2020; Royal College of Speech and Language Therapists 2021a; Royal College of Nursing 2022).

Caring for unvaccinated patients has also placed ethical burdens on fatigued staff. Admissions of unvaccinated patients to ICUs in the UK was high and has fluctuated from 75% (May 2021) to 47% (October 2021) to 61% (December 2021) (Intensive Care National Audit & Research Centre 2021). Overall, ICU staff showed unprecedented bravery, adaptability, and resilience in the face of virus exposure whilst caring for countless sick and distressed patients.

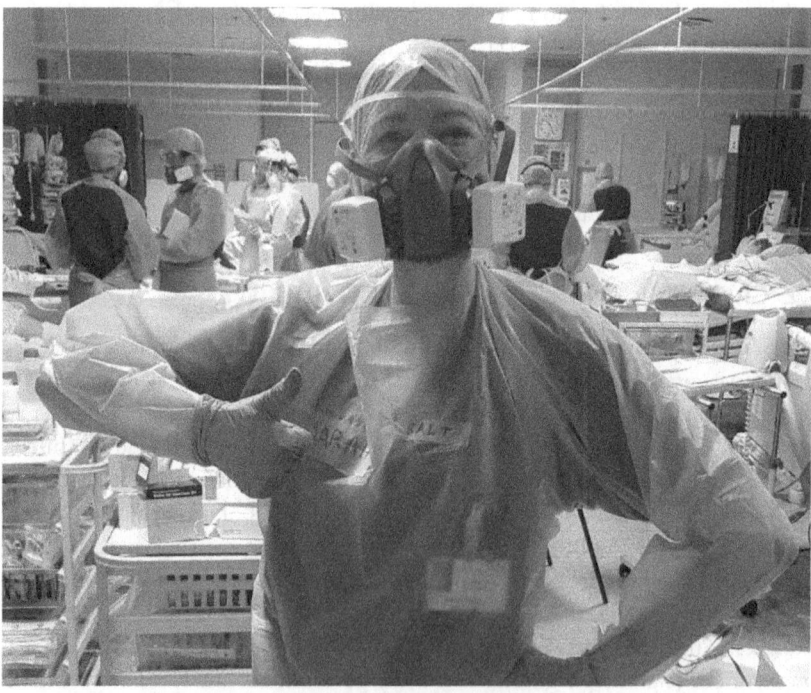

**FIGURE 8.1**   The author in PPE in the COVID ICU

## 8.3 Medical presentation of severe SARS-CoV-2

The SARS-CoV-2 virus causes a myriad of clinical issues in the severe disease state. It has become clear that this is not simply a respiratory virus but a complex multisystemic illness. There are respiratory, neurological, gastro-intestinal, renal, and cardiac symptoms, with severe inflammatory response and coagulopathy also features. Hypoxaemic respiratory failure is the most common reason for artificial mechanical ventilatory support and admission to ICU. Studies suggest 61%–81% of ICU patients develop Acute Respiratory Distress Syndrome (ARDS), a condition in which the alveolar sacs in the lungs become filled with fluid, as COVID-19 related pneumonia progresses (Gibson et al. 2020), with septic shock, multi-organ failure, and death being common consequences. Ventilatory support for respiratory failure involves non-invasive high-flow nasal cannulae oxygen therapy (HFNC), continuous positive airway pressure (CPAP), or invasive tracheal intubation. Previous studies show that dysphagia is associated with both HFNC and CPAP, with choking at 40L–50L/min flow and inhibition of the swallow reflex (Oomagari et al. 2015; Teramoto 2013). These fragile patients often need SLT intervention to prevent further aspiration-related respiratory complications. The effectiveness and optimal timing of respiratory interventions is unclear, but emerging studies suggest that early CPAP may reduce the need for invasive ventilation (National Institute for Health Research 2021). Intubation for ongoing ventilatory support leads to primary extubation, endotracheal tube (ETT) removal, ETT reinsertion, and/or insertion of a tracheostomy tube. Prolonged cardiac and respiratory life support via extracorporeal membrane oxygenation (ECMO) surged, and UK services scaled up to 990% of usual demand (Jooste et al. 2021). In total, SARS-CoV-2 gave rise to a vast increase in extubated and tracheostomised patients requiring SLT.

This multi-systemic disease requires critical care SLTs to utilise an array of knowledge, from neurology, ENT, and respiratory specialities. For example, neurological impairments result from viral invasion via the olfactory nerve, trans-synaptic transfer, vascular infection, or leukocyte migration across the blood-brain barrier. Neurological manifestations of COVID-19 in ICU include acute confusion, encephalopathy, myopathy, and cerebrovascular events, all of which can contribute to dysphagia and cognitive communication impairment (Abenza-Abildúa et al. 2020). Dysphagia and dysarthria symptoms vary according to cranial nerves, stroke, encephalopathies, or Guillain-Barre syndrome manifestation (Aoyagi et al. 2021; Regan et al. 2022).

The aetiology of communication and swallowing impairments in ICU are known to be complex and multifactorial (Zuercher et al. 2019). Determining iatrogenic factors (result of critical care intervention, e.g., intubation), comorbidities, medical and psychological features is essential for effective management. Critical illness myopathy occurs in 70% of people in ICU over seven days and causes severe weakness-related dysphagia in 91% (Ponfick et al. 2015). COVID-19 adds a range of issues affecting oromotor and laryngopharyngeal functions such as fatigue, laryngeal hypersensitivity, altered taste/smell, and persistent respiratory compromise. Swallowing and communication trajectory and outcomes are not yet fully understood.

## 8.4 Critical care cohorts

In 2020, hospitals scrambled to reconfigure and increase capacity to deal with large volumes of hospital and ICU admissions. Studies report a range of 14.2% to 26% of hospitalised patients received ICU care (Wang et al. 2019; Richardson et al. 2020). Discharged alive data reports 41% of 20,133 hospitalised patients and 28% (826/3001) (Docherty et al. 2020) to 61.6% of 25,849 patients requiring ICU admission survived (Intensive Care National Audit & Research Centre 2021). Various studies report comorbidities of significance for dysphagia risk indicating a need for SLT intervention (Brodsky, Gellar et al. 2014; Brodsky, González-Fernández et al. 2014; Brodsky et al. 2017; Zuercher et al. 2019). In the COVID-19 cohort, these include hypertension (56.6%); obesity (11%–41.7%); diabetes (21%–33.8%); chronic cardiac disease (31%); chronic obstructive pulmonary disease (COPD; 18%); acute and chronic kidney disease (16–78%); asthma (15%); dementia (14%); and chronic neurological disorder (11%) (Richardson et al. 2020; Docherty et al. 2020; Argenziano et al. 2020). However, Docherty et al. (2020) also found a lack of major comorbidity in 23% of patients. Dysphagia is linked to increasing age and male sex, which are common features of SARS-CoV-2 ICU patients (Wang et al. 2019).

Geographical variation in ICU cohorts is inevitable due to differences in capacity, resources, and admission criteria. But generally, ICU patients with COVID-19 faced major morbidity and mortality, especially those severely ill undergoing ECMO (Vuylsteke 2021). People of Black Asian and Minority Ethnic (BAME) groups were also disproportionately affected due to health inequalities (35% of ICU admissions) (House of Commons Women and Equalities Committee 2020). Despite young cohorts in each subsequent COVID-19 wave, the need for SLT input remains very high.

## 8.5 Intubation trauma, post-extubation dysphagia, dysphonia, and dysarthria in COVID-19

Overall, studies show 10%–15% of hospitalised SARS-CoV-2 patients require invasive mechanical ventilation due to disease severity. For a significant proportion, ventilation is much longer than for other viral pneumonias (Argenziano et al. 2020; Williams and McGrath 2021). Laryngeal complications due to trans-laryngeal intubation are common and previously well documented, with post-extubation laryngeal injury reported in up to 83% (average intubation 8.2 days), occurring even after short periods of intubation (Mota et al. 2012;

Brodsky et al. 2018; Kelly et al. 2020). Apart from duration, risk factors for laryngeal injury include larger ETT size, diabetes, emergency intubation, and reintubation. SARS-CoV-2 related laryngeal oedema is a common reason for failed extubation (Wallace and McGrath 2021; McGrath, Wallace and Goswamy 2020). Evidence suggests that prolonged intubation and tracheostomy, both common in COVID-19, are associated with a high prevalence of extubation failure, laryngeal injury (57–83%), dysphonia (76%), and dysphagia (49%) (Tadié et al. 2010; Skoretz et al. 2010; Mota et al. 2012; Brodsky et al. 2018).

Whilst common, the exact incidence and underlying mechanisms of post-extubation dysphagia (PED) are not fully understood. Brodsky et al. (2017) reported PED in 60% with 50% aspirating. Female sex and intubation duration were associated with the need for swallowing assessment (Brodsky et al. 2014). PED causes increased aspiration and aspiration pneumonia risk, delayed oral intake, malnutrition, prolonged ICU and hospital length of stay, higher morbidity and mortality (Zuercher et al. 2019), and adverse clinical outcomes and worse quality of life persist post ICU (Macht et al. 2013; Zielske et al. 2014). Prognostic indicators for dysphagia include intubation duration, reintubation, severity at initial swallow assessment, amount of SLT treatment and age (Moraes et al. 2013).

Evidence is emerging that PED is exacerbated in SARS-CoV-2 due to reduced lung function and prolonged intubation, a feature of ECMO survivors (Félix et al. 2021; Frajkova et al. 2020). Regan et al. (2021) found 66% of extubated patients referred to SLT in ICU presented with dysphonia and dysphagia. Ninety percent required altered oral intake, 36% were nil by mouth, and dysphagia and dysphonia persisted at hospital discharge (37% and 27%, respectively). Age, proning, and pre-existing respiratory disease were predictors of oral intake status. A further report by Regan et al. (2022) stated history of intubation was predictive of voice quality and oral intake status and neurological manifestations were predictive of dysarthria. Significant improvements in severity were noted but problems with need for modified oral intake (59%); dysphonia (23%); and dysarthria (14%) persisted at hospital discharge. These figures suggest a significant need for SLT in ICU and beyond.

## 8.6 Laryngeal complications in ICU patients with SARS-CoV-2

Laryngeal complications in ICU patients with SARS-CoV-2 are common, wide-ranging, and multifactorial (see Table 8.1). Mechanisms include ETT effects (insertion, removal, pressure on delicate structures) and recurrent laryngeal nerve compression from cuff. In addition, lack of trans-laryngeal airflow due to cuff inflation causes laryngopharyngeal hypoaesthesia, swallow downregulation, and prevention of voicing (Wallace and McGrath 2021). Concomitant factors in ICU impact also on swallowing and communication such as sedatives, ARDS, and COVID-19 neurological manifestations. It may be difficult to be certain

**TABLE 8.1** Laryngeal complications in SARS-CoV-2

| Mechanism | Potential effects |
| --- | --- |
| **Direct laryngeal injury from intubation**<br>– ETT insertion<br>– Presence of tube: pressure, cuff compression of recurrent laryngeal nerve<br>– ETT removal<br>– Emergency intubation<br>– Reintubation<br>– Prolonged intubation leading to pressure necrosis of perichondrium and cartilages | – Laryngeal oedema<br>– Vocal fold and laryngeal mucosal trauma (e.g., ulcerations)<br>– Granulomas<br>– Erythema<br>– Vocal cord palsy/paresis – unilateral or bilateral immobility<br>– Vocal fold atrophy<br>– Arytenoid dislocation, subluxation<br>– Anterior/posterior glottic web<br>– Laryngopharyngeal hyper or hyposensitivity<br>– Odynophagia<br>– Dysphagia, aspiration<br>– Stridor, hoarseness<br>– Dysphonia, vocal fatigue<br>– Laryngotracheal malacia<br>– Laryngotracheal stenosis (due to scarring) and airway patency concern – long-term tracheostomy, ENT intervention |
| **Cuff inflation: ETT or tracheostomy**<br>– Disrupted trans-laryngeal/upper airway airflow<br>– Dependence on mechanical ventilatory support | – Laryngopharyngeal desensitisation<br>– Disuse atrophy<br>– Dysphagia<br>– Aspiration, aspiration pneumonia<br>– Impaired saliva secretion management<br>– Weak cough<br>– Impaired Laryngeal Adductor Reflex<br>– Respiratory/swallow asynchrony<br>– Laryngeal hypersensitivity – food sticking sensation, fear of choking, excessive coughing, poor tolerance of cuff deflation/one-way valve<br>– Inability to speak<br>– Aphonia/dysphonia<br>– Anxiety/depression<br>– Loss of taste, smell, and appetite |
| **Concomitant factors**<br>– Prolonged intubation and/or tracheostomy<br>– Prolonged need for paralysing and sedative medications<br>– Hypo/hyperactive delirium | – Laryngeal injury<br>– Delayed vocalisation and oral intake<br>– Dysphagia – laryngopharyngeal weakness, reduced pharyngeal constriction, residue, aspiration risk<br>– Impaired secretion management<br>– Aspiration pneumonia |

| Mechanism | Potential effects |
|---|---|
| – Prolonged corticosteroid use (dexamethasone)<br>– ARDS, acute lung injury<br>– Sepsis<br>– ICU acquired weakness, polyneuropathy/myopathy<br>– Fatigue<br>– Proning – cranial nerve (CN) injury<br>– Pre-existing dysphagia<br>– Co-morbidities | – Bulbar weakness<br>– Dysarthria<br>– Cognitive behavioural features – reduced bolus awareness, impulsive feeding, poor insight<br>– Swallow fatigue<br>– Poor appetite/oral intake, dependence on tube feeding<br>– Malnutrition<br>– Increased length of stay, mortality risk |
| **SARS-CoV-2 virus** | – Severe/persistent laryngeal oedema<br>– Erythema<br>– Increased frequency/severity -granulomas, cystic lesions, vocal cord immobility<br>– Laryngitis<br>– Dysphonia<br>– Laryngopharyngeal reflux (related to gastro-intestinal symptoms, obesity)<br>– Neurogenic dysphagia (embolic strokes, GBS) |

of the impact of each factor, but SLT investigation is essential for their effective treatment.

Emerging evidence suggests that patients with SARS-CoV-2 exhibit a significantly higher incidence of laryngeal abnormalities (Boggiano et al. 2021; Naunheim et al. 2020). The virus binds to ACE-2 receptors which are particularly dense in respiratory epithelial cells, leading to upper airway manifestations including sore throat, anosmia, aguesia, dysphagia, laryngopharyngeal erythema, and subglottic and tracheal oedema (Özçelik Korkmaz et al. 2020; El-Anwar et al. 2020). Laryngeal oedema in the critically ill is common and can be detected by a cuff – leak test, ultrasound, or laryngoscopy (Pluijms et al. 2015). In SARS-CoV-2 laryngeal oedema, laryngo-tracheitis and subglottic granulations appear prolonged, leading to failed extubation (Oliver et al. 2020; McGrath, Wallace and Goswamy 2020).

Inevitably, laryngeal complications increase laryngeal dysfunction, dysphagia, and dysphonia (Brodsky et al. 2018; Wallace and McGrath 2021). It is difficult to determine how much laryngeal abnormalities are due to intubation trauma or the virus itself, but some issues seem atypical (see Figure 8.2).

Naunheim et al. (2020) found 100% of patients had laryngeal abnormalities impacting on voice, airway, and swallowing on flexible laryngoscopy; 65% had prolonged intubation (average duration 22 days); and 69% had been proned.

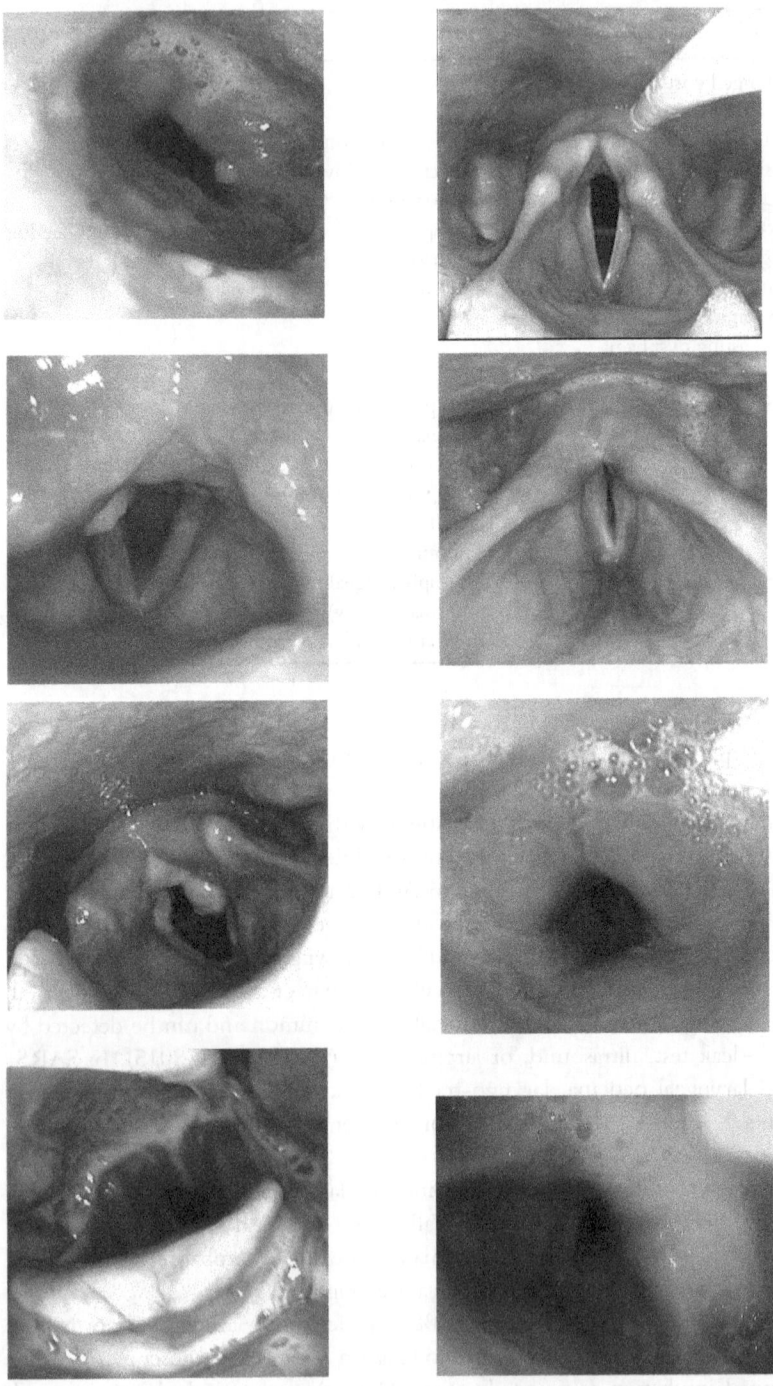

**FIGURE 8.2** Flexible endoscopic evaluation of swallowing (FEES) in ICU patients with SARS–CoV-2

Further, 40% had unilateral vocal fold immobility; 15% posterior glottic stenosis; 10% subglottic stenosis; and 45% required ENT/otolaryngologist procedural intervention. Laryngotracheal lesions were detected in 40% of patients undergoing videoendoscopy, with severe stenosis in 6% (grade 3 or 4). All patients had been intubated and proned, with tube size a significant risk factor for lesion development (Félix et al. 2021). Similarly, Boggiano et al. (2021) identified a median of three laryngeal abnormalities per patient on FEES in ICU patients with COVID-19, of which 63% were considered clinically significant. Laryngeal oedema (75%); impaired vocal fold mobility (75%); atypical lesions (69%); and erythema (38%) were the most common abnormalities (see Figure 8.2). Dexamethasone is often used to treat laryngeal oedema in ICU. But despite routine use to reduce mortality in SARS-CoV-2, oedema still persists, and therefore, discussion by the MDT on the risks versus benefits of further use of steroids is warranted in individual cases. The use of FEES positively influences patient management by identifying silent aspiration (88% of overall aspirators) and airway patency issues impacting tracheostomy weaning and by targeting dysphagia therapy, optimising reflux management, and signalling ENT referral (Boggiano et al. 2021).

Dysphagia in severe COVID-19 in ICU is due to multiple aetiologies, including primary damage to central and peripheral neurological networks, brainstem and cranial nerves, and prolonged intubation and mechanical ventilation (Frank and Frank 2021). Osbeck Sandblom et al. (2021) used FEES to investigate dysphagia in patients with COVID-19 in ICU and found pooled laryngeal secretions (92%); silent aspiration (44%); and pharyngeal residue (100%) with impaired vocal fold mobility, oedema, and erythema in over 60%. A UK study found ICU patients admitted with COVID-19 exhibited delirium (hyper- and hypoactive), laryngeal compromise (vocal cord palsy, laryngeal oedema), respiratory-swallow incoordination, secretion burden and fatigue (Dawson et al. 2020). 67% of ICU patients were kept nil by mouth following initial assessment and those with a tracheostomy were more likely to need modified diet than those without (87% vs 59%), with a significant correlation between duration of intubation and days to oral intake (Dawson et al. 2021). Similar findings have emerged from an international data set reporting high rates of dysphagia and dysphonia in ICU patients. This manifested in poor secretion management, poor cough, impaired swallow, hoarse voice, and inability to protect the airway (Miles et al. 2022).

The pandemic resulted in a surge of patients with ARDS. Prone positioning has often been used to optimise oxygenation in ARDS, but there may be negative consequences for laryngeal function. Limited evidence exists on the direct effects of proning on the larynx, however inevitably intubation is prolonged with subsequent increased risks of laryngeal injury. Several case reports have described proning leading to lower cranial nerve paralysis and injuries to lips, jaw, tongue, palate, and laryngeal structures with impaired secretion clearance (Trejo-Gabriel-Galan et al. 2017; Le et al. 2020). Facial swelling, oropharyngeal oedema, and ETT pressure injuries may be worse in the presence of obesity, a common comorbidity of COVID-19. Proned patients require more sedation. As sedation is weaned, patients may develop hyperactive delirium and agitation, with head movements and pulling at the ETT potentially worsening laryngeal injury. Proning also hinders the practice of oral hygiene, which may lead to aspiration of micro-organisms in pooled saliva secretions, a risk factor for aspiration and ventilator-associated pneumonias. Delirium and resultant hallucinations, anxiety, and fear can also delay SLT assessment and resumption of oral intake. The intricate relationship between respiration and swallowing also makes patients with COVID-19 and ARDS vulnerable to incoordination of breath-swallow patterns and dysphagia (Mohan and Mohapatra 2020). ARDS itself is known to increase the likelihood of dysphagia and one-third of orally intubated ARDS survivors exhibit dysphagia symptoms persisting beyond ICU (Brodsky et al. 2017).

Medications commonly used for sedation and anaesthesia, such as midazolam, are known to cause pharyngeal dysfunction and increase risks of penetration and aspiration (Hårdemark Cedborg et al. 2015). In patients with SARS-CoV-2, who frequently require prolonged sedation, this is a likely contributing factor for dysphagia. Severe sepsis, common in severe SARS-CoV-2, is a risk factor for long-term dysphagia in survivors of critical illness (Zielske et al. 2014). Additionally, up to 6% of usual patients admitted to ICU have pre-existing difficult airways which pose further risks of laryngeal intubation trauma and difficult intubation in SARS-CoV-2 (Higgs et al. 2018). Overall, dysphagia is common and the need for modified diets in ICU is high (55%), and SLTs need to consider multiple contributory factors (Catlow et al. 2021).

## 8.7 Tracheostomy and COVID-19

The pandemic led to a global surge in critically ill patients with COVID-19 disease requiring tracheostomy. Data suggests that pre-pandemic, approximately 8%–13% of patients in ICU were tracheostomised for a median of 28 days and spent 23 days in ICU. This equated to 15,000 tracheostomies per year in the UK (Williams and McGrath 2021). Rates of tracheostomy during the pandemic vary (16%–61%) but are significantly higher than usual, and determining which SARS-CoV-2 patients benefit from tracheostomy and optimal timing remains controversial (Rozenblat et al. 2021). International protocols showed that timing of tracheostomy insertion varied from 3–21 days (Williams and McGrath 2021). One large UK centre found 30-day survival was higher and ICU stay shorter in patients receiving tracheostomy irrespective of severity of critical illness (Queen Elizabeth Hospital Birmingham COVID-19 airway team 2020).

Tracheostomy is considered a safe procedure if it is conducted with additional aerosol precautions (Mehta and Kochar 2021). Delaying tracheostomy insertion lowers the risk of staff infection but may increase length of stay, with slow weans doubling duration in ICU and reducing the likelihood of liberation from ventilation (Kwak et al. 2021; Olanipekun and Ezeagu 2021). These are important factors impacting on dysphagia and communication. It has been shown that early tracheostomy may reduce laryngeal injury and dysfunction, enabling earlier return to oral intake and vocalisation (Ng et al. 2019; McGrath, Wallace, Lynch et al. 2020). One study showed that tracheostomy facilitated sedation and ventilator weaning in patients with COVID-19 after prolonged ventilation (median 24 days), with a median time from tracheostomy to decannulation of 36 days (Long et al. 2021). There has been a significant rise in surgical versus percutaneous tracheostomies during COVID-19, and Long et al. (2021) found no difference in outcomes. Overall, the majority of tracheostomised COVID-19 patients survive, wean from ventilation, and are successfully decannulated, which may reflect patient-selection processes.

Dysphagia often co-exists in tracheostomy due to anatomical location and shared respiratory and swallowing pathways, with a reported incidence of between 11%–93% (Skoretz et al. 2020). Tracheostomy is an independent risk factor for long-term dysphagia in the critically ill (Zielske et al. 2014). A study by Archer et al. (2021) of hospitalised patients with COVID-19 in a London hospital found 71% of tracheostomised patients were eventually decannulated (median time to decannulation 19 days) but had marked impairments in voice and swallowing. Time to commencing oral intake was much longer in ICU tracheostomised patients than in those undergoing primary extubation (28 days vs 15.8 days). A study pooling international data reports high rates of dysphagia, dysphonia, and laryngeal injury in ICU patients, with a median tracheostomy duration of 19–38 days (Miles et al. 2022). Patients can present with hypoesthesia but more atypically show signs of laryngeal hypersensitivity, leading to sensations of residue, choking, and coughing in the absence of a trigger. Hypersensitivity along with altered taste sensation can increase patient anxiety and delay establishment of oral intake. FEES can assist with biofeedback and can provide reassurance that aspiration and residue are less of a risk than perceived by the patient.

Tracheostomy weaning practice presented a unique challenge in COVID-19 due to aerosol risks. A global and multidisciplinary collaborative response reviewed protocols and produced guidance (Vergara et al. 2020a; Zaga et al. 2020; McGrath, Ashby et al. 2020; McGrath, Brenner et al. 2020; Brenner et al. 2021; Bier-Laning et al. 2021). Various strategies to reduce aerosol generation such as prolonging cuff inflation were initially recommended. However, delayed vocalisation compounds patient anxiety and communication difficulties reduce engagement in all aspects of rehabilitation. Accurate assessment of swallowing with the cuff inflated would usually require FEES, but endoscopy was avoided during the first wave. Staff trust in the effectiveness of PPE has seen weaning and FEES practice return to business as usual in later waves, promoting early cuff deflation and one-way valve use for voice restoration and laryngeal rehabilitation (Brenner et al. 2021; Royal College of Speech and Language Therapists 2021b).

## 8.8 Early SLT intervention, FEES, and rehabilitation of laryngeal function in ICU

National and international guidelines support early SLT intervention and FEES as essential to assessment, proactive management, and optimisation of functional recovery (National Confidential Enquiry into Patient Outcome and Death 2014; Faculty of Intensive Care Medicine and Intensive Care Society 2019; Wallace et al. 2020). Laryngeal injury, for example, frequently remains undetected without the use of direct visualisation using nasendoscopy or FEES (McGrath, Wallace, Lynch et al. 2020; Wallace and McGrath 2021). Early in 2020, nasendoscopy was halted by ENT, subsequently preventing the use of FEES in ICU. This delayed oral trials and impacted the ability of SLTs to accurately assess and treat prevalent and severe dysphonia and dysphagia issues and to advise the MDT on tracheostomy weaning and decannulation decisions. The RCSLT worked with expert advisors to urgently develop guidance on SLT-led nasendoscopy, enabling safe recommencement of FEES by June 2020 with business as usual by October 2020 and ongoing supportive statements (Royal College of Speech and Language Therapists 2021b). Suspension of FEES also led to an interest in laryngeal ultrasound and an international expert group published a rapid review of evidence (Allen et al. 2021). Current recommendations are that the literature does not support ultrasound use as a clinical swallowing assessment tool (Miles et al. 2022). It remains to be seen whether lack of FEES affected patient outcomes and whether timely FEES-guided interventions in later waves reduced durations of dysphonia and dysphagia.

Laryngeal rehabilitation is vital for recovery of swallowing and communication functions. A national data-collection strategy – using the PICUPS screening tool to identify swallowing, voice, airway, and cognitive-communication problems – is essential to understanding SLT rehabilitation needs and service demands going forward. Multidisciplinary management of intubation-related dysphagia and dysphonia is key to improving patient-centred outcomes, such as earlier vocalisation and safe resumption of oral intake (Brodsky et al. 2020; McGrath and Wallace 2014, 2020). Dawson et al. (2020) found that providing intensive dysphagia rehabilitation in ICU led to the majority of SARS-CoV-2 patients with dysphagia regaining near normal swallow function prior to hospital discharge. SLT interventions were provided for an average of 11.3 days for those extubated and 12.9 days for those tracheostomised, much longer than the non-ICU COVID-19 group (8.6 days). Swallow rehabilitation techniques for COVID-19 in ICU do not differ from non-COVID-19 and include individualised compensatory strategies, with diet modification, swallowing, and voice exercises being frequent options (Archer et al. 2021). One case report showed successful treatment of severe COVID-related neurogenic dysphagia using pharyngeal electrical stimulation (Traugott et al. 2021). Optimal treatment interventions for COVID-19 related dysphagia are still not fully understood.

## 8.9 Post–intensive care syndrome (PICS) and swallowing, voice, and airway issues

SARS-CoV-2 patients can suffer persistent swallowing, voice, and airway effects related to post–intensive care syndrome, which require ongoing rehabilitation (Turner-Stokes et al. 2021). One report suggests that 40% of patients requiring rehabilitation post-ICU have dysphagia (Wiertz et al. 2021). Another study found a high prevalence of dysphagia (90%) detected on videofluoroscopy in patients recovering from ARDS two weeks post-ICU (Lagier et al. 2021). Miu et al. (2021) found higher rates of prolonged airway (59% vs 44% vs 31%); voice (40% vs 19% vs 19%); and swallowing (21% vs 6% vs 12%) dysfunction in ICU COVID-19 patients with respiratory failure versus patients with non–COVID-19 respiratory failure versus non-respiratory patients. Similar findings by Neevel et al. (2021) found fixed upper airway obstruction (22%); dysphonia (53%); and self-reported dysphagia (30%) persisted at two-month follow-up for ICU patients. Impaired vocal fold mobility (50%); glottic injury (39%); subglottic/tracheal stenosis (22%); and posterior glottic stenosis (17%) were frequent.

The European Laryngological Society issued a warning in 2020 concerning potential unprecedented increases in airway stenosis as a result of long-term intubation for SARS-CoV-2 (Piazza et al. 2020). Whilst the incidence of laryngotracheal stenosis (LTS) is not yet certain, risk factors have been described, with intubation >10 days (average 24 days, median 14 days), cuff pressure>30mm $H_2O$, and obesity associated with greater rates of LTS post-tracheostomy (Li et al. 2018; Tsehaye et al. 2021; Rouhani et al. 2020; Neevel et al. 2021). Studies to date indicate a high frequency of laryngeal sequelae and SLT rehabilitation needs for respiratory COVID-19 patients recovering from critical illness.

## 8.10 Summary

This chapter has examined the clinical challenges and presentation of patients with COVID-19 in critical care, in particular the communication, swallowing, and airway problems related to intubation and tracheostomy. As the pandemic continues, our understanding of the clinical picture is still evolving, and whilst the true prevalence is not yet known, it is clear that ICU patients develop significant laryngeal dysfunction. Aetiology is multifactorial and relates to the increased need for prolonged intubation and tracheostomy, comorbidities, and the virus itself causing laryngeal, neurological and respiratory complications.

The trajectory of recovery of laryngeal function is variable, but indications suggest that early SLT intervention with integrated MDT rehabilitation improves outcomes. Severe ARDS may be an important prognostic indicator for more persistent dysphagia, dysphonia, and airway issues, as this increases intubation, proning, tracheostomy, illness severity, and ICU acquired weakness. Collaborative research on effective treatments must continue to ensure SLTs can optimise patient outcomes with scarce workforce resources. Symptom monitoring should be built in to COVID pathways as rehabilitation needs persist post-ICU. COVID-19 presents a growing healthcare and economic burden, but early SLT intervention within the ICU MDT is crucial to optimising patient recovery and quality of life.

## References

Abenza-Abildúa, M. J., Ramírez-Prieto, M. T., Moreno-Zabaleta, R., Arenas-Valls, R., Salvador-Maya, R. A., Algarra-Lucas, C., et al. (2020). Neurological complications in critical patients with COVID-19. *Neurología*, 35(9), 621–627.

Allen, J. E., Clunie, G. M., Slinger, C., Haines, J., Mossey-Gaston, C., Zaga, C. J., Scott, B., Wallace, S., & Govender, R. (2021). Utility of ultrasound in the assessment of swallowing and laryngeal function: A rapid review and critical appraisal of the literature. *International Journal of Language & Communication Disorders*, 56(1), 174–204.

Aoyagi, Y., Inamoto, Y., Shibata, S., Kagaya, H., et al. (2021). Clinical manifestation, evaluation, and rehabilitative strategy of dysphagia associated with COVID-19. *American Journal of Physical Medicine & Rehabilitation*, 100(5), 424–431.

Archer, S., Iezzi, C., & Gilpin, L. (2021). Swallowing and voice outcomes in patients hospitalised with Covid-19: An observational cohort study. *Archives of Physical Medicine and Rehabilitation*, 102(6),1084–1090.

Argenziano, M. G., Bruce, S. L., Slater, C. L., Tiao, J. R., et al. (2020). Characterization and clinical course of 1,000 patients with coronavirus disease in New York: Retrospective case series. *BMJ*, 369, m1996. doi:10.1136/bmj.m1996.

Bier-Laning, C., Cramer, J. D., Roy, S., Palmieri, P. A., Amin, A., Añon, J. M., et al. (2021). Tracheostomy during the COVID-19 pandemic: Comparison of international perioperative care protocols and practices in 26 countries. *Otolaryngology-Head and Neck Surgery*, 164(6), 1136–1147.

Boggiano, S., Williams, T., Gill, S., Alexander, P., Khwaja, S., Wallace, S., & McGrath, B. A. (2021). Multidisciplinary management of laryngeal pathology identified in patients with COVID-19 following translaryngeal intubation and tracheostomy. *Journal of the Intensive Care Society*. https://journals.sagepub.com/doi/full/10.1177/17511437211034699.

Bolton, L., Mills, C., Wallace, S., & Brady, M. (2020). Aerosol generating procedures, dysphagia assessment and COVID-19: A rapid review. *International Journal of Language & Communication Disorders*, 55(4), 629–636.

Bonvento, B., Wallace, S., Lynch, J., Coe, B., & McGrath, B. A. (2017). Role of the multidisciplinary team in the care of the tracheostomy patient. *Journal of Multidisciplinary Healthcare*, 10, 391–398.

Brenner, M. J., McGrath, B. A., & Pandian, V. (2021). Small steps towards better tracheostomy care during the evolving COVID-19 pandemic. *Journal of Intensive Care Medicine*, 36(12), 1513–1515.

British Society of Rehabilitation Medicine and Intensive Care Society (2020). Responding to COVID-19 and beyond: A framework for assessing early rehabilitation needs following treatment in intensive care. National Post-Intensive Care Rehabilitation Collaborative. Version 1. www.bsrm.org.uk/downloads/2020.06.23 – icsframework-for-assessing-early-reha-(1).pdf. Accessed 8 December 2021.

Brodsky, M. B., Gellar, J. E., Dinglas, V. D., Colantuoni, E., et al. (2014). Duration of oral endotracheal intubation is associated with dysphagia symptoms in acute lung injury patients. *Journal of Critical Care*, 29(4), 574–579.

Brodsky, M. B., González-Fernández, M., Mendez-Tellez, P. A., Shanholtz, C., Palmer, J. B., & Needham, D. M. (2014). Factors associated with swallowing assessment after oral endotracheal intubation and mechanical ventilation for acute lung injury. *Annals of the American Thoracic Society*, 11(10), 1545–1552.

Brodsky, M. B., Huang, M., Shanholtz, C., Mendez-Tellez, P. A., Palmer, J. B., Colantuoni, E., & Needham, D. M. (2017). Recovery from dysphagia symptoms after oral endotracheal intubation in acute respiratory distress syndrome survivors. A 5-year longitudinal study. *Annals of the American Thoracic Society*, 14(3), 376–383.

Brodsky, M. B., Levy, M. J., Jedlanek, E., et al. (2018). Laryngeal injury and upper airway symptoms after oral tracheal intubation with mechanical ventilation during critical care: A systematic review. *Critical Care Medicine*, 46, 2010–2017.

Brodsky, M. B., Pandian, V., & Needham, D. M. (2020). Post-extubation dysphagia: A problem needing multidisciplinary efforts. *Intensive Care Medicine*, 46(1), 93–96.

Catlow, R., Cheeseman, C., & Newman, H. (2021). Covid-19: Nutrition and functional outcomes for critical care survivors in a 400-bedded district general hospital in North London. *Journal of the Intensive Care Society*. https://journals.sagepub.com/doi/full/10.1177/17511437211025420.

Dawson, C., Capewell, R., Ellis, S., et al. (2020). Dysphagia presentation and management following COVID-19: An acute care tertiary Centre experience. *Journal of Laryngology and Otology*. https://doi.org/10.1017/S0022215120002443.

Docherty, A. B., Harrison, E. M., Green, C. A., Hardwick, H. E., et al. (2020). Features of 20,133 UK patients in hospital with covid-19 using the ISARIC WHO Clinical Characterisation Protocol: Prospective observational cohort study. *BMJ*, 369, m1985. doi:10.1136/bmj.m1985.

El-Anwar, M. W., Elzayat, S., & Fouad, Y. A. (2020). ENT manifestation in COVID-19 patients. *Auris, Nasus, Larynx*, 47(4), 559–564.

Faculty of Intensive Care Medicine and Intensive Care Society (2019). Guidelines for the provision of intensive care services. Edition 2. https://ficm.ac.uk/sites/ficm/files/documents/2021-10/gpics v2.pdf. Accessed 9 December 2021.

Félix, L., Tavares, T. L., Almeida, V. P. B., & Tiago, R. S. L. (2021). Incidence of laryngotracheal lesions after orotracheal intubation in coronavirus disease patients. *Laryngoscope*. doi:10.1002/lary.29862.

Frajkova, Z., Tedla, M., Tedlova, E., Suchankova, M., & Geneid, A. (2020). Postintubation dysphagia during COVID-19 outbreak – contemporary review. *Dysphagia*, 35(4), 549–557.

Frank, U., & Frank, K. (2021). Covid-19 – new challenges in dysphagia and respiratory therapy. *Nervenartz*. doi:10.1007/s00115-021-01162-5.

Freeman-Sanderson, A., Ward, E. C., Miles, A., et al. (2021). A consensus statement for the management and rehabilitation of communication and swallowing function in the ICU: A global response to COVID-19. *Archives of Physical Medicine and Rehabilitation*, 2(5), 835–842.

Gibson, P. G., Qin, L., & Puah, S. H. (2020). COVID-19 acute respiratory distress syndrome (ARDS): Clinical features and differences from typical pre-COVID-19 ARDS. *Medical Journal of Australia*, 213(2), 54–56.

Hårdemark Cedborg, A. I., Sundman, E., Bodén, K., et al. (2015). Effects of morphine and midazolam on pharyngeal function, airway protection, and coordination of breathing and swallowing in healthy adults. *Anesthesiology*, 122(6), 1253–1267.

Higgs, A., McGrath, B. A., Goddard, C., Rangasami, J., Suntharalingam, G., Gale, R., Cook, T. M., Difficult Airway Society, Intensive Care Society, Faculty of Intensive

Care Medicine, Royal College of Anaesthetists (2018). Guidelines for the management of tracheal intubation in critically ill adults. *British Journal of Anaesthesia*, 120(2), 323–352.

House of Commons Women and Equalities Committee (2020). Unequal impact? Coronavirus and BAME people. https://committees.parliament.uk/publications/3965/documents/39887/default/. Accessed 9 December 2021.

Intensive Care National Audit & Research Centre (ICNARC) (2021). ICNARC report on COVID-19 in critical care: England, Wales and Northern Ireland. 31 December 2021. www.icnarc.org/our-audit/audits/cmp/reports. Accessed 28 January 2022.

Intensive Care Society (2020). Speech and language therapy for Covid-19 patients in ICU and beyond. www.ics.ac.uk/Society/COVID-19/PDFs/Speech_and_language_therapy_for_COVID-19_patients. Accessed 28 January 2022.

Intensive Care Society (2021). The speech and language therapy pillar: A supplementary resource of the Allied Health Professionals (AHP) Critical Care Professional Development Framework (CCPDF). www.ics.ac.uk/Society/Guidance/PDFs/SLT_Pillar. Accessed 9 December 2021.

Jooste, R., Rowan, K. M., Symes, N., & Vuylsteke, A. (2021). Scaling up a national extracorporeal membrane oxygenation referral service for adult patients in acute severe respiratory failure at the time of a pandemic. *Journal of the Intensive Care Society*. https://journals.sagepub.com/doi/10.1177/17511437211022129.

Kelly, E., Wallace, S., & Puthucheary, Z. (2020). Prolonged intubation and tracheostomy in Covid-19 survivors: Consequences and recovery of laryngeal function. *ICU Management and Practice*, 20(4), 243–249.

Kwak, P. E., Connors, J. R., Benedict, P. A., et al. (2021). Early outcomes from early tracheostomy for patients with COVID-19. *JAMA Otolaryngology – Head & Neck Surgery*, 147(3), 239–244.

Lagier, A., Melotte, E., Poncelet, M., Remacle, S., & Meunier, P. (2021). Swallowing function after severe COVID-19: Early videofluoroscopic findings. *European Archives of Otorhinolaryngology*, 278(8), 3119–3123.

Le, M. Q., Rosales, R., Shapiro, L. T., & Huang, L. Y. (2020). The down side of prone positioning: The case of a coronavirus 2019 survivor. *American Journal of Physical Medicine & Rehabilitation*, 99(10), 870–872.

Li, M., Yiu, Y., Merrill, T., Yildiz, V., deSilva, B., & Matrka, L. (2018). Risk factors for post tracheostomy tracheal stenosis. *Otolaryngology – Head & Neck Surgery*, 159(4), 698–704.

Long, S. M., Chern, A., Feit, N. Z., Chung, S., Ramaswamy, A. T., Li, C., et al. (2021). Percutaneous and open tracheostomy in patients with COVID-19: Comparison and outcomes of an institutional series in New York City. *Annals of Surgery*, 273(3), 403–409.

Macht, M., King, C. J., Wimbish, T., Clark, B. J., et al. (2013). Post-extubation dysphagia is associated with longer hospitalization in survivors of critical illness with neurologic impairment. *Critical Care*, 17(3), R119. doi:10.1186/cc12791.

McGrath, B. A. (Ed.). (2014). *Comprehensive tracheostomy care: The national tracheostomy safety project manual*. Chichester, West Sussex: Wiley Blackwell.

McGrath, B. A., Ashby, N., Birchall, M., Dean, P., Doherty, C., Ferguson, K., et al. (2020). Multidisciplinary guidance for safe tracheostomy care during the COVID-19 pandemic: The NHS National Patient Safety Improvement Programme (NatPatSIP). *Anaesthesia*, 75(12), 1659–1670.

McGrath, B. A., Brenner, M. J., Warrillow, S. J., Pandian, V., et al. (2020). Tracheostomy in the COVID-19 era: Global and multidisciplinary guidance. *The Lancet. Respiratory Medicine*, 8(7), 717–725.

McGrath, B. A., & Wallace, S. (2014). The UK national tracheostomy safety project and the role of speech and language therapists. *Current Opinion in Otolaryngology & Head and Neck Surgery*, 22(3), 181–187.

McGrath, B., Wallace, S., & Goswamy, J. (2020). Laryngeal oedema associated with COVID-19 complicating airway management. *Anaesthesia*, 75(7), 972. https://doi.org/10.1111/anae.1509.

McGrath, B. A., Wallace, S., Lynch, J., Bonvento, B., Coe, B., Firn, M., et al. (2020). Improving tracheostomy care in the United Kingdom: Results of a guided quality improvement programme in 20 diverse hospitals. *British Journal of Anaesthesia*, 125(1), e119–e129. https://doi.org/10.1016/j.bja.2020.04.064.

Mehta, Y., & Kochar, G. (2021). Tracheostomy in COVID times. *Journal of Cardiac Critical Care*, 5(2), 82–83.

Miles, A., McRae, J., Clunie, G., Gillivan-Murphy, P., Inamoto, Y., Kalf, H., Pillay, M., Pownall, S., Ratcliffe, P., Richard, T., Robinson, U., Wallace, S., & Brodsky, M. (2022). An international commentary on dysphagia and dysphonia during the COVID-19 pandemic. *Dysphagia*. https://doi.org/10.1007/s00455-021-10396-z.

Miu, K., Miller, B., Tornari, C., Slack, A., Murphy, P., Ahmed, I., Burnay, V., & Karagama, Y. (2021). Airway, voice and swallow outcomes following endotracheal intubation and mechanical ventilation for COVID-19 pneumonitis: Preliminary results of a prospective cohort study. *British Journal of Surgery*, 108(Suppl 2). https://doi.org/10.1093/bjs/znab134.049.

Mohan, R., & Mohapatra, B. (2020). Shedding light on dysphagia associated with Covid-19: The what and why. *OTO Open*, 4(2), 1–2.

Moraes, D. P., Sassi, F. C., Mangilli, L. D., et al. (2013). Clinical prognostic indicators of dysphagia following prolonged orotracheal intubation in ICU patients. *Critical Care*, 17(5), R243. doi:10.1186/cc13069.

Mota, L., de Cavalho, G., & Brito, V. (2012). Laryngeal complications by orotracheal intubation: Literature review. *International Archives of Otorhinolaryngology*, 16(2), 236–245.

National Confidential Enquiry into Patient Outcome and Death (NCEPOD) (2014). On the right trach: A review of the care received by patients who underwent a tracheostomy. www.ncepod.org.uk/2014report1/downloads/OnTheRightTrach_FullReport.pdf. Accessed 9 December 2021.

National Institute for Health Research (2021). RECOVERY-RS trial finds continuous positive airway pressure (CPAP) reduces need for invasive ventilation in hospitalised COVID-19 patients. www.nihr.ac.uk/news/recovery-rs-trial-finds-continuous-positive-airway-pressure-cpap-reduces-need-for-invasive-ventilation-in-hospitalised-covid-19-patients/28366. Accessed 8 December 2021.

Naunheim, M. R., Zhou, A. S., Puka, E., Franco, R. A., et al. (2020). Laryngeal complications of COVID-19. *Laryngoscope Investigative Otolaryngology*, 5(6), 1117–1124.

Neevel, A. J., Smith, J. D., Morrison, R. J., Hogikyan, N. D., et al. (2021). Postacute COVID-19 laryngeal injury and dysfunction. *OTO Open*, 5(3), 1–8. https://doi.org/10.1177/2473974X211041040.

Ng, F. K., Wallace, S., Khallil, U., & McGrath, B. A. (2019). Duration of trans-laryngeal intubation before tracheostomy is associated with laryngeal injury when assessed using fibreoptic endoscopic evaluation of swallow. *British Journal of Anaesthesia*, 123(3), e447. www.bjanaesthesia.org/article/S0007-0912(19)30412-X/fulltext.

Olanipekun, T., & Ezeagu, R. (2021). Outcomes and safety of early percutaneous tracheostomy in coronavirus disease 2019 patients admitted to the ICU. *Critical Care Medicine*, 49(6), e653–e654. doi:10.1097/CCM.0000000000004925.

Oliver, C. M., Campbell, M., Dulan, O., Hamilton, N., & Birchall, M. (2020). Appearance and management of COVID-19 laryngo-tracheitis: Two case reports. *F1000Res*, 9, 310. doi:10.12688/f1000research.23204.2.

Oomagari, M., Fujishima, I., Katagiri, N., Arizono, S., et al. (2015). Swallowing function during high-flow nasal cannula therapy. *European Respiratory Journal*, 46, PA4199. doi:10.1183/13993003.congress-2015.

Osbeck Sandblom, H., Dotevall, H., Svennerholm, K., Tuomi, L., & Finizia, C. (2021). Characterization of dysphagia and laryngeal findings in COVID-19 patients treated in the ICU – an observational clinical study. *PLoS One*, 16(6), e0252347. doi:10.1371/journal.pone.0252347.

Özçelik Korkmaz, M., Eğilmez, O. K., Özçelik, M. A., & Güven, M. (2020). Otolaryngological manifestations of hospitalised patients with confirmed COVID-19 infection. *European Archives of Oto-Rhino-Laryngology*, 278(5), 1675–1685.

Piazza, C., Filauro, M., Dikkers, F. G., et al. (2020). Long-term intubation and high rate of tracheostomy in COVID-19 patients might determine an unprecedented increase of airway stenoses: A call to action from the European Laryngological Society. *European Archives of Oto-Rhino-Laryngology*, 278(1), 1–7.

Pluijms, W. A., van Mook, W. N., Wittekamp, B. H., et al. (2015). Postextubation laryngeal edema and stridor resulting in respiratory failure in critically ill adult patients: Updated review. *Critical Care*, 19, 295. https://doi.org/10.1186/s13054-015-1018-2.

Ponfick, M., Linden, R., & Nowak, D. A. (2015). Dysphagia – a common, transient symptom in critical illness polyneuropathy: A fiberoptic endoscopic evaluation of swallowing study. *Critical Care Medicine*, 43(2), 365–372.

Puthucheary, Z., Brown, C., Corner, E., Wallace, S., Highfield, J., Bear, D., et al. (2021). The Post-ICU presentation screen (PICUPS) and rehabilitation prescription (RP) for intensive care survivors. Part II: Clinical engagement and future directions for the national post-intensive care rehabilitation collaborative. *Journal of the Intensive Care Society*. doi:10.1177/1751143720988715.

Queen Elizabeth Hospital Birmingham COVID-19 airway team (2020). Safety and 30-day outcomes of tracheostomy for COVID-19: A prospective observational cohort study. *British Journal of Anaesthesia*, 125(6), 872–879.

Regan, J., Walshe, M., Lavan, S., Horan, E., et al. (2021). Post-extubation dysphagia and dysphonia amongst adults with Covid-19 in the Republic of Ireland: A prospective multi-site observational cohort study. *Clinical Otolaryngology*, 46(6), 1290–1299.

Regan, J., Walshe, M., Lavan, S., Horan, E., et al. (2022). Dysphagia, dysphonia and dysarthria outcomes among adults hospitalised with Covid-19 across Ireland. *The Laryngoscope*. https://doi.org/10.1002/lary.29900.

Richardson, S., Hirsch, J. S., Narasimhan, M., et al. (2020). Presenting characteristics, comorbidities, and outcomes among 5700 patients hospitalized with COVID-19 in the New York City area. *JAMA*, 323(20), 2052–2059.

Rouhani, M. J., Clunie, G., Thong, G., Lovell, L., et al. (2020). A prospective study of voice, swallow and airway outcomes following tracheostomy for Covid-19. *The Laryngoscope*, 131(6), e1918–e1925. doi:10.1002/lary.29346.

Royal College of Nursing (2022). Covid-19 workplace risk assessment toolkit. www.rcn.org.uk/clinical-topics/infection-prevention-and-control/covid-19-workplace-risk-assessment-toolkit. Accessed 29 January 2022.

Royal College of Speech and Language Therapists (2021a). Advice to RCSLT members on reducing the transmission of COVID-19. www.rcslt.org/wp-content/uploads/2021/07/Advice-to-RCSLT-members-on-reducing-the-transmission-of-COVID-02072021.pdf. Accessed 8 December 2021.

Royal College of Speech and Language Therapists (2021b). Speech and language therapist-led endoscopic procedures: Considerations for all patients during the COVID-19 pandemic. www.rcslt.org/wp-content/uploads/2020/11/RCSLT_COVID-19_SLT-led_endoscopic_procedure_guidance_April21.pdf. Accessed 8 December 2021.

Rozenblat, T., Reifen, E., Benov, A., Shaul, C., Neuman, U., Karol, D., et al. (2021). The value of tracheostomy of critically ill COVID-19 patients – a multicentral study. *American Journal of Otolaryngology*, 43(1), 103230. doi:10.1016/j.amjoto.2021.103230.

Skoretz, S. A., Anger, N., Wellman, L., Takai, O., & Empey, A. (2020). A systematic review of tracheostomy modifications and swallowing in adults. *Dysphagia*, 35(6), 935–947.

Skoretz, S. A., Flowers, H. L., & Martino, R. (2010). The incidence of dysphagia following endotracheal intubation: A systematic review. *Chest*, 137(3), 665–673.

Tadié, J., Behm, E., Lecuyer, L., et al. (2010). Post-intubation laryngeal injuries and extubation failure: A fiberoptic endoscopic study. *Intensive Care Medicine*, 36(6), 991–998.

Teramoto, S. (2013). Swallowing, gastroesophageal reflux and sleep apnoea. In C. Idzikowski (Ed.), *Sleep and its disorders affect society*. InTech Open. www.intechopen.com/chapters/46441.

Traugott, M., Hoepler, W., Kitzberger, R., Pavlata, S., Seitz, T., et al. (2021). Successful treatment of intubation-induced severe neurogenic post-extubation dysphagia using pharyngeal electrical stimulation in a COVID-19 survivor: A case report. *Journal of Medical Case Reports*, 15(1), 148. doi:10.1186/s13256-021-02763-z.

Trejo-Gabriel-Galan, J. M., Perea-Rodriguez, M. E., Aicua-Rapun, I., & Martinez-Barrio, E. (2017). Lower cranial nerves paralysis following prone-position mechanical ventilation. *Critical Care Medicine*, 45(8), e865–e866. doi:10.1097/CCM.0000000000002411.

Tsehaye, M. T., Kelly, E., & Thomas, A. J. (2021). Identification of laryngotracheal stenosis during weaning from tracheostomy – a clinical conundrum. *Journal of Experimental Pathology*, 2(2), 67–74. www.scientificarchives.com/admin/assets/articles/pdf/identification-of-laryngotracheal-stenosis-during-weaning-from-tracheostomy – a-clinical-conundrum-20210526050509.pdf.

Turner-Stokes, L., Corner, E., Siegert, R., Brown, C., Wallace, S., et al. (2021). The post-ICU presentation screen (PICUPS) and rehabilitation prescription (RP) for intensive care survivors. Part I: Development and preliminary clinimetric evaluation. *Journal of the Intensive Care Society*. https://journals.sagepub.com/doi/full/10.1177/1751143720988715.

Twose, P., Jones, U., Bharal, M., Bruce, J., & Wallace, S. (2021). Exploration of therapist's views of practice within critical care. *BMJ Open Respiratory Research*, 8(1), e001086. doi:10.1136/bmjresp-2021-001086.

Twose, P., Terblanche, E., Jones, U., Bruce, J., Firshman, P., Highfield, J., Jones, G., Newman, H., Rock, C., & Wallace, S. (2022). Therapy professionals in critical care: A UK wide workforce survey. *Journal of the Intensive Care Society*. doi:10.1177/17511437221100332.

Vergara, J., Starmer, H., Wallace, S., Bolton, L., et al. (2020a). Assessment, diagnosis, and treatment of dysphagia in patients infected with SARS-CoV-2: A review of the literature and international guidelines. *American Journal of Speech-Language Pathology*, 29(4), 2242–2253.

Vergara, J., Starmer, H. M., Wallace, S., Bolton, L., et al. (2020b). Swallowing and communication management of tracheostomy and laryngectomy in the context of COVID-19: A review. *JAMA Otolaryngology – Head & Neck Surgery*. doi:10.1001/jamaoto.2020.3720.

Vuylsteke, A. (2021). ECMO in Covid-19: Do not blame the tool. *The Lancet*, 398(10307), 1197–1199.

Wallace, S., & McGrath, B. A. (2021). Laryngeal complications after tracheal intubation and tracheostomy. *BJA Education*, 21(7), 250–257.

Wallace, S., McLaughlin, C., Clayton, J., Coffey, M., et al. (2020). *Fibreoptic endoscopic evaluation of swallowing (FEES): The role of speech and language therapy*. London: Royal College of Speech and Language Therapists.

Wang, D., Hu, B., Hu, C., Zhu, F., et al. (2019). Clinical characteristics of 138 hospitalized patients with novel coronavirus-infected pneumonia in Wuhan, China. *JAMA*, 323(11), 1061–1069.

Wiertz, C. M. H., Vints, W. A. J., Maas, G. J. C. M., Rasquin, S. M. C., et al. (2021). COVID-19: Patient characteristics in the first phase of post intensive care rehabilitation. *Archives of Rehabilitation Research and Clinical Translation*, 3(2), 100108. doi:10.1016/j.arrct.2021.100108. Epub Feb 4.

Williams, T., & McGrath, B. A. (2021). Tracheostomy for COVID-19: Evolving best practice. *Critical Care*, 25, 316. doi:10.1186/s13054-021-03674-7.

Zaga, C., Pandian, V., Brodsky, M., Wallace, S., et al. (2020). Speech-language pathology guidance for tracheostomy during the COVID-19 pandemic: An international multidisciplinary perspective. *American Journal of Speech-Language Pathology*, 29(3), 1320–1334.

Zielske, J., Bohne, S., Brunkhorst, F., Axer, H., & Guntinas-Lichius, O. (2014). Acute and long-term dysphagia in critically ill patients with severe sepsis: Results of a prospective controlled observational study. *European Archives of Oto-Rhino-Laryngology*, 271(11), 3085–3093.

Zuercher, P., Moret, C. S., Dziewas, R., & Schefold, J. C. (2019). Dysphagia in the intensive care unit: Epidemiology, mechanisms, and clinical management. *Critical Care*, 23(1), 103. doi:10.1186/s13054-019-2400-2.

# 9

# SWALLOWING DIFFICULTIES IN ADULTS AFTER COVID-19

*Anna Miles*

## 9.1 Introduction

The first 12 months of the pandemic brought about a range of guidance from otolaryngology associations, speech-language therapy associations, and dysphagia societies on minimising viral spread in dysphagia services (Vergara et al. 2020). Frequent surveys explored the impact of the pandemic on dysphagia care (Miles et al. 2021). As it became clear that COVID-19 was spread by aerosols, debates arose regarding the current definition of aerosol generating procedures (AGPs). Many associations challenged the exclusion of speech, voice, and swallowing activities as listed AGPs and advocated for enhanced infection control protocols for speech-language therapists to prevent viral transmission. Dysphagia services were significantly impacted, in comparison to other areas of medicine, due to the need for direct contact with the aerodigestive tract known to hold high viral load (Miles et al. 2022). Many common dysphagia practices in those with laryngectomies and tracheostomies were considered aerosol generating (Miles et al. 2022; Freeman-Sanderson et al. 2021). The Dysphagia Research Society COVID-19 Taskforce published a list of low-, medium-, and high-risk dysphagia activities for aerosol generation (Miles et al. 2022). Early guidance banned cough reflex testing and flexible endoscopic evaluation of swallowing (FEES) (Bolton et al. 2020). Telehealth was strongly recommended with a number of key publications to support the use of telehealth in dysphagia management across the lifespan (Malandraki et al. 2021).

By September 2020, the Centres for Medicare & Medicaid Services (CMS) had released a statement recommending *not* delaying endoscopic procedures. Associations gradually released guidance to reinstate in-person evidence-based best practice in dysphagia care, including endoscopic evaluations with enhanced

DOI: 10.4324/9781003257318-9

personal protective equipment (PPE) to optimally treat patients safely during the pandemic. Ku and colleagues describe practical solutions for videofluoroscopic swallowing study (VFSS) and FEES during the pandemic for patients with head and neck cancer. Their guidance includes patient pre-screening, triaging for urgency, PPE, and ventilation (Ku et al. 2020). Goldman and colleagues offered adaptations to VFSS suite management, including HEPA filtration and sanitation procedures (Goldman et al. 2021). Implementation strategies to minimise the spread of COVID-19 whilst maximising dysphagia care were rapidly published to support clinicians worldwide (Fritz et al. 2021; Miles et al. 2022). At the time of writing this chapter, the debate on the classification of AGPs and aerosol-generating behaviours persists, with a recent report in the *Lancet* stating that close proximity for prolonged periods of time in poorly ventilated spaces in addition to speaking and coughing hold greater risk than any of the currently listed AGPs (Hamilton et al. 2021). This is a strong reminder of the risk our dysphagia teams endure as they care for patients with COVID-19 and dysphagia.

The Dysphagia Research Society Taskforce provides a clear explanation of why dysphagia teams have been at such a heightened risk during the pandemic (Miles et al. 2022). Dysphagia teams needed to work with patients with COVID-19 and are often involved in the care of those with open airways (tracheostomy, laryngectomy). Dysphagia assessment and treatments regularly evoke aerosol generating behaviours such as coughing, speaking, singing, and forced expiratory acts such as Lee Silverman Voice Treatments and Expiratory Muscle Strength Training (EMST). However, this is coupled with other higher-risk exposure activities: an inability of the patient to wear a face mask or face covering during the procedure, close proximity to the airway which both increases aerosol exposure as well as exposure to secretions, and the longer duration of exposure for many dysphagia activities. With this knowledge, dysphagia teams have needed a cautious approach to in-person consultations. This requires careful attention to PPE and sanitation when treating patients with COVID-19 but also during periods of community spread to avoid catching the virus themselves in order to protect patients who have been admitted with other conditions such as stroke. Well-being surveys reflect the stressors of those working in dysphagia care, with ~60% of clinicians screening positive for depression, anxiety, stress, and post-traumatic stress disorder in Ireland in mid-2020 (Rouse and Regan 2021).

## 9.2 Risk factors for dysphagia

As hospitalisations and deaths rapidly rose in early 2020, researchers and clinicians moved quickly to publish primary data to support those working with patients. Early large hospital cohorts from China (Zhou et al. 2020; Guan et al. 2020; Wang et al. 2020; Yang et al. 2020; Tian et al. 2020); Italy (Grasselli et al. 2021); and New York (Richardson et al. 2020) offered trends in those patients most likely to develop more severe COVID-19 symptoms. A meta-analysis found chronic obstructive pulmonary disease, cardiovascular disease, and malignancy comorbidities resulting in poorer clinical outcome (Ahmed et al. 2021). Clinicians soon began to realise that many of these comorbidities also make patients more at risk of pre-morbid dysphagia or developing dysphagia during an acute illness or hospitalisation, and with this realisation came research into dysphagia and COVID-19.

Miles and colleagues were invited by the journal *Dysphagia* to provide an overview of current evidence published in December 2021. The resulting paper offers a thorough review of the dysphagia trajectory in over 1,700 patients (Miles et al. 2021). Current evidence suggests that a third of patients hospitalised with COVID-19 will require dysphagia services (Printza et al. 2021; Miles et al. 2021; Dawson et al. 2020; Boggiano et al. 2021; Bordejé Laguna et al. 2021; Lagier et al. 2021; Lima et al. 2020; Regan et al. 2021; Wang et al. 2020; Webler et al. 2021), and our understanding of swallowing symptoms and trajectory of recovery is slowly building.

The huge numbers of confirmed cases of COVID-19 worldwide have allowed large cohort analysis of risk factors for the development of swallowing difficulties (Printza et al. 2021; Miles et al. 2021; Mohan and Mohapatra 2020). Table 9.1 lists risk factors reported in the literature for the development of dysphagia and/or poor functional swallowing outcomes. Premorbid comorbidities such as increased age and chronic neurological and respiratory conditions inherently predispose patients to swallowing difficulties and poorer swallowing outcomes.

**TABLE 9.1** Risk factors for dysphagia after COVID-19 (Printza et al. 2021; Miles et al. 2021; Can et al. 2021)

| *Risk factors for dysphagia after COVID-19* | |
| --- | --- |
| **Pre-admission factors** | Increased age |
| | Pre-admission dysphagia |
| | Pre-admission neurological conditions |
| | Pre-admission respiratory conditions including COPD and asthma |
| | Increased BMI |
| **Hospital factors** | New onset neurological symptoms |
| | Extracorporeal membrane oxygenation (ECMO) |
| | Acute respiratory distress syndrome (ARDS) |
| | Vasopressor treatment for septic shock |
| | Increased duration of intubation |
| | Tracheostomy insertion |
| | Prone ventilation |
| | Significant respiratory compromise |
| | Severe and long-lasting delirium |
| | Sarcopenia and general deconditioning due to prolonged intubation, long-term analgesics, neuromuscular locking agents, and sedation |
| | Laryngeal pathology caused by prolonged intubation |
| | Requirements for sedative medications |

These should be considered in screening for swallowing difficulties in acute care. Like many patient populations who are at risk of severe illness and require critical care, medical interventions such as intubation, tracheostomy, and ventilation can result in laryngeal injury and contribute to swallowing difficulties. Severe respiratory compromise offers challenges to respiratory-swallow coordination and comes with implications for airway safety and mealtime endurance. Prolonged illness and hospitalisation result in secondary problems such as delirium, sarcopenia, and general deconditioning resulting in cognitive-behavioural eating and drinking difficulties as well as fatigue and generalised weakness of the swallowing muscles. As risk factors increase for a patient, the chances of developing dysphagia and having persisting dysphagia that requires speech-language therapy (and potentially otolaryngology) interventions increases. Speech-language therapists need to be available in intensive care units (ICUs) as well as acute hospital wards to identify and manage patients recovering from COVID-19.

## 9.3 Acute care ICU

Laryngeal pathology is a well-known complication of prolonged intubation, and patients with COVID-19 are intubated for longer than non-COVID-19 patients admitted to ICU (Vasanthan et al. 2021; McGrath et al. 2020; Boggiano et al. 2021). The reader is referred to Chapter 8 regarding tracheostomised patients and Chapter 7 regarding management of voice disorders for further information on these topics. Laryngeal pathology has implications for dysphagia management particularly in terms of airway protection mechanisms. Table 9.2 lists common laryngeal pathologies reported after COVID-19 and their potential impact on eating and drinking.

Laryngeal pathologies appear to be more common in patients after COVID-19 in comparison to other ICU populations (Boggiano et al. 2021). It is still unknown whether this relates to neural injuries from the virus itself, the prolonged intubation times or perhaps some of the typical medical interventions required during a patient's ICU journey such as proning and high-pressure ventilation for those recovering from COVID-19. Since endoscopy was re-established in ICUs, a number of papers have described the pathologies present and their prevalence. Vocal cord movement disorders are common both bilateral and unilateral (Boggiano et al. 2021). Oedema, granulomas, ulcerations, and stenosis have been regularly reported. Sandblom and colleagues report on 25 patients with dysphagia and found 92% had pooled secretions, 44% had silent aspiration, 76% had vocal cord movement impairments, and 60% had laryngeal oedema (Sandblom et al. 2021). Figures 9.1 and 9.2 provide examples of laryngeal presentations and associated swallowing difficulties.

There is a clear need for FEES in treating patients with COVID-19 to identify and then treat laryngeal pathology alongside managing swallowing and voice complaints (Boggiano et al. 2021). Identification of and interventions for

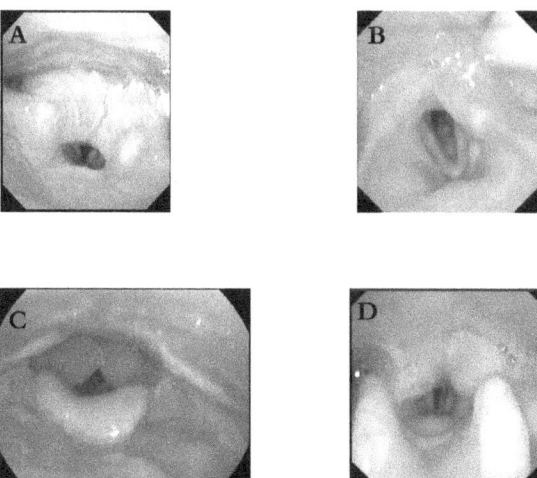

**FIGURE 9.1**    Laryngeal pathologies in patients with COVID-19 (A=severe oedema and severe sensory deficits leading to silent aspiration of saliva and bolus trials. Required to be nil-by-mouth for safety; B=generalised weakness and unilateral vocal cord immobility leading to aspiration on thin drinks; C=oedema leading to reduced holding capacity in pyriforms. Volume control and pacing required for safety; D=oedema and poor secretion clearance. Slow return to oral intake required with progressive oral trials)

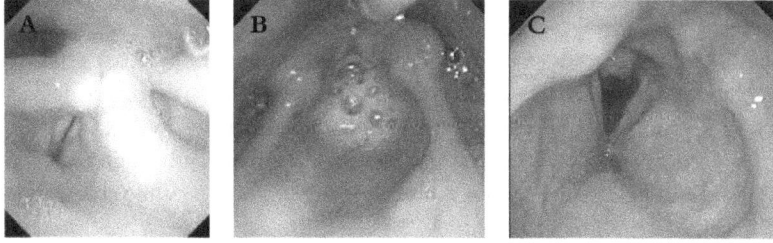

**FIGURE 9.2**    Laryngeal pathologies and associated swallowing difficulties in patients with COVID-19 (A=muscle tension and anxiety leading to persistent coughing with oral trials. After education following FEES, the patient was able to recommence oral intake; B=generalised weakness, poor respiratory function, and poor secretion clearance. Slow tracheostomy wean. Once able to tolerate cuff down, the patient was able to slowly increase oral intake. Strengthening exercises provided; C=granuloma affecting tracheostomy wean. Required surgical excision prior to tracheostomy decannulation and return to oral intake)

**TABLE 9.2** Common laryngeal pathologies after COVID-19 and their impact on swallowing function (Boggiano et al. 2021; Miles et al. 2021; Piazza et al. 2021; Printza et al. 2021)

| *Laryngeal pathologies* | *Effect on eating and drinking* |
|---|---|
| Granulation | Poor pharyngeal constriction |
| Cystic lesions | Reduced space for secretions and bolus in |
| Laryngeal webs |     vallecular and pyriform sinus |
| Stenosis | Impaired airway closure – multiple levels |
| Malacia | Impaired cough strength |
| Oedema | Impaired secretion clearance |
| Erythema | Airway obstruction/compromise affecting |
| Laryngitis |     swallow-respiratory coordination |
| Posterior glottic ulceration | Silent aspiration of secretions, food, drinks |
| Subglottic ulceration | Lack of awareness of pharyngeal residue/ |
| Vocal cord mobility impairment including |     secretion accumulation |
|     vocal cord paralysis | Odynophagia and/or globus leading to |
| Arytenoid collapse |     reluctance to eat |
| Pseudosulcus vocalis | Respiratory-swallow coordination |
| Pharyngo-laryngeal atrophy/weakness |     impairments |
| Sensory impairments | |

laryngeal pathology are critical for successful extubation and tracheostomy decannulation as well as swallowing management in terms of secretion clearance and airway protection. Both sensory and motor implications of laryngology pathology need to be considered in managing dysphagia in the ICU. Motor impairments of the vocal cords impair airway closure and can result in aspiration. Non-organic masses such as granulomas and ulcerations can affect airway closure and/or affect respiratory-swallowing coordination if they cause airway issues. Laryngeal and pharyngeal oedema can lead to reduced holding capacity in pyriforms for secretions and residue and affect swallow safety. Laryngeal and pharyngeal oedema also results in sensory alterations, affecting secretion clearance, swallowing motor-sensory feedback loops, spontaneous clearance of residue, and cough responsiveness. Without FEES, these aspects of swallowing difficulties cannot be identified and managed appropriately.

## 9.4 Dysphagia recovery

Reassuringly, many studies report high recovery rates of swallowing function during hospitalisation. Dawson et al. (2020) found the majority of their 208 patients referred to speech-language therapy subsequently regained near normal swallow function prior to discharge, regardless of intubation duration or tracheostomy status (Dawson et al. 2020). Miles and colleagues reported over 90% of patients had returned to a normal diet by discharge across a number of UK hospital sites (Miles et al. 2021; Dawson et al. 2020), with patients who required a tracheostomy having longer on texture-modified diets than those without a tracheostomy (Dawson et al. 2020). Webler and colleagues in the US offer a closer observation of 40 patients admitted to an inpatient rehabilitation ward and referred to videofluoroscopy. Eighty-five percent of patients had been intubated and five had suffered a stroke alongside their COVID-19 diagnosis. Thirty percent of patients had a penetration-aspiration scale score of 6+ (27% silently aspirated), and with every additional day of intubation, there was a 15% greater likelihood of airway invasion (Webler et al. 2021). Interestingly, the authors compared the Mann Assessment of Swallowing Ability (MASA) clinical swallowing evaluation total score and likelihood of aspiration ratio with presence of aspiration during videofluoroscopy and found that the clinical swallowing evaluation was a poor predictor of aspiration. This is likely due to high silent aspiration rates and again adds to the evidence that instrumental assessment is needed in the management of patients after COVID-19 wherever possible.

Despite this trend towards return-to-normal diet at discharge, there is interestingly ongoing self-reports of dysphagia in outpatient clinics. In mixed cohorts of intubated and non-intubated patients, persisting self-reported dysphagia in those referred to outpatient appointments is reported at ~30% (Neevel et al. 2021; Naunheim et al. 2020; Rouhani et al. 2020). Grilli and colleagues in Germany followed 41 non-intubated hospitalised patients for six months. Eight presented with swallowing difficulties at admission (assessed using the Volume-Viscosity Swallow Test (VVST) and Swallowing Disturbance Questionnaire), with only two reporting persisting problems at six months (Grilli et al. 2021). Martin-Martinez and colleagues in Spain conducted a similar study and followed up 205 patients admitted to general wards in the spring wave of 2020. At admission, 52% of patients had swallowing difficulties and 46% developed malnutrition (using Volume-Viscosity Swallowing Test and NRS2002 Nutrition Screen). At six months, 23% still had swallowing difficulties and 7% had malnutrition, with oropharyngeal dysphagia an independent risk factor for survival (Martin – Martinez et al. 2021).

Across 11 hospitals in Ireland, a similar pattern is reported. A third of ICU patients referred to speech-language therapy with swallowing difficulties required rehabilitation for their swallowing prior to discharge (Regan et al. 2021). Importantly, 27% continued to have swallowing difficulties on hospital discharge, indicating that for those who do develop significant dysphagia as part of their COVID-19 sequalae, outpatient as well as inpatient services may be required to support rehabilitation. This combined data suggests that intensive therapy is required for those with persisting dysphagia in order to achieve successful outcomes. With oropharyngeal dysphagia associated with comorbidities, neurological symptoms, and poor function (Martin – Martinez et al. 2021; Langton-Frost and Brodsky 2021) and the additional associated symptoms of COVID-19, these patients are complex to treat. Premorbid swallowing difficulties and neurological and/or respiratory conditions in addition to COVID-19 recovery is challenging. Generalised deconditioning, fatigue, depression, and anxiety need consideration. The additional effects of reduced taste, smell, appetite, and gastrointestinal

**TABLE 9.3** Considerations and barriers to rehabilitation of swallowing difficulties after COVID-19

| Considerations/Barriers | Strategies |
| --- | --- |
| Fatigue | Short, regular sessions throughout the day |
| Reduced exercise tolerance | Incorporating swallow exercises into physical therapy sessions |
| | Timing dysphagia treatments before physical therapies |
| | Generalised strengthening programmes to build endurance |
| Generalised weakness affecting ability to perform swallow exercises | Short, regular sessions throughout the day |
| | Slow progressive exercise programmes |
| | Generalised strengthening programmes to build endurance, including direct and indirect swallow exercises, EMST, and progressive oral trials |
| | Selecting swallow exercises with reduced trunk/neck muscle requirements. For example, some patients have struggled with Shaker head lift |
| Co-existing premorbid or new-onset cognitive and communication impairments | Supported communication strategies |
| | Use of easy to read/pictographic written exercise programmes |
| | Use of therapy assistants to support adherence of therapy |
| Reduced taste/smell/ appetite | Working with dietitian to find motivating, safe food options |
| | Exploring temperature, carbonation, and texture for enhanced enjoyment |
| | Focus on visual appeal |
| | Enhancing mealtime enjoyment with other patients and family/friends where infection control procedures allow (including via video call) |
| Gastrointestinal dysfunction | Close collaboration with dietitian and gastroenterology |
| Respiratory-swallow coordination impairments/ breathlessness/respiratory instability | Frequent monitoring of vital signs and oxygen saturation |
| | Pacing and adjusting volume |
| | Optimising respiratory rehabilitation and cough strength |
| | Timing meals to avoid times of greater fatigue |
| | Respiratory-swallow coordination training |
| | Avoiding airway protection strategies that exacerbate breathlessness. For example, some patients have struggled with supraglottic swallow/super supraglottic swallow |
| Anxiety | Psychology input |
| Depression/low motivation | Relaxation and mindfulness techniques |
| | Cognitive-behavioural therapies/psychotherapies |
| | Setting small goals with focus on positive gains rather than areas for improvement |
| | Adherence charts |
| | Patient-led goals and choice/empowerment |

| Considerations/Barriers | Strategies |
|---|---|
| Isolation from clinicians/ family/friends secondary to infection control restrictions | Finding connections/building rapport despite physical distancing |
| | Once COVID negative and medically stable, conduct therapy outside of ward for increased opportunity for socialisation |
| | Group therapy |
| | Psychology input |
| | iPads for family connection |
| Restrictions of physical distancing/PPE | Rehabilitation with family present via video link |
| | Recording exercise demonstrations (without PPE on) to send to patient's phones for exercises that require visual demonstrations |

dysfunction all hinder progress. Multidisciplinary teamwork is critical, and dysphagia teams need to regularly brainstorm solutions to rehabilitation barriers. Table 9.3 provides a list of considerations and barriers to rehabilitation and possible solutions.

## 9.5 Outpatient presentations and long COVID

Our understanding of Long COVID (defined as prolonged symptoms beyond 28 days) is now building (Ladds et al. 2020). We now see that Long COVID does not always follow severe illness and even those with a mild initial illness may have more symptoms post-COVID-19 (Groff et al. 2021). The trajectory of post-COVID-19 symptoms can be unpredictable, with improving symptoms, progressive symptoms, new symptoms, and relapsing/remitting symptoms all possible (Nalbandian et al. 2021; Groff et al. 2021). Common symptoms that have an impact on eating and drinking include fatigue, muscle weakness, cough, dyspnea, anxiety, depression, and cognitive disturbances (Nalbandian et al. 2021; Groff et al. 2021). The neurological consequences of COVID-19 are also relevant to swallowing function, with many symptoms reported: neuroinflammation; loss of consciousness/cognition; haemorrhages; meningitis/meningeal irritation; hypoxia; cerebrovascular disease; encephalitis; neuromuscular agitation; and dysexecutive syndrome (Jarrahi et al. 2020). All these have implications for dysphagia care and need to be considered in assessment and treatment planning.

In relation to swallowing, Davis and colleagues surveyed 3,762 patients after COVID-19 across 56 countries. More than 91% of patients reported that time to recover exceeded 35 weeks, with ~100% reporting fatigue, over 30% reporting lump in throat/difficulties swallowing and ~30% reporting changes in voice

(Davis et al. 2021). In addition to the swallowing difficulties, 85% reported gastrointestinal issues and ~60% reported persistent taste/smell symptoms. Relapsing-remitting symptom trajectories were common. Neevel and colleagues report that "[p]atients may develop significant voice, airway, and/or swallowing issues post-acute COVID-19. These complications are not limited to patients requiring intubation or tracheostomy. Multidisciplinary laryngology clinics will continue to play an integral role in diagnosing and treating patients with COVID-19–related laryngeal sequelae." (Neevel et al. 2021, p. 1)

This early data on outpatient presentations is critical in view of the high numbers of people who have survived COVID-19 worldwide. With a reasonable proportion of people recovering from COVID-19 potentially suffering from swallowing difficulties or associated upper and middle airway disorders and voice disorders, speech-language therapy services are critical. In Table 9.4, some of the swallowing and swallowing-associated presentations reported by clinicians internationally are presented, with the likely effects on eating and drinking listed. Speech-language therapists and dysphagia teams/outpatient teams will need to be ready to receive discharged patients still recovering from long inpatient stays with deconditioning and residual laryngology pathologies from their ICU stays. They also need to be ready to accept new referrals for non-hospitalised outpatients with continuing abnormal respiratory patterns, muscle tension, hypersensitive larynx syndrome and globus, and viral vocal cord mobility disorders. Those more vulnerable due to age or pre-existing comorbidities will be most at risk and most complex to rehabilitate. Swallowing disorders will need to be managed alongside

TABLE 9.4 Outpatient presentations after COVID-19 and their impact on swallowing function (Printza et al. 2021; Piazza et al. 2021; McGrath et al. 2020; Miles et al. 2021; Boggiano et al. 2021; Meng and Yuandan 2021)

| Outpatient presentations | Effect on swallowing safety, efficiency, and mealtime enjoyment |
| --- | --- |
| Continuing abnormal respiratory patterns | Respiratory-swallow coordination |
| Globus | impairments |
| Muscle tension dysphonia | Poor nutritional intake/malnutrition |
| Chronic cough | Psychogenic dysphagia/fear of swallowing |
| Hypersensitive larynx syndrome | Airway compromise |
| Vocal cord mobility impairment including vocal cord paralysis | Risk of aspiration and aspiration pneumonia Choking risk |
| Reduced smell | Reluctance to eat |
| Reduced texture | Mealtime fatigue with poor mealtime |
| Fatigue | endurance: |
| Poor appetite | – leading to reduced intake |
| Gastrointestinal issues | – increased weakness and therefore residue |
| Mood disorders and anxiety | as meal progresses |
| Socioeconomic impact if unable to work | – reduced swallow safety as meal progresses |

the other physical, mental, and psychosocial implications of Long COVID as well as the burden of living in a pandemic.

## 9.6 Future directions

Whilst we appear to have learnt a huge amount about swallowing difficulties in this complex disease over the past two years, there is still much to learn as the pandemic continues. Much of our data is on unvaccinated people in 2020 when intensive care teams were only just understanding how to manage acute COVID-19. As 2021 comes to an end, we now have some countries with extremely high vaccination rates, and we have new treatments on the horizon which are looking promising. In contrast, we also have the looming anxiety of new variants and how the vaccines will protect against each new variant as it emerges. We do not know what the impact of vaccines and treatments will be on severity of dysphagia. It is highly likely that vaccine protection against severe disease and new pharmaceutical treatments may reduce ICU stays and in turn reduce the number of patients suffering ICU-related swallowing sequelae. The likely pattern in Long COVID-related swallowing difficulties and associated upper and middle airway disorders and voice disorders is less certain.

The pathophysiology of COVID-related dysphagia symptoms is still unknown. The extent that COVID-specific neurological impairments contribute to swallowing difficulties is unknown in comparison to generalised weakness from recovery. Langton-Frost and Brodsky provide an interesting reflection on neuroplasticity and its role in dysphagia rehabilitation after COVID-19. They encourage early and frequent swallowing interventions to capitalise on neuroplasticity (Langton-Frost and Brodsky 2021). Vergara and colleagues reflect on our lack of understanding of olfactory and gustatory alterations and pharyngolaryngeal sensation and how this affects swallowing function (Vergara et al. 2021). They describe the need for new approaches to sensory system examination in patients with COVID-19 and new approaches in therapeutic sensory stimulation. Extrapolating peripheral viral recurrent laryngeal nerve injuries from ICU-related laryngeal injuries is difficult, and so we will not understand this fully until more non-hospitalised endoscopic data is collected.

From a dysphagia team perspective, COVID-19 has highlighted the role of the speech-language therapist in ICU, and this will hopefully lead to better resourcing of speech-language therapists in ICU in the future. PPE in the presence of droplet and airborne diseases is probably going to be permanent for all those working in dysphagia care. Speech-language therapists need to continue to work with the best assessment tools available to us and use our knowledge across all our population groups (neurological, ICU, respiratory, aged care, trauma) and our best clinical reasoning to continue to provide flexible and innovative clinical support to patients with dysphagia in the future. Everything that we have learnt prepares us for the next virus and develops our understanding of dysphagia in severe illness and across all the patient populations that we serve.

## 9.7 Summary

In this chapter, I have described our current understanding of the types of swallowing problems seen in patients with COVID-19 and the possible causes of each symptom. Swallowing difficulties are most definitely multifactorial in nature and are related to comorbidities that predispose patients to developing dysphagia, the SARS-CoV-2 virus itself, and the medical interventions required to treat COVID-19. From a dysphagia team perspective, COVID-19 has highlighted the role of the speech-language therapist in ICU, and this will hopefully lead to better resourcing of speech-language therapists in ICU in the future. PPE in the presence of droplet and airborne diseases is probably going to be permanent for all those working in dysphagia care. Speech-language therapists need to continue to work with the best assessment tools available to us and use our knowledge across all our population groups (neurological, ICU, respiratory, aged care, trauma) and our best clinical reasoning to continue to provide flexible and innovative clinical support to patients with dysphagia in the future. Everything that we have learnt prepares us for the next virus and develops our understanding of dysphagia in severe illness and across all the patient populations that we serve.

## Acknowledgements

Thank you to all the clinicians who have worked throughout the pandemic and shared their experiences to support all those working with patients with dysphagia after COVID-19.

## References

Ahmed, Y., Cao, A., Thal, A., Shah, S., Kinkhabwala, C., Liao, D., et al. (2021). Tracheotomy outcomes in 64 ventilated COVID-19 patients at a high-volume center in Bronx, NY. *Laryngoscope*, 131(6), e1797–e1804. doi:10.1002/lary.29391.

Boggiano, S., Williams, T., Gill, S. E., Alexander, P. D. G., Khwaja, S., Wallace, S., et al. (2021). Multidisciplinary management of laryngeal pathology identified in patients with COVID-19 following trans-laryngeal intubation and tracheostomy. *Journal of the Intensive Care* Society. doi:10.1177/17511437211034699.

Bolton, L., Mills, C., Wallace, S., & Brady, M. C. (2020). Aerosol generating procedures, dysphagia assessment and COVID-19: A rapid review. *International Journal of Language & Communication Disorders*, 55(44), 629–636.

Bordejé Laguna, L., Marcos-Neira, P., de Lagrán Zurbano, I. M., Marco, E. M., Guisasola, C. P., Viñas Soria, C. D., et al. (2021). Dysphagia and mechanical ventilation in SARS-COV-2 pneumonia: It's real. *Clinical Nutrition*, S0261–5614(21)00527–6. https://doi.org/10.1016/j.clnu.2021.11.018.

Can, B., İsmagulova, N., Enver, N., Tufan, A., & Cinel, İ. (2021). Sarcopenic dysphagia following COVID-19 infection: A new danger. *Nutrition in Clinical Practice*, 36(4), 828–832.

Davis, H. E., Assaf, G. S., McCorkell, L., Wei, H., Low, R. J., Re'em, Y., et al. (2021). Characterizing Long COVID in an international cohort: 7 months of symptoms and their impact. *MedRexIv*, 38. doi:10.1016/j.eclinm.2021.101019.

Dawson, C., Capewell, R., Ellis, S., Matthews, S., Adamson, S., Wood, M., et al. (2020). Dysphagia presentation and management following coronavirus disease 2019: An acute care tertiary Centre experience. *The Journal of Laryngology & Otology*, 134(11), 981–986.

Freeman-Sanderson, A., Ward, E. C., Miles, A., de Pedro Netto, I., Duncan, S., Inamoto, Y., et al. (2021). A consensus statement for the management and rehabilitation of communication and swallowing function in the ICU: A global response to COVID-19. *Archives of Physical Medicine and Rehabilitation*,102(5), 835–842.

Fritz, M. A., Howell, R. J., Brodsky, M. B., Suiter, D. M., Dhar, S. I., Rameau, A., et al. (2021). Moving forward with dysphagia care: Implementing strategies during the COVID-19 pandemic and beyond. *Dysphagia*, 36(2), 161–169.

Goldman, A. R., Parade, J. K., Langton-Frost, N. A., Hodges, C. A., Taylor, A. M., Bova, G., et al. (2021). Adapting the modified barium swallow: Modifications to improve safety in the setting of airborne respiratory illnesses like COVID-19. *Abdominal Radiology*, 46(7), 3058–3065.

Grasselli, G., Zangrillo, A., & Zanella, A. (2021). Baseline characteristics and outcomes of 1591 patients infected with SARS-CoV-2 admitted to ICUs of the Lombardy Region, Italy. *JAMA*, 323(16), 1574–1581.

Grilli, G. M., Giancaspro, R., Del Colle, A., Quarato, C. M. I., Lacedonia, D., Foschino Barbaro, M. P., et al. (2021). Dysphagia in non-intubated patients affected by COVID-19 infection. *European Archives of Otorhinolaryngology*. https://doi.org/10.1007/s00405-021-07062-3.

Groff, D., Sun, A., & Ssentongo, A. E. (2021). Short-term and long-term rates of post-acute sequelae of SARS-CoV-2 infection: A systematic review. *JAMA Netw Open*, 4(10), e2128568. doi:10.1001/jamanetworkopen.2021.28568.

Guan, W., Ni, Z., & Hu, Y. (2020). Clinical characteristics of coronavirus disease 2019 in China. *New England Journal of Medicine*, 382(18), 1708–1720.

Hamilton, F., Arnold, D., Bzdek, B. R., Dodd, J., Reid, J., & Maskell, N. (2021). Aerosol generating procedures: Are they of relevance for transmission of SARS-CoV-2? *The Lancet Respiratory Medicine*, 9(7), 687–689.

Jarrahi, A., Ahluwalia, M., & Khodadadi, H. (2020). Neurological consequences of COVID-19: What have we learned and where do we go from here? *Journal of Neuroinflammation*, 17(1), 286. doi:10.1186/s12974-020-01957-4.

Ku, P., Holsinger, F. C., Chan, J., Yeung, Z., Chan, B., Tong, M., et al. (2020). Management of dysphagia in the patient with head and neck cancer during COVID-19 pandemic: Practical strategy. *Journal of the Sciences and Specialities of the Head and Neck*, 42(7), 1491–1496.

Ladds, E., Rushford, A., & Wieringa, S. (2020). Persistent symptoms after Covid-19: Qualitative study of 114 "long Covid" patients and draft quality principles for services. *BMC Health Services Research*, 20(1), 1144. doi:10.1186/s12913-020-06001-y.

Lagier, A., Melotte, E., Poncelet, M., Remacle, S., & Meunier, P. (2021). Swallowing function after severe COVID-19: Early videofluoroscopic findings. *European Archives of Oto-Rhino-Laryngology*, 278(8), 3119–3123.

Langton-Frost, N., & Brodsky, M. B. (2021). Speech-language pathology approaches to neurorehabilitation in acute care during COVID-19: Capitalizing on neuroplasticity. *PM&R*. doi:10.1002/pmrj.12717.

Lima, M. S., Sassi, F. C., Medeiros, G. C., Ritto, A. P., & Andrade, C. (2020). Preliminary results of a clinical study to evaluate the performance and safety of swallowing in critical patients with COVID-19. *Clinics (Sao Paulo)*, 75, e2021. doi:10.6061/clinics/2020/e2021.

Malandraki, G. A., Arkenberg, R. H., Mitchell, S. S., & Malandraki, J. B. (2021). Telehealth for dysphagia across the life span: Using contemporary evidence and expertise to guide clinical practice during and after COVID-19. *American Journal of Speech-Language Pathology*, 30(2), 532–550.

Martin-Martinez, A., Ortega, O., Viñas, P., Arreola, V., Nascimento, W., Costa, A., et al. (2021). COVID-19 is associated with oropharyngeal dysphagia and malnutrition in hospitalized patients during the spring 2020 wave of the pandemic. *Clinical Nutrition*, S0261–5614(21)00297–1. doi:10.1016/j.clnu.2021.06.010.

McGrath, B. A., Wallace, S., & Goswamy, J. (2020). Laryngeal oedema associated with COVID-19 complicating airway management. *Anaesthesia*, 75(7), 972. doi:10.1111/anae.15092.

Meng, X., & Yuandan, P. (2021). COVID-19 and anosmia: The story so far. *Ear, Nose, & Throat Journal*. doi:10.1177/01455613211048998.

Miles, A., Connor, N. P., Desia, R., Jadcherla, S., Allen, J., Brodsky, M., et al. (2021). Dysphagia care across the continuum: A multidisciplinary Dysphagia Research Society taskforce report of service-delivery during the COVID-19 global pandemic. *Dysphagia*, 36(2), 170–182.

Miles, A., McRae, J., Clunie, G., Gillivan-Murphy, P., Inamoto, Y., Kalf, H., et al. (2022). An international commentary on dysphagia and dysphonia during the COVID-19 pandemic. *Dysphagia*. doi:10.1007/s00455-021-10396-z.

Mohan, R., & Mohapatra, B. (2020). Shedding light on dysphagia associated with COVID-19: The what and why. *OTO Open*, 4(2), 2473974X20934770. doi:10.1177/2473974X20934770.

Nalbandian, A., Sehgal, K., & Gupta, A. (2021). Post-acute COVID-19 syndrome. *Nature Medicine*, 27(4), 601–615.

Naunheim, M. R., Zhou, A. S., Puka, E., Franco, R. A., Carroll, T. L., Teng, et al. (2020). Laryngeal complications of COVID-19. *Laryngoscope Investigative Otolaryngology*, 5(6), 1117–1124.

Neevel, A. J., Smith, J. D., Morrison, R. J., Hogikyan, N. D., Kupfer, R. A., & Stein, A. P. (2021). Postacute COVID-19 laryngeal injury and dysfunction. *OTO Open*, 5(3), 2473974X211041040. doi:10.1177/2473974X211041040.

Piazza, C., Filauro, M., Dikkers, F. G., Nouraei, S., Sandu, K., Sittel, C., et al. (2021). Long-term intubation and high rate of tracheostomy in COVID-19 patients might determine an unprecedented increase of airway stenoses: A call to action from the European laryngological society. *European Archives of Oto-Rhino-Laryngology*, 278(1), 1–7.

Printza, A., Tedla, M., Frajkova, Z., Sapalidis, K., & Triaridis, S. (2021). Dysphagia severity and management in patients with COVID-19. *Current Health Sciences Journal*, 47(2), 147–156.

Regan, J., Walshe, M., & Lavan, S. (2021). Post-extubation dysphagia and dysphonia amongst adults with COVID-19 in the Republic of Ireland: A prospective multi-site observational cohort study. *Clinical Otolaryngology*, 46(6), 1290–1299.

Richardson, S., Hirsch, J. S., Narasimhan, M., Crawford, J. M., McGinn, T., Davidson, K. W., et al. (2020). Presenting characteristics, comorbidities, and outcomes among 5700 patients hospitalized with COVID-19 in the New York City area. *JAMA*, 323(20), 2052–2059.

Rouhani, M. J., Clunie, G., Thong, G., Lovell, L., Roe, J., Ashcroft, M., et al. (2020). Prospective study of voice, swallow, and airway outcomes following tracheostomy for COVID-19. *Laryngoscope*, 131(6), e1918–e1925. doi:10.1002/lary.29346.

Rouse, R., & Regan, J. (2021). Psychological impact of COVID-19 on speech and language therapists working with adult dysphagia: A national survey. *International Journal of Language & Communication Disorders*, 56(5), 1037–1052.

Sandblom, O. H., Dotevall, H., Svennerholm, K., Tuomi, L., & Finizia, C. (2021). Characterization of dysphagia and laryngeal findings in COVID-19 patients treated in the ICU-An observational clinical study. *PLoS One*, 16(6), e0252347. doi:10.1371/journal.pone.0252347.

Tian, S., Hu, N., & Lou, J. (2020). Characteristics of COVID-19 infection in Beijing. *The Journal of Infection*, 80(4), 401–406.

Vasanthan, R., Sorooshian, P., Sri Shanmuganathan, V., & Al-Hashim, M. (2021). Laryngotracheal stenosis following intubation and tracheostomy for COVID-19 pneumonia: A case report. *Journal of Surgical Case Reports*, 2021(1), rjaa569. doi:10.1093/jscr/rjaa569.

Vergara, J., Lirani-Silva, C., Brodsky, M. B., Miles, A., Clavé, P., Nascimento, W., et al. (2021). Potential influence of olfactory, gustatory, and pharyngolaryngeal sensory dysfunctions on swallowing physiology in COVID-19. *Otolaryngology-Head and Neck Surgery*, 164(6), 1134–1135.

Vergara, J., Skoretz, S. A., Brodsky, M. B., Miles, A., Langmore, S. E., Wallace, S., et al. (2020). Assessment, diagnosis, and treatment of dysphagia in patients infected with SARS-CoV-2: A review of the literature and international guidelines. *American Journal of Speech-Language Pathology*, 29(4), 2242–2253.

Wang, D., Hu, B., Hu, C., Zhu, F., Liu, X., Zhang, J., et al. (2020). Clinical characteristics of 138 hospitalized patients with 2019 novel coronavirus-infected pneumonia in Wuhan, China. *JAMA*, 323(11), 1061–1069.

Webler, K., Carpenter, J., Hamilton, V., Rafferty, M., & Cherney, L. R. (2021). Dysphagia characteristics of patients post SARS-CoV-2 during inpatient rehabilitation. *Archives of Physical Medicine and Rehabilitation*, S0003–9993(21)01517–3. doi:10.1016/j.apmr.2021.10.007.

Yang, W., Cao, Q., & Qin, L. (2020). Clinical characteristics and imaging manifestations of the 2019 novel coronavirus disease (COVID-19): A multi-center study in Wenzhou city, Zhejiang, China. *Journal of Infection*, 8(4), 388–393.

Zhou, F., Yu, T., Du, R., Fan, G., Liu, Y., Liu, Z., et al. (2020). Clinical course and risk factors for mortality of adult inpatients with COVID-19 in Wuhan, China: A retrospective cohort study. *Lancet*, 28(395), 1054–1062.

# 10

# TELEPRACTICE IN ADULT SPEECH-LANGUAGE PATHOLOGY DURING COVID-19

*Elizabeth C. Ward and Ashley E. Cameron*

## 10.1 Introduction

The day of 11 March 2020 saw the world hit by a global pandemic of unimaginable proportions, and humanity was profoundly affected at every level from the individual to the collective. Coronavirus 2 (SARS-CoV-2), the virus that causes COVID-19, shook the foundations on which life had been built. In the fight to contain the virus, organisations and individuals were required to rapidly adapt usual processes to maintain safety, meet evolving demands, and manage widespread uncertainty. Almost overnight, speech-language pathology (SLP), alongside many other professions, was forced to re-evaluate how to provide services and maintain continuity of care whilst meeting social distancing and isolation measures. A key part of these service adaptations was the uptake and more widespread use of telepractice within the SLP profession. As a result of these unprecedented times, a new healthcare landscape has emerged, with the use of telepractice becoming a pragmatic option for SLPs to support the delivery of patient care and connect health professionals.

## 10.2 What is telepractice?

Telepractice is a versatile service delivery model. It facilitates the management of numerous conditions, enables easy access to expert support, and empowers patients to self-manage their health using various telecommunication technologies (e.g., video, telephone, email, messaging, web-based services). The application of telepractice in adult SLP practice is broad. It can be employed across a wide range of settings such as hospitals, outpatient clinics, residential aged care facilities, community settings, private practice, and home environments. It also

DOI: 10.4324/9781003257318-10

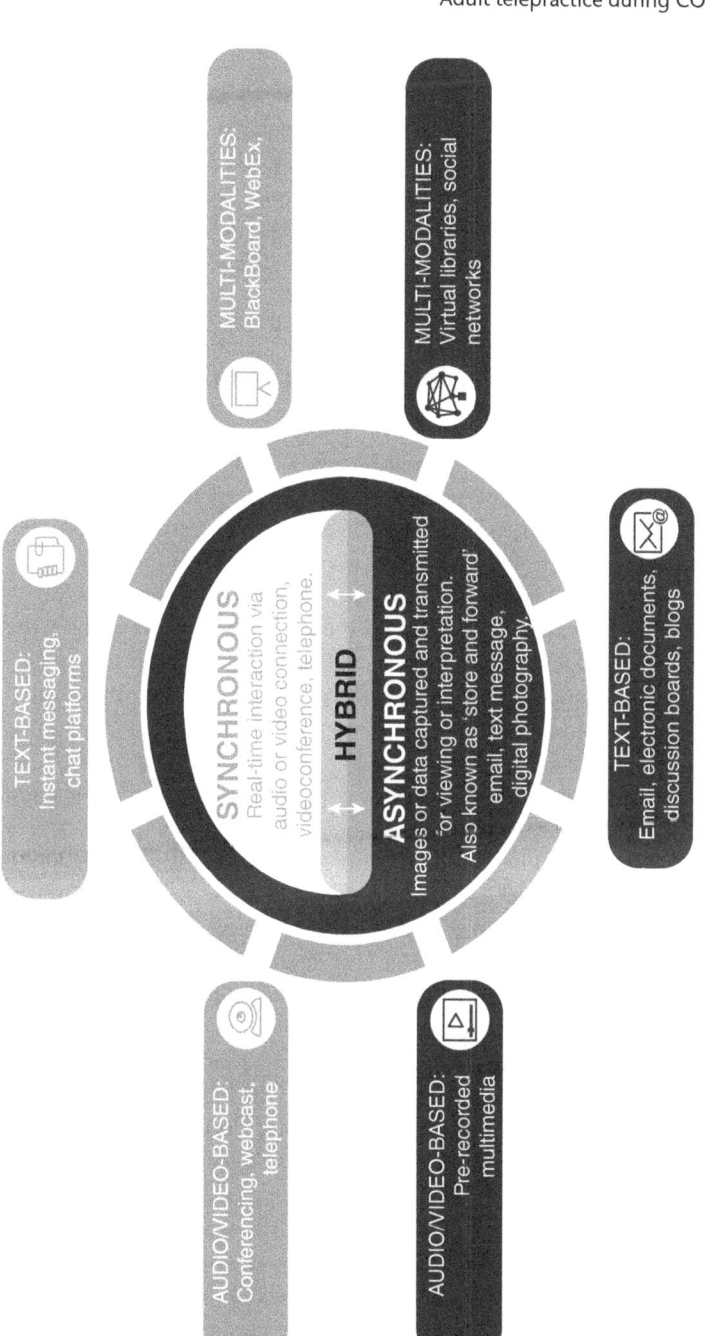

**FIGURE 10.1**   Telepractice modes of delivery

can be used for most clinical and administrative tasks including evaluations, interventions, group sessions, consultations, education, monitoring, supervision, meetings, and multidisciplinary management. Although the term "telepractice" is most commonly associated with videoconferencing, it is critical to acknowledge that there is no single method of delivering telepractice services, with synchronous (live interaction), asynchronous (store and forward), or hybrid methods (including virtual and in-person) providing multiple solutions for service delivery across different clinical contexts (Figure 10.1).

## 10.3 Telepractice in SLP: considerations prior to and since COVID-19

Like many clinical areas, there was a small but growing body of evidence supporting telepractice within the SLP profession prior to the pandemic. Across that body of work, there is evidence to support telepractice as a feasible, clinically sound, and cost-effective means of delivering personalised care to patients across many different clinical populations and practice settings (e.g., Burns et al. 2019; Fisk et al. 2020; Ward et al. 2021). Yet despite the evidence compiled over the decade prior to the pandemic, the majority of SLP services continued to be delivered in person, with telepractice options reserved mainly for remote and isolated patients, groups, or communities.

Barriers to the uptake of telepractice established prior to the pandemic are well documented in the literature and include negative clinician perceptions and attitudes, operational barriers, and lack of training, along with the perception of a lack of available evidence (Fisk et al. 2020; Miles et al. 2020; Ward et al. 2021). In addition, it is recognised that establishing telepractice services adds a layer of inherent complexity that takes time to master (Ben-Aharon 2019; Malandraki et al. 2021; Weidner and Lowman 2020). Developing tele-based services can also be costly and challenging due to the equipment and infrastructure required, ongoing technical support, licensure, funding, reimbursement, and policies.

Many of these barriers remain. However, during the pandemic, such barriers had to be addressed as services were faced with a limited set of options – from ceasing services altogether, providing only limited services with high levels of personal protective equipment (PPE), or utilising telepractice. The global demand for telepractice as a pandemic care solution forced many practice owners, services, and organisations to finally invest in the infrastructure and equipment needed to support telepractice, providing many clinicians with the capacity to deliver telepractice for the very first time. Equally, governments in many countries reviewed and incentivised funding for telepractice, allowing reimbursements that were not previously available. Then for many clinicians, this period of "forced adoption" also provided them with their first experience of telepractice and an opportunity to see the potential of this service model. Organisations and professional associations also actively developed, curated, and distributed practice guidelines and key resources and delivered webinars to support clinicians in operationalising telepractice and complying with mandated regulations (e.g., Royal College of Speech and Language Therapists 2021; Speech Pathology Australia 2021). As such, key barriers were lifted for the first time for many clinicians, and the opportunities to develop telepractice services became an actual reality.

However, it is acknowledged that with a lack of time to prepare for service redesign, there were many instances where the adoption of telepractice was made reactively, without the benefit of training, prior experience, awareness of best-care delivery standards, or adequate time to prepare a detailed approach for implementation. Whilst this is not ideal and is recognised as contributing to some negative/less than ideal experiences, there have also been positive outcomes. Many services are now offering a range of telepractice services, and more opportunities are now available for clinicians to develop sustainable telepractice models that meet the ongoing needs of their caseload, not only supporting the care needs of patients during the pandemic.

It must be recognised, though, that the use of telepractice as the "only" care solution offered to many patients during the pandemic is not an ideal situation. Telepractice should never be offered as the "only" option. Rather, it should be offered as part of an integrated care model where both in-person and telepractice options are available for the patient depending on their preference and the nature of the services they need to receive. It is also important that we acknowledge the many benefits of telepractice for patients and services and not view telepractice purely as a pandemic management solution. Telepractice is more than a model of care for infection control. Although it has served this purpose well, it has always been a model used to overcome many other important challenges – such as distance, provider shortages, government mandates, mobility constraints, and practical barriers (e.g., travel, time away from work, childcare, appointments, social distancing, isolation measures). It also enables access to expertise, coordinated scheduling, the opportunity to "check in" with patients, and the capability to engage patients within familiar environments. As such, it needs to be viewed as an integral part of ongoing SLP service delivery.

It is also critical to ensure that any telepractice services established meet key professional standards. A number of SLP organisations worldwide stipulate that the quality of service delivered via telepractice must be equivalent to in-person services with no discernible distinction between the two modalities (e.g., American Speech-Language-Hearing Association 2021; Royal College of Speech and Language Therapists 2021). For example, Speech Pathology Australia's telepractice position statement concludes, "It is critical that the outcomes from speech pathology services using telepractice are at least comparable to current clinical care" (Speech Pathology Australia 2014, p. 7). To achieve this, it is important to recognise that telepractice involves more than simply delivering services as you would in person. It is also much more than just learning to use technology. It is a service model that requires careful planning across multiple domains and clarity regarding *how best* to use technology to support the task at hand.

Key principles of developing effective telepractice services have been discussed in detail within the literature. These should be adhered to when developing any new telepractice service. These include consideration of (1) patient suitability and eligibility; (2) the development of a detailed service plan; (3) preparation and training of both staff and patients; (4) consideration of appropriate technology, equipment, and infrastructure; (5) clear identification of roles and responsibilities; (6) appropriate documentation; (7) adherence to ethical legal and local policy; and (8) ongoing service monitoring (Galpin et al. 2021; Riegler 2021). In a recently published study, the experiences of 16 allied health departments (including four SLP departments) from a hospital network in Australia were examined and used to create a framework to guide telehealth service implementation and sustainability (Thomas et al. 2022). Developed by exploring the experiences of 80 allied health clinicians, managers and administration staff involved in telepractice services during the first wave of the pandemic, the framework provides valuable insights into the factors that must be considered when establishing and sustaining quality telepractice services.

## 10.4  Changing drivers for telepractice within SLP

Pre-pandemic the primary driver for the use of telepractice was to help overcome the challenges of distance and improve service access. However, it is noteworthy that in the COVID-19 context, telepractice was used to *create distance* rather than overcome it. Creating a safe distance between the clinician and patient became a key aspect of service redesign, as services became more aware of the risks of aerosol generating procedures (AGPs), the need to protect vulnerable populations, and significant patient and clinician concerns regarding exposure/infection risk. As such, telepractice suddenly became a service delivery model needed by most SLP services, not only those serving rural and remote populations.

It rapidly became evident that COVID-19 was a highly communicable virus spread through airborne transmission and as a result, minimising the risks associated with AGPs became a key driver for telepractice. AGPs are usually medical or dental procedures that produce a large aerosolisation volume, contributing to viral transmission (Chacon et al. 2021). According to preliminary research, there is a high viral load of SARS-CoV-2 in the oropharynx and nasopharynx (Chacon et al. 2021). Consequently, there was much discussion regarding the classification of SLP tasks and aerosolisation-causing behaviours. In the intervening months following March 2020, AGP recommendations had a significant impact on SLP services (e.g., Bolton et al. 2020; Freeman-Sanderson et al. 2020). AGP concerns led to considerable disruptions to the in-person care for patients with a tracheostomy or a laryngectomy and the assessment and management of patients for voice, swallowing, and communication. This included disruptions to assessment processes (e.g., videofluoroscopy and endoscopic evaluations) and key aspects of SLP management such as oral cares, triggering vegetative reflexes (e.g., reflexive or voluntary cough), and conducting performance tasks (Araújo et al. 2020; McGrath et al. 2020; Miles et al. 2020). A lack of consensus and limited research explicitly investigating the aerosolisation of procedures and activities performed by SLPs caused widespread hesitation in the profession. Immediate concerns for clinician and patient safety led to many services being cancelled or, in urgent cases, being conducted under rigorous infection prevention and control measures (Chacon et al. 2021; Fritz et al. 2020). However, stopping services or limiting services to the prioritised few was not a sustainable solution. Encouragingly, telepractice provided an opportunity for many of these AGP tasks to be performed virtually, enabling the continuation of care.

It also became recognised that medically vulnerable groups were at the greatest risk of serious consequences from the virus. As such, another key driver for telepractice adoption during the pandemic became the need to support safe, ongoing care for vulnerable/at risk populations. The widespread closure of services within the residential aged care sector was a key example, with many settings limiting access to medical professionals only. Some disability services introduced similar restrictions, ceasing in-person SLP services due to infection risk fears. In order to sustain necessary SLP services, telepractice became the only way that management could be continued.

The desire to reduce the risk of viral contact also became a key driver for patients, with many seeking telepractice services rather than attending in-person care. Even when there were no longer specific lockdown requirements, many individuals preferred to limit their exposure risks by staying away from hospitals and health services unless it was absolutely necessary. This subgroup of patients specifically sought out telepractice services, creating patient demand for more services and opportunities to be provided via telepractice.

## 10.5  Growth of telepractice during COVID-19

With the onset of COVID-19 and multiple new drivers for telepractice, the challenge faced by SLPs globally was to rapidly grasp telepractice evidence and acquire the necessary skills and knowledge to deliver virtual interventions during a dynamic, stressful, and high-pressured situation. Since 2020, a number of papers have emerged from SLP groups across the world, outlining the early experiences and engagement with telehealth during those first months of the pandemic. For example, Chadd et al. (2021) surveyed clinicians in the United Kingdom 6 weeks and 22 weeks after the pandemic onset. Rapid uptake in telepractice was evident from the first survey, and by the second survey, clinicians estimated that on average 46.2% of individuals on their caseloads were receiving some services via telepractice. Survey data of SLPs in Hong Kong showed similar uptake patterns, with 34.8% of clinicians reporting providing services via telepractice, the majority of which was conducted via videoconferencing (Fong et al. 2021). Within Quebec, Canada, the uptake rates were even higher, with 84% of respondents reporting they began using telepractice during the pandemic (Macoir et al. 2021). As expected, this rapid uptake did not come without its challenges. As Fong et al. (2021) noted from their data, 60% of clinicians stated they had had no prior training in how to deliver services via telepractice, and over a quarter still felt there was insufficient evidence to support telepractice delivery of SLP services. This highlighted the challenges of preparing the workforce for such a massive shift in service delivery in a short period.

Although these early experiences highlighted a period of enormous change and challenge, new data emerging in the literature suggests that healthcare providers, patients, and caregivers are becoming more comfortable and confident in using telepractice. In one metropolitan quaternary hospital in Australia, the perceptions of stakeholders involved in tele-based services during COVID-19 and the factors that influenced uptake were explored (Cottrell et al. 2021). A survey completed by 109 patients and 66 allied health professionals from six disciplines (including seven SLPs) found that telepractice was viewed positively, despite best-practice processes for implementation not being consistently followed due to the critical nature of COVID-19. Notably, 80% of patients reported that a hybrid model for accessing services was preferred, with the option for tele-based appointments seen as highly desirable. Similarly, 89% of allied health professionals identified that telepractice was an important component of their role. Twenty-four allied health professionals and 13 administration officers also participated in interviews/focus groups. Overall, their responses echoed that of the survey, with 92% of allied health professionals stating they would provide virtual services post-pandemic. Further, dedicated administrative staff were deemed critical to navigate non-clinical tasks and manage logistical considerations. The work also highlighted that maintaining telepractice requires an ongoing commitment to support this service delivery model, with areas of ongoing concern including infrastructure and technical support, training and adaptations, adequate staffing, environmental and patient factors, confidence, and general preparedness (Cottrell et al. 2021).

## 10.6  Delivery of SLP services via telepractice

Across adult health services, telepractice was introduced as a means to triage potential patients with COVID-19 to appropriate services, enhance and support ongoing care, monitor patients in quarantine, and facilitate improved patient experience through increased service options whilst maintaining safety (Fisk et al. 2020; Galpin et al. 2021). Within SLP services, widespread adoption of telepractice has seen changes to models of care across many areas. The following sections will present telepractice service adaptations across three clinical service areas (critical care, dysphagia management, head and neck cancer) to highlight different ways in which telepractice has been integrated into care since COVID-19.

## 10.6.1 *Critical care*

On 28 April 2020, the World Health Organisation (WHO) recognised the need for SLP services for COVID-19 patients (World Health Organisation/Europe 2020). Patients with the virus were more likely to require a tracheostomy during their intensive care unit (ICU) admission and experience ICU-acquired weakness due to mechanical ventilation, prolonged weaning, failed extubation, or laryngeal complications (Freeman-Sanderson et al. 2020; McGrath et al. 2020; Miles et al. 2020). COVID-19 was also found to dramatically increase the number of patients in ICU who presented with communication barriers such as cognitive-linguistic changes related to the virus. However, although the service need was recognised, providing SLP care for this population posed several challenges. The need to minimise the viral exposure risk of staff and concerns over tracheostomy management and dysphagia assessments and their potential as AGPs, alongside shortages of PPE supplies, created multiple barriers to in-person models and required SLPs to rapidly adopt remote models of care to continue providing services within the ICU.

Telepractice is not a new phenomenon in critical care. For well over a decade, medical and nursing professionals have used telepractice to provide remote consultations, seek expert consultations with other experts, and monitor patient care. However, prior to the pandemic, SLP services within critical care have traditionally been delivered purely via in-person care models. As such, for many SLPs working in critical care environments, the need to adopt telepractice with COVID-19 patients within the ICU was a completely new method of care delivery and one which initially many were poorly prepared to deliver. This was recognised in work conducted early in the pandemic, which developed core recommendations for preparing the SLP workforce to manage COVID-19 in the ICU setting. Involving 35 SLPs from 12 countries across six continents, core strategies to support workforce preparation for managing COVID patients in critical care, as well as supporting communication and swallowing practices with this caseload were formed. The resulting document, "A Consensus Statement for the Management and Rehabilitation of Communication and Swallowing Function in the ICU: A Global Response to COVID-19," provided much-needed structure in an ambiguous and volatile landscape (Freeman-Sanderson et al. 2020). Within that document, assisting staff in the acquisition of telehealth capabilities and the use of telehealth to support swallowing and communication management were part of the core set of consensus statements.

During the pandemic, virtual assessment and management by SLPs ensured timely and appropriate swallowing and communication evaluation of patients in critical care and facilitated communication between patients, health professionals, interpreters, and family/significant others (Freeman-Sanderson et al. 2020; Vergara et al. 2020). Moreover, it has enabled SLPs and patients to communicate without wearing PPE, ensuring that facial expressions and oral musculature movement were visible and protective face coverings did not affect the ability to view facial expressions or limit additional information from lip-reading in the loud and busy ICU environment. However, although it is recognised clinically that telepractice has become a key element in supporting patients within the critical care environment, at present there is a dearth of published information explicitly documenting the practice changes and adaptations undertaken by SLPs during the pandemic.

One example from the United States highlights the successful integration of existing ICU technology to provide SLP services to confirmed COVID-19 patients. To provide clinical swallow evaluations to patients in isolation, a group of critical care SLPs modified a high-definition camera system called *Tele-ICU* (Khurrum et al. 2020), typically used for tele-based medical consultation and monitoring vital signs (Kurtz 2020). Following a checklist to determine patient suitability to participate in a virtual assessment, a nurse assumed the role of facilitator, and sessions were scheduled to correspond with existing nursing care to limit exposure risks and minimise the use of PPE. The modifications allowed SLPs to operate the system's camera from a separate control room and obtain a clear view of the patient to support remote oromotor examinations and swallowing evaluations. The system also enabled caregivers to attend sessions via a remote link. The main barriers reported for using *Tele-ICU* included background noise from the negative pressure rooms and the presence of dysphonia (attributable to prolonged intubation) (Kurtz 2020).

SLPs have identified several challenges when preparing for telepractice sessions in the ICU. These include identifying clinicians with critical care specific skills, issues accessing resources and equipment, timely referrals and consultation with care teams; staff availability to provide in-room facilitation or troubleshooting (i.e., nurse or allied health assistant); environmental factors (e.g., acoustics); and patient variables (e.g., level of alertness, access to glasses, hearing aids, call bells, assistive devices) (Riegler 2021; Weidner and Lowman 2020).

However, telepractice has enabled SLP services to adapt and continue to provide necessary support in the critical care environment. In turn, this has allowed other professionals to progress their own management. For example, the use of telepractice allowed the oral prescription of medication as SLPs were able to complete swallow evaluations and clear patients for oral intake. Telepractice also assisted families in navigating visitor restrictions to communicate with loved ones in ICU and with members of the care team. These opportunities to connect virtually underscored the value of tele-based services introduced during this rapid state of change. In particular, connecting patients with their significant others was a unique outcome of the use of telepractice in the ICU setting during COVID-19. Further examples of ways that introducing technology into management created tangible "value adds" for patient care included patients having easy access to alternative communication devices (e.g., text-to-speech application, digital whiteboard) when they could not progress cuff deflation trials or having carers/significant others record messages to re-play for their loved ones in ICU when they were more alert.

## 10.6.2 Dysphagia management

COVID-19 presented an array of unique challenges for SLPs working in the area of dysphagia management. There were multiple AGP concerns related to triggering coughing during food/fluid trials, the inability to maintain physical distancing when conducting the assessment, and in many settings, both videofluoroscopy (VFSS) and fiberoptic endoscopic assessments (FEES) were also ceased due to AGP concerns. One positive factor was that there was existing evidence to support the use of telepractice to conduct clinical swallow examinations (CSEs) available prior to the pandemic (Borders et al. 2021; Burns et al. 2019; Morrell et al. 2017; Ward et al. 2012, 2014). Although the diagnostic limitations of a CSE (conducted either in-person or via telepractice) are fully acknowledged, within the context of COVID restrictions and limited access to instrumental swallowing assessments, the telepractice CSE model at least provided a means for making some clinical decisions regarding dysphagia risk. It also helped clinicians form interim management plans until an instrumental assessment was able to be conducted.

The implementation of telepractice to manage dysphagia requires a systematic approach, ongoing training, upskilling, awareness of available technology, and the use of an evidence-based model of care that includes appropriate safety measures and appropriate patient support. Depending on the service need, existing models were able to be adapted during the pandemic to provide CSEs via telepractice to inpatients within a healthcare service, other healthcare facilities, or patients' homes, as discussed further here.

The inpatient model was used when swallowing assessments were required for COVID-19 patients within the critical care environment or with any "suspected" COVID-19 (awaiting confirmation from testing) patients (e.g., in the emergency department setting). In this model, the speech-language pathologist conducted the assessment from either their office/another room or outside the patient's room, connecting with the patient using videoconferencing via a tablet or phone as per published studies (Morrell et al. 2017; Ward et al. 2012, 2014) or other ICU camera systems (Khurrum et al. 2020). If the patient was located within a room with an observation window, then having the SLP located on the other side of the observation window enabled further visual connection and interaction between those involved in the assessment. Located with the patient is their nurse, who was on hand to facilitate the session, monitor patient safety, and provide in-room assistance when necessary. Engaging the assistance of a nurse facilitator who was already in PPE and who was scheduled to be in the room with the patient to complete the assessment as well as other routine care tasks meant reduced PPE use and limited exposure risks for staff (Kurtz 2020). Patients were also encouraged to self-feed whenever possible to maintain an appropriate level of social distance between themselves and the facilitator.

The CSE via telepractice model was also adapted to administer assessments to non-COVID patients located within other facilities, similar to the service model described by Burns et al. (2019). In that context, social distancing requirements (e.g., during lockdown restrictions) or the vulnerable health state of the patient meant that the speech-language pathologist was unable to see the patient in person and instead had to provide a remote CSE via telehealth from a distant location. During the pandemic this model was often used within the aged care sector when facilities limited (or prevented) health professionals from attending on-site to reduce the exposure risk for residents. In that model, local nursing and care staff from within the facility assisted at the patient end during the trials, enabling the online clinician to conduct the assessment without any contact with the patient.

For dysphagic patients accessing community and outpatient services, many actively sought the use of telepractice to receive services in their own homes during the pandemic. For many this helped manage concerns about travelling to a health service and the potential risk of viral exposure from community transfer during these visits. For these individuals, completing a CSE via telepractice from their own home became a useful model to ensure they remained in regular contact with their speech-language pathologist and their dysphagia progress was able to be monitored from the safety of their own homes. In this context, a carer or family member was present in the home to assist the patient and provide support if a medical emergency arose. As the connection was being made into the home, videoconferencing was conducted using the patient's home device (e.g., phone, tablet, laptop). Studies have shown that various device types can be successfully used for home assessments (Morrell et al. 2017). In some circumstances additional preparation prior to the session was organised to ensure patients had appropriate foods/fluids available for the assessment. Equally, having the opportunity to observe how patients prepared and managed food and fluid items at home provided valuable insights into their daily management.

Telepractice offers flexible service delivery options for direct patient management of dysphagia. It can also facilitate virtual mentoring opportunities, provide clinicians with access to experts to support complex dysphagia management, and enable sessions to be recorded and used for ongoing education and training. It can also help expedite access to SLP services (e.g., in a residential aged care setting). This has an immediate impact on resident safety and potentially avoids additional travel, call-out expenses, or delays due to lockdowns. Telepractice can also ensure patients receive consistent and responsive dysphagia management, which in turn can facilitate oral intake and therapeutic input and support the overall maintenance of swallow function. As multiple aspects of dysphagia care can be provided safely and effectively via telepractice, it can feasibly become part of the ongoing management options for all patients with swallowing difficulties, not only those impacted by COVID.

### 10.6.3 Head and neck cancer

Establishing new and practical workflow solutions for managing patients with head and neck cancer (HNC) was crucial during the pandemic to ensure the efficient and safe provision of services (Ku et al. 2020; Spelten et al. 2021). Due to the diverse negative impacts of HNC and its management, practice guidelines for this population advocate for regular supportive care by SLP and the wider multidisciplinary team during active treatment, as well as during the post-acute and long-term recovery stages. However, with the onset of the pandemic, providing this level of support and monitoring required extensive service reimagining. It was recognised early on that limiting the risk of exposure to infection for this group was crucial, as their immunocompromised health state made them more susceptible to the virus and more likely to have higher morbidity and mortality rates (Paleri et al. 2020). Hence, rapid transition to virtual solutions to deliver care became critical to ensure patients within the hospital setting and those living in the community could continue receiving necessary individual and group support (Nilsen et al. 2020; Spelten et al. 2021).

Effective use of telepractice to support patient care following HNC management had been established in the pre-pandemic literature, and various models were available for implementation. Models with demonstrated efficacy for providing SLP and multidisciplinary support to patients within their homes post-treatment via telepractice (Collins et al. 2017) were implemented to support ongoing care. A study published post-pandemic demonstrated how this type of home-based model enabled patients to remain supported by weekly videoconferencing sessions with a speech-language pathologist whilst receiving treatment (Nilsen et al. 2020). There is also evidence for models which use videoconferencing to link in with other expert clinicians from another facility to help troubleshoot and guide local care (Burns et al. 2017; Burns and Wall 2017), which was used for clinical support. Positive outcomes have also been achieved through asynchronous digital solutions for supporting therapy (Wall et al. 2020), which provided effective ways to support therapy remotely.

In addition to these approaches, electronic monitoring via email or other systems to collect online surveys, self-evaluation tools, and checklists to stay updated on how patients are progressing has also been supported by published evidence (e.g., Wall et al. 2016). This sort of monitoring enabled teams to identify when patients needed care and escalate issues of greater urgency. Multidisciplinary videoconferencing models such as the one reported by Collins et al. (2017) were also used to conduct meetings between patients and multiple health professionals involved in their care (e.g., speech-language pathologist, dietitian, radiation oncologist), allowing multidisciplinary consultation and opportunities to discuss concerns and manage/mitigate the impacts of cancer treatment. The opportunity to use group videoconferencing to provide education sessions to groups of patients simultaneously (e.g., for delivery of education sessions prior to commencing radiotherapy) or to provide support groups for survivors of HNC was also a key part of this reimagined model of care. These multiple different telepractice solutions all provided new opportunities to ensure patients received their required regular monitoring and opportunities for engagement with support groups without the need to travel to the cancer service.

For some services that required more time to get their digital solutions ready to use with their patients, there were anecdotal reports of early issues and some negative consequences associated with missed care and loss of regular follow-up monitoring. There were also early concerns that there would be poor acceptance of telepractice by this clinical population. Fortunately, for the majority of patients, this was not the case. Once services had telepractice solutions ready for patient use and patients were supported to engage with these telepractice solutions, it was found that flexibly connecting with patients via telepractice helped identify issues as they arose (Paleri et al. 2020). Some SLPs also found that telepractice enabled more responsive and time-sensitive care, particularly relating to patient triaging and waitlists.

Although the vulnerable health state of patients with HNC was a key driver for service redesign for this population, finding ways to ensure the safe and responsible management of the AGPs associated specifically with laryngectomy care (e.g., prosthesis changes, stoma care) was also a significant discussion area. It was recommended that individuals already caring for patients should be delegated these tasks to minimise the risk of exposure and contain the virus (Miles et al. 2020). Patients were also encouraged to self-manage their voice prosthesis where possible (e.g., within their home environment) and troubleshoot with a speech-language pathologist via a virtual consultation on the phone or via video (Bolton et al. 2020). Again, support models via telepractice were able to be established based on existing evidence for supporting laryngectomy care (Burns et al. 2017; Ward et al. 2009).

Overall, it has been reassuring to observe the willingness and capacity of health services and providers to adapt to telepractice-based solutions necessitated by COVID-19 (Spelten et al. 2021). Unsurprisingly, it has also highlighted the notable influence providers and patient groups have on the utility and acceptability of a service. It is imperative that quality assurances are reviewed and processes are implemented to safeguard the acceptability, adaptability, and sustainability of telepractice (including hybrid offerings) in the HNC population post-pandemic (Spelten et al. 2021).

## 10.7 Summary

As stated by Roy (2020), "Historically pandemics have forced humans to break with the past and imagine their world anew. [COVID-19] is a portal, a gateway between one world and the next" (p. 239). Indeed, this pandemic has intensified the need for healthcare providers to push boundaries, manage change, adapt, and reimagine how services can be accessed and delivered. The growth of telepractice in SLP services is a key example of this. Across services globally, the sudden disruption to routine practice forced health services to shift their perceptions and implement telepractice to sustain care, and the scope of telepractice has grown exponentially as a direct result. Importantly, this shift provided individuals with first-hand experience of tele-based delivery and management, which in turn provided them with greater clarity regarding (1) *how* telepractice could be used; (2) *what* training, upskilling, resources, and supports were required; (3) *who* was able to administer and engage in telepractice; and (4) *what* workflow practices were needed. As providers have become more aware of and comfortable with operating in the virtual space, a greater understanding of the capabilities, situations, and opportunities to employ telepractice has become evident. Through shared experience, a culture of learning and adaptation has been fostered.

Telepractice is a high-value model of care that continues to develop, evolve, and change. During this global emergency, there have been valuable lessons learnt and recognition that telepractice models can enhance the holistic management of patients. As momentum builds within the health service system, ongoing barriers to implementation including infrastructure, training, technology, eligibility, and financial considerations will need to be continually reviewed and addressed. This will ensure meaningful and targeted telepractice models can be established and supported. As we move towards a "new world," future studies are needed to investigate the real-world challenges SLPs faced during COVID-19 and unpack what was done to provide services via telepractice during the pandemic. Understanding the *what* and *how* will help inform future telehealth service delivery models, enhance patient-centred care, and improve practice efficiency. Critical to the success of telepractice services is training and education. SLPs must continue to develop, consolidate, and maintain their currency of telepractice knowledge to facilitate the integration and expansion of tele-based services. Ultimately, it is not just about understanding how telepractice has been used to respond to the pandemic but rather how the profession will distil what it has learnt from this period and embed this into the telepractice services that evolve into future *business as usual* care.

# References

American Speech-Language-Hearing Association (2021). Telepractice. Resource document. American Speech-Language-Hearing Association. www.asha.org/practice-portal/professional-issues/telepractice/. Accessed 20 August 2021.

Araújo, B. C. L., Lima, T. R. C. D. M., Gois-Santos, V. T. D., Santos, V. S., Simões, S. D. M., & Martins-Filho, P. R. (2020). Speech therapy practice in hospital settings and COVID-19 pandemic. *Revista Da Associação Médica Brasileira*, 66(Suppl 2), 10–12.

Ben-Aharon, A. (2019). A practical guide to establishing an online speech therapy private practice. *Perspectives of the ASHA Special Interest Groups*, 4(4), 712–718.

Bolton, L., Mills, C., Wallace, S., & Brady, M. C. (2020). Aerosol generating procedures, dysphagia assessment and COVID-19: A rapid review. *International Journal of Language and Communication Disorders*, 55(4), 629–636.

Borders, J. C., Sevitz, J. S., Malandraki, J. B., Malandraki, G. A., & Troche, M. S. (2021). Objective and subjective clinical swallowing outcomes via telehealth: Reliability in outpatient clinical practice. *American Journal of Speech-Language Pathology*, 30(2), 598–608.

Burns, C. L., & Wall, L. R. (2017). Using telepractice to support the management of head and neck cancer: Key considerations for speech-language pathology service planning, establishment and evaluation. *Perspectives of the ASHA Special Interest Groups*, 2(SIG13), 139–146.

Burns, C. L., Ward, E. C., Gray, A., Baker, L., Cowie, B., Winter, N., et al. (2019). Implementation of speech pathology telepractice services for clinical swallowing assessment: An evaluation of service outcomes, costs and consumer satisfaction. *Journal of Telemedicine and Telecare*, 25(9), 545–551.

Burns, C. L., Ward, E. C., Hill, A. J., Kularatna, S., Byrnes, J., & Kenny, L. M. (2017). Randomised controlled trial of a multisite speech pathology telepractice service providing swallowing and communication intervention to patients with head and neck cancer: An evaluation of service outcomes. *Head and Neck*, 39(5), 932–939.

Chacon, A. M., Nguyen, D. D., McCabe, P., & Madill, C. (2021). Aerosol generating behaviours in speech pathology clinical practice: A systematic literature review. *PLoS One*, 16(4), e0250308. doi:10.1371/journal.pone.0250308.

Chadd, K., Moyse, K., & Enderby, P. (2021). Impact of COVID-19 on the speech and language therapy profession and their patients. *Frontiers in Neurology*, 12. doi:10.3389/fneur.2021.629190.

Collins, A., Burns, C. L., Ward, E. C., Comans, T., Blake, C., Kenny, L., et al. (2017). Home-based telehealth service for swallowing and nutrition management following head and neck cancer treatment. *Journal of Telemedicine and Telecare*, 23(10), 866–872.

Cottrell, M., Burns, C. L., Jones, A., Rahmann, A., Young, A., Sam, S., et al. (2021). Sustaining allied health telehealth services beyond the rapid response to COVID-19: Learning from patient and staff experiences at a large quaternary hospital. *Journal of Telemedicine and Telecare*, 27(10), 615–624.

Fisk, M., Livingstone, A., & Pit, S. W. (2020). Telehealth in the context of COVID-19: Changing perspectives in Australia, the United Kingdom, and the United States. *Journal of Medical Internet Research*, 22(6), e19264. doi:10.2196/19264.

Fong, R., Tsai, C. F., & Yiu, O. Y. (2021). The implementation of telepractice in speech language pathology in Hong Kong during the COVID-19 pandemic. *Telemedicine and E-Health*, 27(1), 30–38.

Freeman-Sanderson, A., Ward, E. C., Miles, A., de Pedro Netto, I., Duncan, S., Inamoto, Y., et al. (2020). A consensus statement for the management and rehabilitation of communication and swallowing function in the ICU: A global response to COVID-19. *Archives of Physical Medicine and Rehabilitation*, 102(5), 835–842.

Fritz, M. A., Howell, R. J., Brodsky, M. B., Suiter, D. M., Dhar, S. I., Rameau, A., et al. (2020). Moving forward with dysphagia care: Implementing strategies during the COVID-19 pandemic and beyond. *Dysphagia*, 36(2), 161–169.

Galpin, K., Sikka, N., King, S. L., Horvath, K. A., Shipman, S. A., Evans, N., et al. (2021). Expert consensus: Telehealth skills for health care professionals. *Telemedicine and E-Health*, 27(7), 820–824.

Khurrum, M., Asmar, S., & Jospeh, B. (2020). Telemedicine in the ICU: Innovation in the critical care process. *Journal of Intensive Care Medicine, 36*(12), 1377–1384.

Ku, P. K. M., Holsinger, F. C., Chan, J. Y. K., Yeung, Z. W. C., Chan, B. Y. T., Tong, M. C. F., et al. (2020). Management of dysphagia in the patient with head and neck cancer during COVID-19 pandemic: Practical strategy. *Head and Neck, 42*(7), 1491–1496.

Kurtz, M. (2020). Making instrumental assessments work in a COVID-19 world. *The ASHA Leader.* https://leader.pubs.asha.org/do/10.1044/leader.OTP.25082020.40/full/. Accessed 5 August 2021.

Macoir, J., Desmarais, C., Martel-Sauvageau, V., & Monetta, L. (2021). Proactive changes in clinical practice as a result of the COVID-19 pandemic: Survey on the use of telepractice by Quebec speech-language pathologists. *International Journal of Language and Communication Disorders, 56*(5), 1086–1096.

Malandraki, G. A., Arkenberg, R. H., Mitchell, S. S., & Malandraki, J. B. (2021). Telehealth for dysphagia across the life span: Using contemporary evidence and expertise to guide clinical practice during and after COVID-19. *American Journal of Speech-Language Pathology, 30*(2), 532–550.

McGrath, B. A., Ashby, N., Birchall, M., Dean, P., Doherty, C., Ferguson, K., et al. (2020). Multidisciplinary guidance for safe tracheostomy care during the COVID-19 pandemic: The NHS National Patient Safety Improvement Programme (NatPatSIP). *Anaesthesia, 75*(12), 1659–1670.

Miles, A., Connor, N. P., Desai, R. V., Jadcherla, S., Allen, J., Brodsky, M., et al. (2020). Dysphagia care across the continuum: A multidisciplinary dysphagia research society taskforce report of service-delivery during the COVID-19 global pandemic. *Dysphagia, 36*(2), 170–182.

Morrell, K., Hyers, M., Stuchiner, T., Lucas, L., Schwartz, K., Mako, J., et al. (2017). Telehealth stroke dysphagia evaluation is safe and effective. *Cerebrovascular Diseases, 44*(3–4), 225–231.

Nilsen, M. L., Clump II, D. A., Kubik, M., Losego, K., Mrozek, A., Pawlowicz, E., et al. (2020). Prevision of multidisciplinary head and neck cancer survivorship care during the 2019 novel coronavirus pandemic. *Journal of the Sciences and Specialties of the Head and Neck, 42*(7). doi:10.1002/hed.26256.

Paleri, V., Hardman, J., Tikka, T., Bradley, P., Pracy, P., & Kerawala, C. (2020). Rapid implementation of an evidence-based remote triaging system for assessment of suspected referrals and patients with head and neck cancer on follow-up after treatment during the COVID-19 pandemic: Model for international collaboration. *Head and Neck, 42*(7), 1674–1680.

Riegler, L. (2021). Health care telepractice success is all about the prep. *The ASHA Leader.* https://leader.pubs.asha.org/do/10.1044/2021-0621-va-telehealth-facilitators/full/. Accessed 5 August 2021.

Roy, A. (2020). *Azadi: Freedom. Fascism. Fiction. (Penguin specials).* London, UK: Penguin.

Royal College of Speech and Language Therapists (2021). Telehealth guidance. Resource document. Royal College of Speech and Language Therapists. www.rcslt.org/members/delivering-quality-services/telehealth/telehealth-guidance/. Accessed 25 September 2021.

Speech Pathology Australia (2014). Telepractice in speech pathology. Resource document. Speech Pathology Australia. www.telemedicine-360.com/wp-content/uploads/2019/02/2015-SPA-0113_Position_Statement_Telepractice_in_Speech.pdf. Accessed 25 September 2021.

Speech Pathology Australia (2021). Telepractice. Resource document. Speech Pathology Australia. www.speechpathologyaustralia.org.au/SPAweb/Resources_for_Speech_Pathologists/Professional_Resources/HTML/Telepractice.aspx. Accessed 25 September 2021.

Spelten, E. R., Hardman, R. N., Pike, K. E., Yuen, E., & Wilson, C. (2021). Best practice in the implementation of telehealth-based supportive cancer care: Using research evidence and discipline-based guidance. *Patient Education and Counseling*, 104(11), 2682–2699.

Thomas, E. E., Taylor, M. L., Ward, E. C., Hwang, R., Cook, R., Ross, J.-A., Webb, C., Harris, M., Hartley, C., Carswell, P., Burns, C., & Caffery, L. J. (2022). Beyond forced telehealth adoption: A framework to sustain telehealth among allied health services. *Journal of Telemedicine and Telecare*. doi:10.1177/1357633X221074499.

Vergara, J., Skoretz, S. A., Brodsky, M. B., Miles, A., Langmore, S. E., Wallace, S., et al. (2020). Assessment, diagnosis, and treatment of dysphagia in patients infected with SARS-CoV-2: A review of the literature and international guidelines. *American Journal of Speech-Language Pathology*, 29(4), 2242–2253.

Wall, L. R., Cartmill, B., Ward, E. C., Hill, A. J., Isenring, E., Byrnes, J., et al. (2016). "ScreenIT": Computerised screening of swallowing, nutrition and distress in head and neck cancer patients during (chemo)radiotherapy. *Oral Oncology*, 54, 47–53.

Wall, L. R., Ward, E. C., Cartmill, B., Hill, A. J., Isenring, E., Byrnes, J., et al. (2020). Prophylactic swallowing therapy for patients with head and neck cancer: A three arm randomised parallel group trial investigating the impact of service delivery model. *Head and Neck*, 42(5), 873–885.

Ward, E. C., Burns, C. L., Gray, A., Baker, L., Cowie, B., Winter, N., et al. (2021). Establishing clinical swallowing assessment services via telepractice: A multisite implementation evaluation. *American Journal of Speech-Language Pathology*, 30(6), 2456–2464.

Ward, E. C., Burns, C. L., Theodoros, D. G., & Russell, T. G. (2014). Impact of dysphagia severity on clinical decision making via telerehabilitation. *Telemedicine and E-Health*, 20(4), 296–303.

Ward, E. C., Crombie, J., Trickey, M., Hill, A., Theodoros, D., & Russell, T. (2009). Assessment of communication and swallowing post-laryngectomy: A telerehabilitation trial. *Journal of Telemedicine and Telecare*, 15(5), 232–237.

Ward, E. C., Sharma, S., Burns, C., Theodoros, D., & Russell, T. (2012). Managing patient factors in the assessment of swallowing via telerehabilitation. *International Journal of Telemedicine and Applications*, 2012, 132719. doi:10.1155/2012/132719.

Weidner, K., & Lowman, J. (2020). Telepractice for adult speech-language pathology services: A systematic review. *Perspectives of the ASHA Special Interest Groups*, 5(1), 326–338.

World Health Organisation/Europe (2020). COVID-19 exposes the critical importance of patient rehabilitation. Resource document. World Health Organisation/Europe. www.euro.who.int/en/health-topics/health-emergencies/coronavirus-covid-19/news/news/2020/4/covid-19-exposes-the-critical-importance-of-patient-rehabilitation. Accessed 5 August 2021.

# 11

# PSYCHOLOGICAL EFFECTS OF COVID-19 ON ADULTS WITH APHASIA AND THEIR CAREGIVERS

## Six-month consequences of COVID-19 lockdowns in Hong Kong

*Anthony Pak-Hin Kong, Dustin Kai-Yan Lau, and Vivian Nga-Ying Chai*

## 11.1 Introduction

In December 2019, the first case of Coronavirus Disease 2019 (COVID-19) was announced in China. The respiratory disease spread quickly around the world, with the World Health Organization (2020) declaring a pandemic on 11 March 2020. The impact of the coronavirus crisis on the lives of families, healthcare systems, and the world economy has been significant (Vernooij-Dassen and Jeon 2016; Ward et al. 2018). Due to the highly contagious nature of SARS-CoV-2 and lack of vaccine in 2020, many governments globally raised their response level and enforced strict public health measures shortly after the outbreak. These measures included city/country lockdowns, stay-at-home orders, home quarantines, suspension of public services, restrictions on public gatherings, and work-from-home arrangements.

The COVID-19 pandemic has also been called the "geriatric emergency of 2020" (Kasai 2020) as it caused worse symptoms and outcomes amongst older people and those with pre-existing/chronic conditions or lowered immunity (Jordan and Adap 2020). Along with worries and even fear of getting infected, the older population had to cope with the distressing experience of quarantine, separation from friends and family, and loss of freedom due to confinement at home (Brooks et al. 2020). All these environmental stressors might have taken a higher psychological toll on older people, as they must also adapt to biological, socioeconomic, and psychosocial risk factors of aging. In fact, one in two women and one in three men aged 60 years or above have self-reported symptoms of emotional distress that they attributed to the pandemic and lockdown (García-Portilla et al. 2020). Concerning populations with clinical disorders, Giebel et al.

DOI: 10.4324/9781003257318-11

(2020) and Roach et al. (2021) examined the negative effects of COVID-19 on well-being in and social support for people with dementia and their caregivers. Psychological conditions such as feeling anxious (or uncertain) and experiencing loss of control over situations were identified. As social support services were gradually closed down, severely restricted, or reformulated in phases, there was a shift from in-person dementia services to remote/virtual care, with reduced weekly hours in social support service usage.

Although reports of the effects of COVID-19 on psychosocial well-being of seniors and some populations with clinical disorders have started to emerge, there is still a lack of research focusing on persons with aphasia (PWAs). Aphasia is a neurological disorder caused by damage to the areas of the brain that are responsible for language processing. It can impair comprehension and expression in verbal, written, and signed modalities (Kong 2016; Worrall et al. 2016). According to Kong (2021a), enhancing social participation and reducing emotional distress is a critical rehabilitation goal for PWAs. Social relationships and meaningful activities performed by PWAs are also crucial to promote positive psychosocial well-being. In a recent webinar conducted by the Royal College of Speech and Language Therapists (2020), stroke survivors' opinions on their unmet needs after COVID-19 were summarised. Specifically, apart from feelings of isolation, loneliness, anxiety, and depression, stroke participants expressed their negative experiences of changes in service delivery in the United Kingdom. Some also reported unexpected cancellations or delay of speech and language therapy service appointments, on top of the need to adjust to digital therapy delivery via phone and video platforms. However, remote therapy might not be suitable for everyone and has caused additional anxieties for some clients because of potential technology accessibility barriers (due to their language deficits), in combination with varying degrees of co-existing age- and cognition-related problems (Brandenburg et al. 2013).

The sudden and dramatic onset of aphasia following stroke is associated with major disruption of everyday life and affects all dimensions of Quality of Life (QoL) (Bury 1982; Code and Herrmann 2003). The psychosocial adjustment process is often complicated and protracted (Parr 2004). PWAs are especially prone to psychosocial problems (e.g., anxiety, depression, reduced social networks, and social isolation/exclusion) because PWAs' communication breakdowns are not only manifested in the impairment of language form and content but also in restrictions of social participation (Davidson et al. 2003). These communication breakdowns can cause various degrees of social limitations (including the number of everyday activities undertaken, the number of communication partners engaged with, and the number of social situations experienced that significantly impact on well-being) that may exacerbate psychosocial problems in PWAs (Bronken et al. 2012). Furthermore, aphasia has been reported to be a significant predictor of emotional distress, social isolation, and negative QoL after stroke (Lee et al. 2015). In 2001, the World Health Organization proposed the

International Classification of Functioning, Disability and Health. It is composed of multiple interdependent domains which dynamically interact and overlap to create QoL. During the pandemic, most people, including PWAs, have predominantly stayed at home and experienced unprecedented social isolation. This is contrary to traditional principles of managing aphasia because community activities amongst PWAs are critical for them to maintain a good mood, psychosocial well-being, and consequently, an acceptable QoL.

## 11.2 Aims of study

People in Hong Kong faced the first round of public health measures in January 2020 when the government announced a work-from-home arrangement for government employees of non-emergency public services and appealed to private sector organisations to make similar arrangements (Information Services Department 2020a). As the city experienced the second wave in March 2020, a regulation prohibiting group gatherings (Hong Kong e-Legislation 2020a) came into operation. These measures were further tightened as the pandemic remained volatile and the city faced the third and fourth waves in July and November 2020, respectively. As Hong Kong was one of the first cities to handle the COVID-19 crisis and commence public health measures, we believe that a systematic examination of the influence of COVID-19 on PWAs in Hong Kong is of high value and relevance to other countries. This chapter aims to summarise and discuss results of a retrospective survey study that examined the following:

1) Did PWAs demonstrate difficulties understanding COVID-19? If so, why?
2) Did communication and social patterns in PWAs change as a result of the COVID-19 outbreak? If so, how?
3) Did COVID-19 affect the psychological wellbeing of PWAs?
4) Did PWAs suffer from negative emotions, including anxiety, depression, and pressure?
5) Over time, how did PWAs experience further impact during the pandemic?

## 11.3 Method

The project has been approved by the Human Subjects Ethics Sub-committee of the Hong Kong Polytechnic University (HSESC Reference Number: HSEARS20200316002).

### 11.3.1 Participants

A total of 131 participants took part in this study. They included 43 PWAs who were at least six months post-onset a stroke and had sufficient receptive and expressive language ability to participate in the interview. They were recruited from two local self-help groups for PWAs in Hong Kong and the Speech Therapy Clinic at a local university. Also, 25 caregivers of PWAs and 63 unimpaired speakers who were naïve about aphasia were recruited by word of mouth. Detailed demographic information of participants is given in Table 11.1.

### 11.3.2 Survey design and item analyses

A 70-item survey questionnaire in Chinese, designed to be completed through a video/audio interview in spoken Cantonese, was devised. It contained questions

**TABLE 11.1** Summary of respondents' demographic information

| | | *PWAs* | *Unimpaired speakers* | *Caregivers* |
|---|---|---|---|---|
| Number (#) | Total=131 | 43 | 63 | 25 |
| Gender (#, %) | Male | 28 (65.1%) | 26 (41.3%) | 9 (36.0%) |
| | Female | 15 (34.9%) | 37 (58.7%) | 16 (64.0%) |
| Age | 18–30 | / | 5 (7.9%) | 1 (4%) |
| (#, %) | 31–40 | 1 (2.3%) | 2 (3.2%) | 1 (4%) |
| | 41–50 | 9 (20.9%) | 5 (7.9%) | 3 (12.0%) |
| | 51–60 | 13 (30.2%) | 38 (60.3%) | 10 (40.0%) |
| | 61–70 | 15 (34.9%) | 11 (17.5%) | 9 (36.0%) |
| | 71 or older | 5 (11.6%) | 2 (3.2%) | 1 (4%) |
| Educational level | Primary | 5 (11,6%) | 6 (9.5%) | 1 (4.0%) |
| (#, %) | Secondary (junior) | 13 (30.2%) | 10 (39.7%) | 4 (16.0%) |
| | Secondary (senior) | 15 (34.9%) | 22 (34.9%) | 11 (44.0%) |
| | Tertiary | 10 (23.3%) | 25 (39.7%) | 9 (36.0%) |
| Age of diagnosis | 18–30 | 3 (7.0%) | | |
| (#, %) | 31–40 | 3 (7.0%) | | |
| | 41–50 | 13 (30.2%) | | |
| | 51–60 | 11 (25.6%) | | |
| | 61–70 | 12 (27.9%) | | |
| | 71 or + | 1 (2.3%) | | |
| Severity | Mild | 13 (30.2%) | | |
| | Moderate | 14 (32.6%) | | |
| | Severe | 16 (37.2%) | | |
| Working status | Full-time | 28 (65.1%) | 33 (52.4%) | 11 (44.0%) |
| (premorbid for | Part-time | 2 (4.7%) | 2 (3.2%) | 2 (8.0%) |
| PWA) | Unemployed | 2 (4.7%) | 3 (4.8%) | / |
| (#, %) | Retired | 6 (14.0%) | 8 (12.7%) | 4 (16.0%) |
| | Never worked | 1 (2.3%) | / | / |
| | Housewife | 3 (7.0%) | 14 (22.2%) | 8 (32.0%) |
| | Students | 1 (2.3%) | 3 (4.8%) | / |

| | | PWAs | Unimpaired speakers | Caregivers |
|---|---|---|---|---|
| Occupation (job industry) (#, %) | Business/financial planners | / | 5 (10.9%) | / |
| | Chefs (catering) | 1 (2.7%) | 1 (2.2%) | / |
| | Civil servants | 4 (10.8%) | / | 2 (12.5%) |
| | Clerks | 2 (5.4%) | 8 (17.4%) | 4 (25.0%) |
| | Construction workers (handyman services) | 4 (10.8%) | 4 (8.7%) | 1 (6.3%) |
| | Drivers | 7 (18.9%) | 1 (2.2%) | / |
| | Education professionals | 2 (5.4%) | 2 (4.3%) | 3 (18.8%) |
| | Insurance representatives | / | 2 (4.3%) | / |
| | Janitors/cleaners | / | 3 (6.5%) | 1 (6.3%) |
| | Managers (management) | 2 (5.4%) | 4 (8.7%) | / |
| | Manufacturing workers | 1 (2.7%) | 2 (4.3%) | / |
| | Other professionals | 6 (16.2%) | 6 (13.0%) | 3 (18.8%) |
| | Customer service representatives/sales | 4 (10.8%) | 2 (4.4%) | 1 (6.3%) |
| | (Not specified) | 1 (2.7%) | 6 (13.0%) | 1 (6.3%) |
| Living status (#, %) | With family | 36 (83.7%) | 58 (92.1%) | 23 (92.0%) |
| | Alone | 4 (9.3%) | 4 (6.3%) | 1 (4.0%) |
| | Others | 3 (7.0%) | 1 (1.6%) | 1 (4.0%) |
| # of cohabitant, including interviewees (mean, s.d.) | | 2.98 (1.49) | 3.35 (1.21) | 3.28 (1.24) |

about participants' (I) demographic information; (II) knowledge about COVID-19; (III) communication and social patterns before and after COVID-19; (IV) psychological well-being; and (V) negative emotions after COVID-19. The types of questions in the questionnaire included rating scales, close-ended questions (e.g., yes/no questions and multiple-choice questions), and open-ended questions. The survey was conducted on a one-to-one basis between April and June 2020. If the participants from the PWA group required assistance, the interviewers would seek support from caregivers to provide responses to the questions in the survey, but only when this was necessary. All participants' responses were recorded for subsequent data analyses.

A major focus of this study was the impact of COVID-19 on the psychological well-being and emotions of PWAs. The questions in section (IV) were adapted and translated from the Scale of Psychological Well-being (SPWB; Ryff 1989), which measures six dimensions of psychological well-being: autonomy, environmental mastery, personal growth, positive relations with others, purpose in life, and self-acceptance. A 7-point scale was adopted for this condensed version of the SPWB Short-Form (containing 24 statements in total). An average score of each of the six dimensions of psychological well-being was obtained (of a maximum sub-score of 28), on top of the total score (of a maximum score of 168). Higher scores indicated greater well-being.

Section (V) of the questionnaire focused on measuring the depressive symptoms or emotional health of the participants. Participants were asked to first indicate the presence or absence of self-perceived anxiety, depression, and stress following the COVID-19 outbreak. Participants who responded "yes" to any of these questions were then asked to self-rate the level of intensity using a 5-point scale (e.g., "slightly anxious" [1] to "highly anxious" [5]). They were also asked to provide examples to illustrate specific symptoms and emotions. Percentage distribution for each degree was then obtained. The participants were also asked about their expectations for the post-outbreak period of COVID-19 in this section.

For responses to all closed-ended questions, there were both mutually exclusive and exhaustive types (Lavrakas 2008). Mutually exclusive answers were used for obtaining demographic information and number of hours for participating in indoor and outdoor activities. Exhaustive answers were used for understanding participants' source of understanding COVID-19 information, communication, and social patterns at home and when going outside. As previously shown, percentage distributions for each question were then obtained.

As for the responses to open-ended questions, they were utilised to understand participants' reasons for encountering difficulties in understanding COVID-19 information, the nature of their indoor and outdoor activities, and the sources of negative emotions. The responses were categorised using a content-analysis approach (Hsieh and Shannon 2005) to quantify and analyse the presence, meanings, and relationships of certain words, themes, or concepts within the given responses.

To measure changes in social and communication patterns in PWAs and their psychosocial well-being over time, re-test interviews were conducted for 17 available participants between June to July 2020, before Hong Kong experienced its third wave of COVID-19. In other words, there was a lapse of two months after the initial interview, conducted between March and June 2020, after the second wave of infection. The same survey was conducted again except for sections (I) and (III). This allowed a longitudinal follow-up of these PWAs to investigate if they had suffered further social or communication complications.

## 11.4  Major findings

### 11.4.1  Participants' demographics

Age of diagnosis in the PWA group was evenly distributed between the age of 41 to 70 years across the three severity levels (Table 11.1). Most participants (75%) were aged between 51 and 70 years. Nearly half of the PWAs (46.5%) and caregivers (40%) fell into the "elderly" category. Around 65% of PWAs were males. Most caregivers were spouses. Concerning living and working status, most participants (>83%) across all three groups lived with their families. A wide range of occupations was also reported.

### 11.4.2  Understanding of COVID-19 information

The most popular means to receive information about COVID-19 (Table 11.2) was through television for all groups, followed by online resources amongst unimpaired speakers (22.7%) and family members/caregivers (19.2%). As for PWAs, both newspapers and online resources were equally popular (17.2%).

Regarding understanding of COVID-19 information (Table 11.3), PWAs demonstrated the highest mean of self-rated understanding (2.95/5) compared to unimpaired speakers (2.28/5) and caregivers (2.30/5). The results of an ANOVA indicated a significant main effect of group, $F(2,128)=8.50$, $p<0.001$. Post hoc multiple comparison analyses with Bonferroni adjustment further revealed a significantly higher score in the PWA group than both the unimpaired speaker and the caregiver groups ($p<.05$). Although PWAs had the highest self-rated score, more of them (i.e., 34.9%) indicated that they had encountered difficulties in comprehending the information compared to caregivers (12%) and unimpaired speakers (10.9%). Amongst participants who encountered difficulties, the majority of PWAs (66.7%) attributed the cause to difficulty in comprehension, whilst unimpaired speakers (42%) and caregivers (75%) expressed that they were overwhelmed by the amount and breadth of new information to process.

**TABLE 11.2** Summary of respondents' ways to receive information about COVID-19

| | # of respondents (%) | | | | | | | |
| --- | --- | --- | --- | --- | --- | --- | --- | --- |
| | Television | Radio | Newspaper | Internet | Self-help organisations | Families | Friends | Others |
| PWAs | 22 (23.7%) | 14 (15.0%) | 16 (17.2%) | 16 (17.2%) | 3 (3.2%) | 11 (11.8%) | 11 (11.8%) | 0 (0%) |
| Unimpaired speakers | 55 (27.8%) | 13 (6.6%) | 28 (14.1%) | 45 (22.7%) | 2 (1.0%) | 26 (13.1%) | 26 (13.1%) | 3 (1.4%) |
| Caregivers | 34 (33.0%) | 10 (9.6%) | 13 (12.5%) | 12 (11.5%) | 3 (2.9%) | 20 (19.2%) | 9 (8.7%) | 3 (2.9%) |

**TABLE 11.3** Summary of respondents' understanding of COVID-19

| | Score of understanding | Participants encountering difficulties | Reasons for encountering difficulties (%) | | | |
|---|---|---|---|---|---|---|
| | Mean (s.d.) | # of respondents (%) | Too much information to process | Unsure of information authenticity | Difficult to comprehend | Others |
| PWAs | 2.95/5 (1.05) | 15 (34.9%) | 6.7% | 6.7% | 66.7% | 20% |
| Unimpaired speakers | 2.28/5 (0.74) | 7 (10.9%) | 42% | 28.6% | 28.6% | 0% |
| Caregivers | 2.30/5 (0.75) | 3 (12%) | 75% | 25% | 0% | 0% |

## 11.4.3 Changes in social and communication pattern after COVID-19

In the first round of interviews, most participants (72.1% of PWAs; 88.9% of unimpaired speakers; 88.0% of caregivers) indicated that they had reduced going out after the outbreak (Table 11.4). Results of paired-sample $t$-tests comparing before and after the outbreak indicated a significant increase of number of days per week at home after the outbreak for PWAs [$t(42)=5.48$, $p<0.001$]; unimpaired speakers [$t(62)-6.29$, $p<0.001$]; and caregivers [$t(24)=3.84$, $p<0.001$].

Concerning activities carried out at home (Table 11.5), PWAs primarily spent time on home-based workouts and home entertainment in pre-outbreak times, whilst unimpaired speakers and caregivers mainly did household chores in addition to entertainment activities. These activities remained relatively consistent after the outbreak.

For activities outside home (Table 11.6), all participants indicated spending only minimal time (1–5 hours weekly) outdoors to carry out essential activities post-outbreak, even for the most common outdoor activities. Leisure activities (such as dining outside and leisure shopping) that were common before the outbreak were all dropped. PWAs typically spent time outside only for outdoor workouts and medical appointments. For unimpaired speakers and caregivers, they primarily went out for work and to buy groceries only. For unimpaired speakers, there was almost a doubling of participants who picked grocery buying as the most common outdoor activities after outbreak (44.4%) compared to 23.8% of them pre-outbreak. Fewer unimpaired speakers (22.2%) and caregivers (24%) indicated the need to go to work compared to pre-outbreak days.

Concerning participants' communication with families and friends (Table 11.7), there were no obvious changes in the communication pattern with families. As for staying connected with friends, the primary way to communicate changed from phone texting (i.e., SMS messaging) to phone talks for all three groups.

**TABLE 11.4** Respondents' reduction of going out under social distancing measures

| | Reduction of going out | No. of days/week at home Mean (s.d.) | |
| --- | --- | --- | --- |
| | # of respondents (%) | Pre-COVID-19 | Post-COVID-19 |
| PWAs | 31 (72.1%) | 2.35 (2.092) | 4.72 (2.622) |
| Unimpaired speakers | 56 (88.9%) | 2.54 (1.974) | 4.03 (2.321) |
| Caregivers | 22 (88.0%) | 2.40 (2.000) | 4.44 (2.162) |

**TABLE 11.5** Percentage changes of respondents' activities at home before and after COVID-19 outbreak

| | Activities of daily living | Exercise | Home entertainment | Household chores | Work | Others | Seldom stay at home |
| --- | --- | --- | --- | --- | --- | --- | --- |
| PWAs | 12.5% → 11.0% | 25.0% → 31.7% | 40.3% → 35.4% | 9.7% → 13.4% | 6.9% → 2.4% | 2.8% → 6.1% | 2.8% → 0% |
| Unimpaired speakers | 9.6% → 4.5% | 4.8% → 11.8% | 40.8% → 39.1% | 22.9% → 28.2% | 6.0% → 9.1% | 8.4% → 7.2% | 0% → 0% |
| Caregivers | 11.4% → 11.1% | 5.7% → 13.3% | 42.9% → 44.4% | 25.7% → 26.7% | 5.7% → 2.2% | 2.9% → 0% | 5.7% → → 2.2% |

**TABLE 11.6** Respondents' activities and numbers of hours spent outside home

*Most common outdoor activities and time spent (# of respondents, %)*

| | Pre-COVID-19 | Post-COVID-19 |
| --- | --- | --- |
| PWAs | Exercise (10, 23.3%) Dining (9, 20.9%) 6–10 hours (12; 27.9%) | Exercise (11, 25.6%) Medical appointment (10, 23.3%) 1–5 hours (23, 53.5%) |
| Unimpaired speakers | Work (19, 30.2%) Buy groceries (15, 23.8%) 6–10 hours (8; 33.3%) | Buy groceries (28, 44.4%) Work (14, 22.2%) 1–5 hours (28, 43.8%) |
| Caregivers | Work (9, 36.0%) 6–10 hours (8; 33.3%) | Buy groceries (8, 32.0%) Work (6, 24.0%) 1–5 hours (9, 37.5%) |

*Second most common outdoor activities and time spent (# of respondents, %)*

| | Pre-COVID-19 | Post-COVID-19 |
| --- | --- | --- |
| PWAs | Dinning (10, 23.3%) Exercise (9, 20.9%) Shopping (9, 20.9%) 1–5 hours (26, 60.5%) | Exercise (10, 23.3%) No activity (10, 23.3%) 1–5 hours (33, 76.7%) |

*(Continued)*

**TABLE 11.6** (Continued)

*Second most common outdoor activities and time spent (# of respondents, %)*

|  | Pre-COVID-19 | Post-COVID-19 |
| --- | --- | --- |
| Unimpaired speakers | Dining (16, 25.6%) Shopping (16, 25.6%) 1–5 hours (33, 51.6%) | Buy groceries (15, 23.8%) Dining (11, 17.5%) 1–5 hours (20, 83.3%) |
| Caregivers | Dining (7, 28%) Shopping (5, 20%) 1–5 hours (12, 50.0%) | Buy groceries (9, 36.0%) 1–5 hours (20, 73.4%) |

*Third most common outdoor activities and time spent (# of respondents, %)*

|  | Pre-COVID-19 | Post-COVID-19 |
| --- | --- | --- |
| PWAs | Dinning (10, 23.3%) Exercise (9, 20.9%) 1–5 hours (32, 74.4%) | No activity (22, 51.2%) 1–5 hours (39, 90.7%) |
| Unimpaired speakers | Dining (13, 20.6%) Exercise (11, 17.5%) 1–5 hours (47, 73.4%) | No activity (22, 51.2%) 1–5 hours (55, 85.9%) |
| Caregivers | Shopping (5, 20%) Exercise (4, 16%) Dining (4, 16%) 1–5 hours (19, 79.2%) | No activity (9, 36.0%) 1–5 hours (22, 91.7%) |

Moreover, all groups opted for face-to-face interaction over the options of email or video/online calls as their third most common method.

## 11.4.4 Psychological well-being

Amongst the six dimensions of psychological well-being across the three participant groups (Table 11.8), the ANOVA results indicated significant difference in environmental mastery [$F(2,128)=5.82$, $p<0.01$]. Results of post hoc multiple comparisons with Bonferroni adjustment further suggested that a significant difference existed between PWAs and unimpaired speakers ($p<0.01$).

## 11.4.5 Negative emotions

Amongst unimpaired speakers, 60.3% indicated feeling anxious, compared to 40% and 35.3% of caregivers and PWAs, respectively (Table 11.9). According to the results of an ANOVA, no significant difference was found for the three groups, $F(2,59)=0.55$, $p=0.58$. PWAs indicated anxiety related to several factors, with the most common reasons being uncertainty about the course of the pandemic (20%); contracting the disease (13.3%); and following social distancing orders (13.3%).

**TABLE 11.7** Respondents' change of communication pattern with families and with friends

| | Communication with families | | Communication with friends | |
|---|---|---|---|---|
| | Pre-COVID-19 | Post-COVID-19 | Pre-COVID-19 | Post-COVID-19 |
| *Most common method; # of respondents (%)* | | | | |
| | Face-to-face | Face-to-face | Phone SMS | Phone talk |
| PWAs | 33 (76.7%) | 31 (72.1%) | 15 (34.9%) | 15 (34.9%) |
| Unimpaired speakers | 50 (78.1) | 45 (70.3%) | 36 (56.3%) | 33 (51.6%) |
| Caregivers | 20 (86.3%) | 19 (79.2%) | 14 (58.3%) | 12 (50.0%) |
| *Second most common method; # of respondents (%)* | | | | |
| | Phone SMS | Phone SMS | Phone talk | Phone talk |
| PWAs | 17 (39.5%) | 17 (39.5%) | 12 (27.9%) | 12 (27.9%) |
| Unimpaired speakers | 33 (51/6%) | 33 (51.6%) | 23 (35.9%) | 25 (39.1%) |
| Caregivers | 12 (50.0%) | 15 (62.5%) | 10 (41.7%) | 13 (54.2%) |
| *Third most common method; # of respondents (%)* | | | | |
| | Phone talk | Phone talk | Phone talk / Face-to-face | Face-to-face |
| PWAs | 13 (30.2%) | 15 (34.9%) | 8 (18.6%) | 7 (16.3%) |
| Unimpaired speakers | 30 (46.9%) | 33 (51.6%) | 13 (20.3%) | 18 (28.1%) |
| Caregivers | 13 (54.2%) | 12 (50.0%) | 14 (58.3%) | 10 (41.7%) |

**TABLE 11.8**  Summary of respondents' self-rating scores for psychological well-being

|  | Ryff total* | Autotomy | Environmental mastery | Personal growth | Positive relationship | Purpose of life | Self-acceptance |
|---|---|---|---|---|---|---|---|
| PWAs |  |  |  |  |  |  |  |
| Mean | 111.88 | 18.98 | 18.19 | 18.74 | 20.91 | 17.40 | 17.67 |
| (s.d.) | 22.312 | 4.234 | 6.134 | 4.408 | 4.623 | 5.399 | 4.460 |
| Unimpaired speakers |  |  |  |  |  |  |  |
| Mean | 119.10 | 19.19 | 21.33 | 18.73 | 21.46 | 19.00 | 19.38 |
| (s.d.) | 15.788 | 3.922 | 3.844 | 3.385 | 4.047 | 3.902 | 3.929 |
| Caregivers |  |  |  |  |  |  |  |
| Mean | 116.66 | 19.64 | 19.20 | 20.32 | 21.56 | 18.84 | 19.20 |
| (s.d.) | 14.356 | 3.108 | 4.340 | 3.172 | 3.959 | 3.923 | 4.123 |

*Note:* * adapted based on Scale of Psychological Well-being (SPWB; Ryff 1989).

Few unimpaired speakers (2.4%) and no caregivers showed concerns about the new social distancing orders. Instead, fear of getting COVID-19 was the greatest concern, followed by caregivers' concerns about economic instability.

Concerning depression, nearly half of PWAs (41.9%) and unimpaired speakers (41.3%) felt depressed. This contrasted with only 28% of caregivers. Results of an ANOVA suggested no significant differences between the three groups, $F(2,48)=1.33$, $p=0.28$, who expanded upon different causes of their negative feelings. For PWAs, the effects of social distancing orders (36.8%) played the major role in causing depression. The immediate health concern of contracting the disease remained the primary source of depression amongst unimpaired speakers. As for caregivers, maintaining environmental hygiene, economic instability, and losing communication/rehabilitation opportunities equally (16.7%) accounted for depression.

Finally, most unimpaired speakers and caregivers indicated a sense of pressure, in contrast to a smaller proportion of PWAs. Results of an ANOVA also indicted a lack of significant differences for the average score of self-rated anxiety amongst the three groups, $F(2,63)=0.60$, $p=0.55$. Avoiding the violation of social distancing rules continued to be the strongest cause of feeling pressured amongst PWAs. Unimpaired speakers felt pressured largely by economic instability. Caregivers were troubled by a more diverse range of reasons: social distancing orders, contracting the disease, maintaining environmental hygiene, and getting protective equipment (e.g., face masks).

### 11.4.6 Longitudinal follow-up of PWAs after outbreak

All 17 re-tested PWAs encountered no difficulties in understanding COVID-19 information, and there was a slight increase of self-rating, from an average score of 3.41 to 3.59 (Table 11.10). As for sources for receiving information (Table 11.11), the top two ways remained television programmes and through family members. However, in the second interview, participants reported a wider range of options

**TABLE 11.9** Summary of respondents' negative emotions (i.e., anxiety, depression, and pressure) and reasons

| | Whether participants felt … | If yes, score of feeling … | For yes, % of reasons for feeling anxious | | | | | | | | | | | | |
| | Yes | | Contracting disease | Pandemic development | Social distancing order | Hygiene | Protective equipment | Economic instability | Sleep quality | Lifestyle | Communication /rehabilitation opportunity | Control of life | Political view | Taking care of families | Others |
| | # of respondents (%) | Mean (s.d.) | % | | | | | | | | | | | | |
| **Anxiety** | | | | | | | | | | | | | | | |
| PWAs | 14 (35.3%) | 2.79/5 (1.25) | 13.3 | 20.0 | 13.3 | 6.7 | 6.7 | 6.7 | 6.7 | – | – | – | – | – | 26.6 |
| Unimpaired speakers | 38 (60.3%) | 2.42/5 (1.27) | 43.9 | 17.1 | 2.4 | 7.3 | 4.9 | 12.2 | 2.4 | 4.9 | – | – | – | – | 4.8 |
| Caregivers | 10 (40.0%) | 2.40/5 (1.11) | 36.8 | 10.5 | – | 15.8 | 10.5 | 26.3 | – | – | – | – | – | – | – |
| **Depression** | | | | | | | | | | | | | | | |
| PWAs | 18 (41.9%) | 2.56/5 (0.856) | – | 13.6 | 31.8 | 13.6 | 4.5 | 9.1 | – | – | 9.1 | 4.5 | – | – | 13.6 |
| Unimpaired speakers | 26 (41.3%) | 2.08/5 (1.197) | 20.0 | 6.7 | 13.3 | 13.3 | – | 10.0 | 3.3 | 6.7 | 6.7 | 6.7 | – | – | 13.3 |
| Caregivers | 7 (28.0%) | 2.00/5 (0.816) | – | 8.3 | 8.3 | 16.7 | – | 16.7 | 8.3 | – | 16.7 | 8.3 | – | – | 16.7 |
| **Pressure** | | | | | | | | | | | | | | | |
| PWAs | 16 (37.2%) | 2.56/5 (1.031) | 12.5 | 18.8 | 25.0 | 18.8 | – | – | – | 6.3 | – | – | – | – | 18.8 |
| Unimpaired speakers | 37 (58.7%) | 2.27/5 (1.262) | 15.9 | 6.8 | 6.8 | – | 11.4 | 31.8 | 2.3 | – | 2.3 | 2.3 | 2.3 | 2.3 | – |
| Caregivers | 13 (52.0%) | 2.62/5 (1.044) | 17.6 | – | 23.5 | 17.6 | 17.6 | 11.8 | – | – | – | – | 5.9 | – | 5.9 |

TABLE 11.10 Changes of understanding information about COVID-19 in retested PWAs

|  |  | 1st interview | 2nd interview |
|---|---|---|---|
| Understanding about COVID-19: | Mean (s.d.) | 3.41/5 (1.06) | 3.59/5 (0.71) |
| Whether participants encountered difficulty | No | 82.4% (14/17) | 100% (17/17) |
|  | Yes | 5.9% (1/17) | 0% (0/17) |
| If yes, % of reason for encountering difficulty | Unsure of information authenticity | 33% (1/3) | – |
|  | Others | 67% (2/3) | – |

TABLE 11.11 Summary of how PWAs received information about COVID-19

|  | 1st interview | 2nd interview |
|---|---|---|
| Television | 30% (15/50) | 24.6% (14/57) |
| Radio | 8% (4/50) | 10.5% (6/57) |
| Newspaper | 14% (7/50) | 14.0% (8/57) |
| Internet | 14% (7/50) | 12.3% (7/57) |
| Self-help organisation | 4% (2/50) | 7.0% (4/57) |
| Family | 18% (9/50) | 17.5% (10/57) |
| Friends | 12% (6/50) | 10.5% (6/57) |
| Others | 0% (0/50) | 3.5% (2/57) |
|  |  | (i.e., elderly community centre; government organisations) |

to obtain information, such as from elderly community centres, government organisations (e.g., Department of Health), and self-help organisations.

Concerning social and communication patterns (Table 11.12), the number of PWAs who reduced going out remained the same (N=12). More participants had spent additional time outdoors (6–10 hours weekly) on their top two common activities. Whilst there were a wider range of tasks PWAs could do outside home, leisure activities appeared to be the most common for only a subset of them. No major changes in their communication pattern were identified, with both families and friends. As for the psychological well-being of PWAs (Table 11.13), the results of paired-sample $t$-tests suggested a further and significant decrease on the score of "environmental mastery" at the time of the second interview, $t(16)=2.70$, $p<0.05$.

Finally, concerning the negative emotion of anxiety (Table 11.14), paired-sample $t$-tests showed an insignificant increase in the self-ratings of PWAs [$t(9)=0.41$, $p=0.69$]. The causes of their worries turned from uncertainty about the course of pandemic (60%) into more immediate concerns about themselves, in terms of practicing social distancing orders (40%) and contracting the disease

**TABLE 11.12** PWAs' changes in social and communication patterns

|  | 1st interview | 2nd interview |
|---|---|---|
| Did reduce going out | 12/17 | 12/17 |
| Number of days/week at home Mean (s.d.) | 4.71 days (2.97) | 4.82 days (2.56) |
| Activities at home (# of respondents) |  |  |
| Activities of daily living | 3 | 4 |
| Exercise | 6 | 6 |
| Home entertainment | 12 | 10 |
| Household chores | 3 | 5 |
| Work | 1 | 1 |
| Activities carried out outdoors (%) |  |  |
| Most common activity | Buy groceries (35.3%) Medical appointment (17.6%) Dining (11.8%) | Buy groceries, dining (23.5%) Medical appointment (11.8%) Leisure activity (11.8%) |
| Time spent for most common activity | 1–5 hours/week (12/17) 6–10 hours/week (11.8%) | 1–5 hours/week (47.1%) 6–10 hours/week (35.3%) |
| 2nd common activity | No activity (29.4%) Exercise (23.5%) Medical appointment (23.5%) | Exercise (29.4%) Medical appointment (23.5%) |
| Time spent for 2nd common activity | 1–5 hours/week (9/17) 6–10 hours/week (1/17) | 1–5 hours/week (11/17) 6–10 hours/week (23.5%) |
| 3rd common activity | No activity (10/17) | No activity (35.3%) |
| Time spent for 3rd common activity | – | – |
| Communication method with family (%) |  |  |
| Most common method | Face-to-face (76.5%) | Face-to-face (64.7%) |
| 2nd common method | Phone SMS (47.1%) | Phone SMS (47.1%) |
| 3rd common method | Phone talk (41.2%) | Phone talk (41.2%) |
| Communication method with friends (%) |  |  |
| Most common method | Phone SMS (76.5%) | Phone SMS (47.1%) |
| 2nd common method | Phone talk (47.1%) | Phone talk (17.6%) |
| 3rd common method | Face-to-face (29.4%) | Face-to-face (11.8%) |

**TABLE 11.13** PWAs' changes in self-rating scores for psychological well-being

|  | Ruff total* | Autotomy | Environmental mastery | Personal growth | Positive relationship | Purpose of life | Self-acceptance |
|---|---|---|---|---|---|---|---|
| 1st interview |  |  |  |  |  |  |  |
| Mean | 117.24 | 19.06 | 20.12 | 18.82 | 21.59 | 18.59 | 19.06 |
| (s.d.) | (21.71) | (4.41) | (5.06) | (4.29) | (4.99) | (5.10) | (4.05) |
| 2nd interview |  |  |  |  |  |  |  |
| Mean | 114.12 | 17.29 | 18 | 19.65 | 20.82 | 18.65 | 18.71 |
| (s.d.) | (17.90) | (3.39) | (4.36) | (3.55) | (4.25) | (5.30) | (5.25) |

Note: *adapted based on Scale of Psychological Well-being (SPWB; Ryff 1989).

**TABLE 11.14** PWAs' changes in negative emotions

| | Whether participants felt ... | If yes, score of feeling ... (out of 5) | For yes, % of reasons for feeling anxious | | | | | | | | | | | | |
| | Yes # of respondents (%) | Mean (s.d.) | % Contracting disease | Pandemic development | Social distancing order | Hygiene | Protective equipment | Economic instability | Sleep quality | Lifestyle | Communication/ rehabilitation opportunity | Control of life | Political view | Taking care of families | Others |
|---|---|---|---|---|---|---|---|---|---|---|---|---|---|---|---|
| **Anxiety** | | | | | | | | | | | | | | | |
| 1st interview | 5/17 (29.4%) | 3.2 (1.48) | 20 | 60 | - | - | - | 20 | - | - | - | - | - | - | - |
| 2nd interview | 6/17 (35.3%) | 2.83 (1.47) | 30 | 10 | 40 | 10 | 10 | - | - | - | - | - | - | - | - |
| **Depression** | | | | | | | | | | | | | | | |
| 1st interview | 8/17 (41.7%) | 2.75 (1.04) | - | 20 | 40 | 20 | - | 10 | - | - | 10 | - | - | - | - |
| 2nd interview | 8/17 (41.7%) | 3 (0.93) | 18 | 18 | 18 | - | 9 | - | - | 18 | 9 | - | - | - | - |
| **Pressure** | | | | | | | | | | | | | | | |
| 1st interview | 9/17 (52.9%) | 2.78 (1.20) | 22 | 22 | 22 | 33 | - | - | - | - | - | - | - | - | - |
| 2nd interview | 12/17 (70.6%) | 2.08 (1.31) | 25 | 12.5 | - | 12.5 | 18.8 | - | - | - | 18.8 | 6.3 | - | 6.3 | - |

(30%). PWAs also displayed an insignificant increase in their mean score for depression, $t(14)=0.51$, $p=0.62$. Interestingly, sources of depression became more diverse. As for pressure that PWAs felt, there was an insignificant decrease in mean self-rating scores, $t(19)=1.24$, $p=0.23$. This seemed to contrast with an increase from about 50% to 70% (in the second interview) of PWAs indicating a sense of pressure. As service receivers, PWAs indicated that their source of pressure originated from concerns about their personal health, in addition to COVID-19's immediate effects on others' health and the environment.

## 11.5  Lessons learnt and implications

As one of the pioneer studies that explored the experiences of PWAs during the COVID-19 pandemic, our findings highlighted a variety of issues concerning how PWAs were navigating this evolving pandemic and its corresponding consequences.

Out of the three participant groups, PWAs demonstrated the highest self-rated understanding of information pertaining to the coronavirus. However, as participants were asked to further elaborate on whether and why they encountered difficulties, PWAs indicated the highest degree (66.7% of total) of self-reported difficulty comprehending these materials (Table 11.3). One possible explanation of this mismatch could be because PWAs had underestimated the amount and complexity of information related to COVID-19. Apart from the inherent impairments in processing linguistic information in various modes, there has been a paucity of aphasia-friendly materials in Chinese. The heavy reliance on television programmes among PWAs decreased their reception of knowledge about the pandemic because aphasia-friendly information is typically not available in this channel. This situation contrasted with most western countries where aphasia-friendly information geared to English-speaking PWAs started to emerge in online aphasia support groups (e.g., Aphasia Center of California 2019). This significant gap between PWAs' need for and accessibility to information in Hong Kong (and possibly other countries in the east) should be addressed.

Consistent across the three participant groups, our respondents demonstrated a sudden and dramatic change in their social and communication patterns since COVID-19 was first reported in January 2020. First, all respondents indicated a significant decrease of time spent outdoors after the second wave of COVID-19 in March 2020. Citizens in Hong Kong have generally been cautious and diligently practiced social distancing. This could be the result of relatively unified responses on taking precautions and measures to reduce the risk of infection (Information Services Department 2020b) after the city's previous experience with the outbreak of severe acute respiratory syndrome (SARS) (Department of Health 2003). Second, all three groups were consistent in the activities that were conducted at home post-outbreak. This included the engagement of PWAs in household chores to maintain better environmental hygiene to prevent the spread of virus, as well as unimpaired speakers' and caregivers' report of doing regular (and in most cases more) workouts and fitting more physical activities into life to keep healthy.

Third, participants showed changes in the pattern and amount of time spent in outdoor activities. After the outbreak, PWAs spent time outdoors mainly for health-related activities whilst unimpaired speakers only maintained minimal essential activities. The decrease in time for work outdoors amongst unimpaired speakers and caregivers might also be the result of the new work-from-home arrangements or, in some cases, the loss of jobs during the economic crisis. This observation did not seem to deviate from reports from overseas (Phillips et al. 2020). Lastly, all three groups indicated changes in the ways they communicated with friends during the pandemic, but not with immediate family members (i.e., face-to-face interactions). Specifically, to stay connected with friends, there was a commonly reported switch to phone conversations from phone messaging/ texting because the former was more interactive. Although in-person meetings were discouraged during the pandemic, this mode of interaction was still reported as the third most common communication method across all three groups. This preference could possibly be related to the less interactive nature of email and lower familiarity with video/online call methods amongst the participants. These findings highlighted the importance of keeping PWAs "physically distant but socially connected" (Ellis and Jacobs 2021).

Regarding the psychological well-being of participants and negative emotions they experienced, PWAs had significantly lower scores in the dimension of "environmental mastery" of the adapted SPWB than their unimpaired counterparts. This finding in the context of a pandemic echoes with Cruice et al. (2011), who reported that the psychological well-being of PWAs is statistically similar to that of the unaffected population, except for a lower degree of environmental mastery and a more negative mood. In other words, the demands of daily life during the pandemic have exerted on PWAs a feeling of loss of control over life activities. In fact, compared with unimpaired individuals (Otu et al. 2020), it was not unexpected that PWAs felt significantly less capable of joining social activities (in a pre-existing state of social isolation due to aphasia) and of building a life and environment that they enjoy (which could have caused even more emotional distress). More importantly, our findings further support the conclusions of Pisano et al. (2020) that PWAs are more affected by (instead of spared from) the pandemic and show more deterioration of their emotional state and communication skills.

Unlike the other two groups in the study, PWAs showed concerns that contributed to their perceived negative emotions during the pandemic. "Social distancing orders" remained their most (or second most) mentioned reason across the three negative emotions, further explaining the association between these measures and the lower environmental mastery of PWAs during the pandemic. For unimpaired speakers and caregivers, their anxiety and pressure were mostly caused by concerns about immediate health hazards (i.e., contracting the disease) and economic instability, respectively. Under the Prevention and Control of Disease (Requirements and Directions) (Business and Premises) Regulation (Hong Kong e-Legislation 2020b), many restaurants and entertainment venues (e.g., karaoke boxes and gyms) were temporarily closed or only provided limited services. There was also a reduction of work hours and/or reduced household income amongst non-PWA respondents.

Caregivers put forward multiple reasons for their feelings of anxiety, depression, and pressure. Besides being worried about economic instability, contracting the disease, and maintaining social distancing orders, they were also concerned about the lack of protective equipment supply (especially at the beginning of the outbreak), environmental hygiene, and their loved ones' loss of rehabilitation services and opportunities for communication. According to the Department of Health (2020), purchase of protective equipment, cleaning products, and other household necessities resulted in great psychological distress during the outbreak. The finding about maintaining environmental hygiene echoes with Nätterlund (2010), who highlighted caregivers' tendency to be emotionally distressed by domestic duties and household labour. As the carer and major communication partner of PWAs, caregivers were also concerned about the suspension of rehabilitation services and decreased social participation of PWAs under various public health measures.

Finally, as we monitored changes in our PWAs on two occasions approximately two months apart during the pandemic, several interesting observations were identified. During the second interview:

1) PWAs showed an increased self-rated understanding of information related to COVID-19, possibly as a result of accumulated information and life experience after months of outbreaks. Related to this was PWAs' shift of reported reasons for their anxiety away from uncertainty about pandemic development (60%) at the first interview to social distancing orders (40%) and contracting the disease (30%) at the second interview.

2) Even with more lenient social distancing orders in place intermittently (and therefore a report of more diverse types of outdoor activities), most PWAs still chose to stay home.

3) Concerning changes in psychological well-being and negative emotions, "environmental mastery" remained the only significant (and diminished) dimension. Prolonged restrictions of social and communication opportunities might have continued to worsen PWAs' feeling of autonomy and their ability to take back control of their lives (Cruice et al. 2011).

4) Relative to negative emotions of depression and pressure, social distancing orders were no longer the major concern. It is likely that this was because precautious and measures had become more lenient in June and July 2020 as the second outbreak improved.

5) Some PWAs reported that they had adjusted to or at least had started to be familiar with the new mode of digital therapy delivery. However, this might have also created additional anxieties due to potential technology accessibility barriers.

## 11.6 Summary

The present investigation identified decreased opportunities for PWAs to communicate and to receive rehabilitation services during the COVID-19 pandemic. The psychosocial burdens in PWAs and their caregivers resulting from COVID-19 remain a major concern. Further studies are needed to address the current knowledge gap regarding short- and long-term impacts of the pandemic on PWAs (Kong 2021b). Moreover, in the wake of the pandemic, it may be a suitable time to review, evaluate, and even reshape our future clinical services for aphasia. This may include the use of digital technologies to improve remote care or to supplement face-to-face social activities (Kong 2021c). Finally, support of psychosocial and communication needs of PWAs in a pandemic can be globally similar, but how it should be implemented will require more careful considerations that are not fully discussed in the literature.

## References

Aphasia Center of California. (2019). Aphasia-friendly emergency kit information. www.aphasiacenter.net/aphasia friendly-emergency-kit-information/. Accessed 12 December 2021.

Brandenburg, C., Worrall, L., Rodriguez, A., & Copland, D. (2013). Mobile computing technology and aphasia: An integrated review of accessibility and potential uses. *Aphasiology*, 27(4), 444–461.

Bronken, B., Kirkevold, M., Martinsen, R., Wyller, T., & Kvigne, K. (2012). Psychosocial well-being in persons with aphasia. *Nursing Research and Practice*, 2012, 568242. https://doi.org/10.1155/2012/568242.

Brooks, S., Webster, R., Smith, L., Woodland, L., Wessely, S., Greenberg, N., et al. (2020). The psychological impact of quarantine and how to reduce it: Rapid review of the evidence. *Lancet*, 395(10227), 912–920.

Bury, M. (1982). Chronic illness as biographical disruption. *Sociology of Health and Illness*, 4(2), 167–182.

Code, C., & Herrmann, M. (2003). The relevance of emotional and psychosocial factors in aphasia to rehabilitation. *Neuropsychological Rehabilitation*, 13(1), 109–132.

Cruice, M., Worrall, L., & Hickson, L. (2011). Reporting on psychological well-being of older adults with chronic aphasia in the context of unaffected peers. *Disability and Rehabilitation,* 33(3), 219–228.

Davidson, B., Worrall, L., & Hickson, L. (2003). Identifying the communication activities of older people with aphasia: Evidence from naturalistic observation. *Aphasiology*, 17, 243–264.

Department of Health (2003). Outbreak of Severe Acute Respiratory Syndrome (SARS) at Amoy Gardens, Kowloon Bay, Hong Kong: Main findings of the investigation. www.info.gov.hk/info/sars/pdf/amoy_e.pdf. Accessed 12 December 2021.

Department of Health (2020). Fight the virus with peace of mind: Psychological adjustments to the COVID-19 outbreak. www.elderly.gov.hk/english/healthy_ageing/mental_health/covid_19.html. Accessed 12 December 2021.

Ellis, C., & Jacobs, M. (2021). The cost of social distancing for persons with aphasia during COVID-19: A need for social connectedness. *Journal of Patient Experience*, 8, 1–3.

García-Portilla, P., de la Fuente Tomás, L., Bobes-Bascarán, T., Jiménez-Treviño, L., Zurrón-Madera, P., Suárez-Álvarez, M., et al. (2020). Are older adults also at higher psychological risk from COVID-19? *Aging & Mental Health*, 25(7), 1297–1304.

Giebel, G., Cannon, J., Hanna, K., Butchard, S., Eley, R., Gaughan, A., et al. (2020). Impact of COVID-19 related social support service closures on people with dementia and unpaid carers: A qualitative study. *Aging & Mental Health*, 25(7), 1281–1288.

Hong Kong e-Legislation (2020a). Cap. 599G Prevention and control of disease (Prohibition on group gathering) regulation. www.elegislation.gov.hk/hk/cap599G!en-zh-Hant-HK?INDEX_CS=N. Accessed 12 December 2021.

Hong Kong e-Legislation (2020b). Cap. 599F Prevention and control of disease (Requirements and directions) (Business and premises) regulation. www.elegislation.gov.hk/hk/cap599F!en?INDEX_CS=N. Accessed 12 December 2021.

Hsieh, H., & Shannon, S. (2005). Three approaches to qualitative content analysis. *Qualitative Health Research*, 15(9), 1277–1288.

Information Services Department (2020a). Gov't staff to work from home. www.news.gov.hk/eng/2020/01/20200128/20200128_114401_545.html. Accessed 12 December 2021.

Information Services Department (2020b). New preventive measures set. www.news.gov.hk/eng/2020/01/20200120/20200120_192835_870.html?type=category&name=covid19&tl=t. Accessed 12 December 2021.

Jordan, R., & Adap, P. (2020). Covid-19: Risk factors for severe disease and death. *BMJ*, 368, 1198. doi:10.1136/bmj.m1198.

Kasai, T. (2020). From the "new normal" to a "new future": A sustainable response to COVID-19. *Lancet Regional Health Western Pacific*, 4, 100043. doi:10.1016/j.lanwpc.2020.100043.

Kong, A. (2016). *Analysis of neurogenic disordered discourse production: From theory to practice*. London: Routledge.

Kong, A. (2021a). The impact of COVID-19 on speakers with aphasia: What is currently known and missing? *Journal of Speech, Language, and Hearing Research*, 64(1), 176–180.

Kong, A. (2021b). COVID-19 and aphasia. *Current Neurology and Neuroscience Reports*, 21, 61. https://doi.org/10.1007/s11910-021-01150-x.

Kong, A. (2021c). Mental health of persons with aphasia during the COVID-19 pandemic: Challenges and opportunities for addressing emotional distress. *Open Journal of Social Sciences*, 9(5), 562–569.

Lavrakas, P. (2008). *Encyclopedia of survey research methods*. Thousand Oaks, CA: Sage Publications, Inc.

Lee, H., Lee, Y., Choi, H., & Pyun, S.-B. (2015). Community integration and quality of life in aphasia after stroke. *Yonsei Medical Journal*, 56(6), 1694–1702.

Nätterlund, B. (2010). Being a close relative of a person with aphasia. *Scandinavian Journal of Occupational Therapy*, 17(1), 18–28.

Otu, A., Charles, C., & Yaya, S. (2020). Mental health and psychosocial well-being during the COVID-19 pandemic: The invisible elephant in the room. *International Journal of Mental Health Systems*, 14, 38. https://doi.org/10.1186/s13033-020-00371-w.

Parr, S. (2004). *Living with severe aphasia: The experience of communication impairment after stroke*. York: Pavilion Publishing (Brighton) Ltd.

Phillips, D., Paul, G., Fahy, M., Dowling-Hetherington, L., Kroll, T., Moloney, B., Duffy, C., Fealy, G., & Lafferty, A. (2020). The invisible workforce during the COVID-19 pandemic: Family carers at the frontline. *HRB Open Research*, 3, 24. doi:10.12688/hrbopenres.13059.1.

Pisano, F., Giachero, A., Rugiero, C., Calati, M., & Marangolo, P. (2020). Does COVID-19 impact less on post-stroke aphasia? This is not the case. *Frontiers in Psychology*, 11, 564717. doi:10.3389/fpsyg.2020.564717.

Roach, P., Zwiers, A., Cox, E., Fischer, K., Charlton, A., Josephson, C., et al. (2021). Understanding the impact of the COVID-19 pandemic on well-being and virtual care for people living with dementia and care partners living in the community. *Dementia*, 20(6), 2007–2023.

Royal College of Speech and Language Therapists (2020). Improving stroke care: The impact of COVID-19 present and future. www.rcslt.org/-/media/docs/RCSLT-Webinar_-Improving-Stroke-Care_V7-21-July.pdf?la=en&hash=94355159156F518F 0F6076D23A6C319BD9DC9090. Accessed 12 December 2021.

Ryff, C. (1989). Happiness is everything, or is it? Explorations on the meaning of psychological well-being. *Journal of Personality and Social Psychology*, 57(6), 1069–1081.

Vernooij-Dassen, M., & Jeon, Y.-H. (2016). Social health and dementia: The power of human capabilities. *International Psychogeriatrics*, 28(5), 701–703.

Ward, R., Clark, A., Campbell, S., Graham, B., Kullberg, A., Manji, K., et al. (2018). The lived neighbourhood: Understanding how people with dementia engage with their local environment. *International Psychogeriatrics*, 30(6), 867–880.

World Health Organization (2020). WHO Director-General's opening remarks at the media briefing on COVID-19–11 March 2020. www.who.int/director-general/speeches/detail/who-director-general-s-opening-remarks-at-the-media-briefing-on-covid-19–11-march-2020. Accessed 12 December 2021.

Worrall, L., Simmons-Mackie, N., Wallace, S., Rose, T., Brady, M., Kong, A., et al. (2016). Let's call it "aphasia": Rationales for eliminating the term "dysphasia." *International Journal of Stroke*, 11(8), 848–851.

# 12

# THE IMPACT OF COVID-19 ON EDUCATION AND TRAINING IN SPEECH-LANGUAGE PATHOLOGY

*Janet Ho-yee Ng*

## 12.1 Introduction

On 31 December 2019, the Wuhan Municipal Health Commission in Wuhan, the capital of Hubei Province of China, reported a cluster of viral pneumonia cases of unknown cause (World Health Organization 2021). The outbreak of the novel coronavirus disease, which was subsequently named COVID-19, took the world by shock. As the COVID-19 outbreak soon developed into a global pandemic, governments worldwide implemented various measures aimed at virus containment, including mandatory mask wearing, school and business closures, restrictions on gatherings, domestic movement restrictions, and international travel restrictions. These public health and social measures have undoubtedly served to limit the spread of the virus. However, they have also affected regular teaching and learning activities in speech-language pathology education.

This chapter explores the impact of COVID-19 on education and training in speech-language pathology. It examines this impact from the perspective of standards in the speech-language pathology profession, lessons that have been learnt from a previous coronavirus disease outbreak, and disruption to and transition in clinical education during the COVID-19 pandemic. Implications of the pandemic for capacity building of educators will also be discussed. Although there is much that we still do not know about the impact of the pandemic on speech-language pathology education, this chapter attempts to draw some preliminary conclusions by examining the impact of the pandemic through the lens of an entry-level master's programme in Hong Kong.

DOI: 10.4324/9781003257318-12

## 12.2 Standards of education and training in speech-language pathology

Training of speech-language pathologists in most industrialised countries takes place in the form of undergraduate or postgraduate education at tertiary institutions. Graduates from accredited education programmes are qualified to practice as speech-language pathologists upon graduation or after completion of additional clinical examinations or fellowships. Whilst the content of curricula can vary, standards of education and training are applied nationally by either statutory regulators or professional bodies. The Health and Care Professions Council in the United Kingdom specifies that "practice-based learning must be integral to the programme" (Health and Care Professions Council 2017, p. 8), whilst Speech Pathology Australia requires education programmes to demonstrate that students have achieved Entry Level competency as defined by their Competency-based Occupational Standards (Speech Pathology Australia 2017, 2019).

Some standards also indicate specific clock hours of supervised clinical practice during study. The national accreditation body in the United States requires entry-level master's programmes in speech-language pathology to provide each student with a minimum of 400 hours of clinical practicum (Council on Academic Accreditation in Audiology and Speech-Language Pathology 2020), whilst the Canadian national coalition of regulators stipulates 350 hours as the minimum clinical practicum component (Canadian Alliance of Audiologists and Speech-Language Pathologists Regulators 2021). The accredited registration system in Hong Kong generally follows the Australian outcome-based standards on Entry Level competency and specifies that 300 hours is the minimum clinical practicum requirement (Hong Kong Institute of Speech Therapists 2017, 2019).

Deemed the most severe education disruption in global history, COVID-19 put more than 1.6 billion learners from over 190 countries out of school at the peak of the pandemic (United Nations Educational Scientific and Cultural Organization 2021). Schools at all levels, including higher education institutions, have been affected by the pandemic. According to a survey conducted by an international non-governmental association serving the global higher education community, 59% of higher education institutions amongst respondents from 109 countries reported cessation of all campus activities in March to April 2020. The majority replaced face-to-face classroom teaching by distance teaching, and many planned to conduct examinations through new measures (Marinoni et al. 2020).

The COVID-19 pandemic deprived medical students of the opportunity to take part in many educational experiences, with thousands of senior students in Europe and North America missing months of training and graduating early to provide extra support to healthcare systems (Gill et al. 2020). A cross-sectional study explored medical students' perception of online teaching during COVID-19 in the United Kingdom. Some 2,721 respondents from 39 medical schools nationwide agreed that online teaching could provide flexibility and save time, yet family distractions and internet connection problems appeared to be obstacles to effective online teaching (Dost et al. 2020). Most medical students in the study also felt that online teaching could not replace clinical teaching through direct patient contact and that practical clinical skills could not be learnt through online teaching. A similar study reported that allied health undergraduates generally found online learning to be convenient and to save time, yet most of them had a negative perception towards online learning for practical and clinical-based subjects (Chandrasiri and Weerakoon 2021).

Whilst the COVID-19 pandemic has undoubtedly disrupted speech-language pathology education, the global community of speech-language pathology educators and stakeholders did not allow it to compromise the education and training of entry-level speech-language pathologists. In view of the responsibility to assure the clinical competency of graduates to fulfil their healthcare and education roles upon graduation, the American accreditation body stated that 400 hours of clinical practicum were to be maintained for postgraduate speech-language pathology programmes (Council on Academic Accreditation in Audiology and Speech-Language Pathology 2021). Clinical hours obtained through telepractice are treated as supervised clinical practicum hours and could be counted towards the required hours of students. Limits on supervised clinical hours obtained through clinical simulation remained the same, with clinical simulation capped at 75 hours and guided observation utilising video recordings capped at 25 hours.

During the COVID-19 pandemic, accreditation site visits for speech-language pathology education programmes have been conducted as virtual site visits. In Hong Kong, despite the establishment of the first entry-level undergraduate programme in speech-language pathology in 1988, the accreditation of local speech-language pathology education programmes did not start until 2018, following the introduction of the accredited registers scheme administered by the government. The COVID-19 pandemic did not prevent local accreditation development. The Hong Kong Institute of Speech Therapists maintained 300 hours as the minimum clinical practicum requirement for entry-level speech-language pathology education programmes, and an accreditation site visit by a panel of overseas and local reviewers for a new speech-language pathology education programme was completed virtually and on schedule in 2020.

The United Kingdom adopted a slightly different approach to maintain entry-level standards. Allied health students in their final years who had completed all clinical placements, or who had demonstrated by their respective universities that the same learning had been achieved, were put on a COVID-19 temporary register by the Health and Care Professions Council (National Health Service 2020). This arrangement allowed final-year students to support the allied health workforce by taking up employment during this time of emergency and prior to graduating. These final-year students could return to their study later or concurrently practise and complete the remaining elements of their academic programmes during the pandemic. They could then join the full register once they fulfilled graduation requirements. Taking up employment through this temporary registration arrangement is voluntary. Allied health students who opt out from temporary registration could explore alternative progression options with their respective universities, such as continuing with their academic studies through different means and taking an authorised break in studies.

## 12.3 Learning from the SARS experience

COVID-19 is not the first infectious disease outbreak to disrupt medical and allied health education. SARS-CoV-2 (the virus that causes COVID-19) is genetically closely related to SARS-CoV (Petersen et al. 2020), and so it is relevant to review the experience of the Severe Acute Respiratory Syndrome (SARS) outbreak in 2003. On 11 February 2003, the Guangdong Health Bureau reported 305 cases of atypical pneumonia of unknown cause in the Guangdong province of China. A third of cases were in health workers who contracted the disease whilst delivering health services (World Health Organization 2006). SARS spread to Hong Kong in February 2003. The World Health Organization issued the first global alert about the virus on 12 March 2003. The outbreak came to an end by 5 July 2003, when all known chains of human transmission of the virus were declared broken. By that stage, there had been 8,098 confirmed cases and 774 deaths in 29 countries and areas. Hong Kong had won the battle against SARS in four months with contact tracing, medical surveillance and quarantine, and port health measures (Tsang and Lam 2003).

SARS alarmed medical and allied health professions in Hong Kong when the first outbreak occurred in a teaching hospital, impacting a large number of hospital staff and medical students (Lee 2003). With the transmission of SARS to medical students subsequent to bedside teaching in hospital wards, both medical schools in Hong Kong ordered the suspension of clinical teaching on 18 March 2003 (Patil and Yan 2003). The authorities later also ordered the closure of primary schools, secondary schools, and universities. Although the availability of online teaching and learning platforms was limited at that time, medical teaching was nevertheless achieved by making narrated PowerPoint available on university websites. Canada's medical education was also impacted by SARS, with some clinical methods skills teaching suspended and clerkships either cancelled or reduced (Rieder et al. 2004). In 2003, there was only one speech-language pathology education programme in Hong Kong. The SARS outbreak brought premature termination of hospital placements for students on this programme.

Notwithstanding the adverse health, social, and economic consequences of SARS, the pandemic served to raise awareness and shape the response of Hong Kong to infectious disease. A case-control study investigating precautions against nosocomial transmission of SARS in Hong Kong found that hospital staff who used masks, gowns, and handwashing appeared less likely to develop SARS after exposure to index patients. The use of surgical masks and N95 masks instead of paper masks significantly reduced the risk of infection (Seto et al. 2003). Another case-control study examining the transmission of SARS amongst hospital workers in Hong Kong further identified that the risk of SARS infection was significantly associated with inconsistent use of personal protection equipment (PPE), perceived inadequate supply of PPE, and inadequate training or knowledge of infection control measures (Lau et al. 2004). A study found that significantly more medical students washed their hands before and after physical examinations and wore masks during history taking and physical examinations one year after the SARS epidemic in Hong Kong than before the epidemic (Wong and Tam 2005).

The SARS outbreak in Hong Kong highlighted the critical need to control the spread of infectious diseases, particularly nosocomial infection. The Centre for Health Protection, a professional arm of the Department of Health, was established in June 2004 with the purpose of preventing and controlling diseases in Hong Kong. At the administration level, the Hong Kong government developed a three-tier plan, with corresponding command structures for Alert, Serious and Emergency response levels in connection with the World Health Organization's call to strengthen the readiness to combat potential novel infectious diseases (Food and Health Bureau 2020). At the hospital level, enhanced isolation facilities, establishment of negative pressure rooms, designated gowning and degowning areas, and provision of sanitary facilities were put in place to prepare for outbreaks of infectious disease. In addition, infection control training has been enhanced in medical and allied health teaching curricula in Hong Kong. For instance, the Hong Kong Training Portal on Infection Control and Infectious Diseases was convened in 2009 to provide infection control training to healthcare and related professionals. The Hospital Authority, a statutory body managing all 43 public hospitals in Hong Kong, requires all allied health students to complete infection control training with specified content prior to their hospital placements.

## 12.4 An era of unforeseen COVID-19 disruptions

The COVID-19 pandemic has undeniably disrupted speech-language pathology education programmes worldwide. In Hong Kong, all four entry-level speech-language pathology education programmes, regardless of bachelor's or master's levels, include clinical placements at Hospital Authority hospitals as part of their clinical education. As a collaborative practice, each of the four local universities arrange hospital placements at different times of the year to facilitate manpower and service planning of hospitals. This section provides a narrative account of the disruption caused by COVID-19 to hospital placements in 2020 as the crisis unfolded.

In view of the geographical proximity of Hong Kong to Mainland China and the high volume of cross-border travellers passing daily through land, sea, and air control points, the Hong Kong government activated the Serious response level for infectious disease on 4 January 2020. This was soon after the report of a cluster of novel viral pneumonia cases in Wuhan. Under the Serious response level, hand hygiene and surgical masks were required for all visitors in patient areas of hospitals. Clinical placement in hospitals was allowed except for high-risk areas. In a regular clinical placement liaison meeting between the Hospital Authority and all local speech-language pathology education programmes on 22 January 2020, universities were reminded that surgical masks and standard precautions, with transmission-based precautions where appropriate, should apply during routine patient care in hospitals. Additionally, the use of N95 respirators, eye protection, gowns, gloves, and caps (optional) should be adopted during aerosol-generating procedures. The list of N95 respirators commonly available in hospitals had been distributed. Universities were told to arrange N95 fit tests and maintain test records for speech-language pathology students before allowing them to be involved in aerosol-generating procedures, including tracheal suctioning during swallowing assessment.

Soon after the confirmation of the first two imported COVID-19 cases on 23 January 2020, the Hong Kong government activated the Emergency response level for infectious disease on 25 January 2020. The corresponding measures of the Emergency response level were a heavy blow to clinical education. All hospital placements were suspended. Hong Kong's first COVID-19 wave occurred between late January to mid-February in 2020. It was of much smaller scale and shorter duration than subsequent waves (Liu et al. 2021). The second wave commenced in mid-March. It reached a peak of 65 daily cases reported on 27 March 2020, followed by a gradual decrease of daily cases (Lam et al. 2020). In view of the improved local COVID-19 situation, the Hospital Authority and universities organised an ad hoc meeting on 21 April 2020 to discuss plans to resume hospital placements gradually in May 2020 to allow speech-language pathology students to catch up with the minimum clinical practicum hours required for graduation. It was the consensus of all parties that hospital placements amongst universities would be prioritised according to intended graduation dates. No training in high-risk areas or on high-risk procedures would be arranged for speech-language pathology students, and students should adhere to all infection control guidelines in addition to completing infection control refresher training.

Hospital placements finally resumed from 10 June 2020. Originally planned placements for students from The University of Hong Kong and The Chinese University of Hong Kong were shortened. After repeated negotiations, hospital placements for students from The Hong Kong Polytechnic University were rescheduled from May–July 2020 to 20 July–4 September 2020. However, just five days before the commencement of hospital placements, they were postponed again due to the arrival of the third wave of COVID-19 in Hong Kong. The Hospital Authority halted all clinical placements at hospitals from 17 July 2020 for at least four weeks to reduce the flow of people in hospitals and to minimise infection control risk. The suspension of clinical placements at Hospital Authority hospitals was extended twice in August 2020. Hospital placements of

**TABLE 12.1** Standards of disposable PPE for speech-language pathology students' hospital placements during COVID-19 (ASTM refers to ASTM International, formerly known as American Society for Testing and Materials; AAMI refers to Association for the Advancement of Medical Instrumentation)

| Type of PPE | Minimum requirements |
| --- | --- |
| Surgical mask | • Comply with ASTM Level 1 standard *or above* |
| Face shield | • Full face covering |
| | • Enable concurrent use of surgical mask, N95 respirator, eyeglasses, or goggles |
| | • Anti-fog |
| | • Comply with ASTM D2457–13 standard (desirable) |
| Isolation gown | • Comply with AAMI PB70 Level 1 or EN 13795 standard *or above* |
| | • The entire gown, including the seams but excluding the cuffs, hems, and bindings, shall achieve claimed barrier performance |
| | • Full back coverage design with Velcro neck closure and waist ties to secure the coverage |
| | • Available in different sizes (desirable) |

all professional-grade students were eventually permitted to restart from 14 September 2020. Students from The Hong Kong Polytechnic University were able to complete a condensed hospital practicum during September–October 2020 within the final semester of their studies. Students at The Education University of Hong Kong experienced less disruption in 2020, as their hospital placements were mainly scheduled between the third and fourth waves of COVID-19 in Hong Kong.

When large-scale COVID outbreaks were observed in many countries in February 2020, the demand for PPE dramatically increased. Together with supply chain disruption, this constituted another crisis of global concern. The World Health Organization accordingly recommended the rationalised and appropriate use of PPE based on the risk of exposure (World Health Organization 2020a). Locally in Hong Kong, in addition to a global procurement approach and prudent use of PPE by hospital staff (Hospital Authority 2021), the Hospital Authority also reached out to a local university to spearhead the design and 3D printing of face shields to ensure stable local supply during this critical time (Han 2020). With an insufficient stockpile of PPE at hospitals, the Hospital Authority requested universities to provide up-to-standard PPE to speech-language pathology students. Table 12.1 illustrates the standards of different types of PPE for students' hospital placements during COVID-19.

## 12.5 Rapid transition of clinical teaching and learning

The impact of COVID-19 on speech-language pathology education is still unclear as the duration of the pandemic remains uncertain. From previous experience of SARS, it is reasonable to assume that some changes in clinical practice and professional education will last beyond the end of the pandemic. The education and training of speech-language pathologists worldwide might be affected by the pandemic to varying extents depending on curriculum design, cohort size and staff ratio. As the COVID-19 pandemic has evolved, speech-language pathology educators from around the world have attempted to innovate by devising methods for students to engage in learning and meet prescribed entry-level standards. This section explores the transition of speech-language pathology education through telepractice and simulation from the perspective of an educator in Hong Kong.

## 12.5.1 Telepractice

Shortly after the emergence of confirmed COVID-19 cases in Hong Kong, the novel coronavirus outbreak was declared a public health emergency of international concern on 30 January 2020 (World Health Organization 2020b). Although the scale and duration of the COVID-19 pandemic were not yet known, the Hong Kong government's announcement to temporarily close schools and the Hospital Authority's decision to suspend all hospital placements in late January put an immediate stop to clinical placements of speech-language pathology students in the territory. The anxiety associated with the progression of students amongst speech-language pathology educators across universities in Hong Kong was further amplified by service suspension of all early education and rehabilitative facilities. To minimise the negative influence on the speech-language pathology workforce, teaching teams at local universities decided to take a bold step and replace face-to-face therapy with telepractice for both adult and paediatric clinical placements.

This was not an easy transition for speech-language pathology educators to make. A study exploring telepractice in Hong Kong found that although speech-language pathologists in pre-school, mainstream and special schools, hospitals, private clinics, nursing homes, and university settings all engaged in telepractice, over 72% of them had only started telepractice in the past three months (Fong et al. 2021). The survey results indicated that telepractice was not only new to practising speech-language pathologists but also to speech-language pathology educators.

In response to COVID-19, our teaching team managed to quickly shift clinical placements to online delivery across a range of practice areas, including paediatric speech and language disorders, adult neurogenic communication disorders, reading and writing disorders, fluency disorder, voice disorder and dysphagia. Telepractice was largely delivered using Zoom, although Skype, WhatsApp Call, and WeChat Call were also possible options for clients. The availability of different online meeting platforms and the provision of written telepractice instructions to clients were found to be crucial for catering for individual circumstances and for enabling successful service delivery. Speech-language pathology students were also engaged in delivering parent-child interaction training for young children over the internet. Qualitative remarks from students revealed that telepractice offered them unique opportunities to consider an indirect treatment approach in addition to a conventional direct treatment approach (Ng et al. 2021). Positive experiences were also shared by university educators who pioneered the development of dysphagia clinical placements via telepractice with the support of old age homes in the community.

The implementation of telepractice in clinical placements at The Hong Kong Polytechnic University started with educator training, followed by student training. The training not only covered the rationale and procedures of telepractice but also included details on telesupervision provided by clinical educators. When clients were approached to participate in online speech-language pathology sessions in 2020, the response from parents of the paediatric population was overwhelmingly positive although most of them had never participated or even heard of telepractice. The enthusiastic response was likely related to the availability of parents due to the work-from-home arrangement and the desire of children to engage in live interactive therapy sessions when many kindergartens and primary schools could only deliver remote teaching through asynchronous mode.

A local study investigating perceptions of telepractice amongst parents of school-age children and speech-language pathology students during the COVID-19 pandemic found that parents were satisfied with speech-language pathology telepractice and its efficacy, yet they preferred in-person service to telepractice. On the contrary, speech-language pathology students expressed satisfaction with telepractice, and they did not show preference for either of the two service delivery modes (Lam et al. 2021). A client survey conducted in Australia also found that most speech-language pathology clients preferred in-person sessions instead of consultation using video or telephone (Filbay et al. 2021).

With high internet penetration in households in Hong Kong, connectivity did not appear to be an issue restricting telepractice for speech-language pathology students and most clients. Some of our speech-language pathology students, however, indicated some specific challenges associated with telepractice. For initial assessment, in view of issues with copyright and the adherence to test administration procedures, students could not make use of standardised assessment tools but had to rely on a restricted selection of criterion-referenced assessment tools and informal assessment approaches to evaluate a client's therapy needs and inform intervention planning. For therapy sessions, since students usually prepared presentation slide decks as treatment materials for a specific client ahead of the session, they found it difficult to amend such materials flexibly should new or changed needs be identified during the session.

Moreover, our teaching team also realised an unanticipated issue when speech-language pathology students were required to deliver telepractice from home. Hong Kong is a highly dense city. The sky-high housing prices have limited the average living space per person. As university-managed accommodations were unavailable to most postgraduate students at The Hong Kong Polytechnic University, most of our students live with their families. Those living in cramped apartments without their own private bedroom found it challenging, if not embarrassing, to play the role of a professional student clinician when delivering telepractice from home. Some students had to invest in a green screen and headsets with noise-cancelling microphone when on-campus clinic rooms became inaccessible during the pandemic.

## 12.5.2 Simulation

Simulation is generally referred to as "the artificial representation of a real-world process to achieve educational goals via experiential learning" (Flanagan et al. 2004, p. 57). Clinical simulation is regarded as supervised clinical practicum hours in accordance with the accreditation standards of postgraduate speech-language pathology programmes in the United States (Council on Academic Accreditation in Audiology and Speech-Language Pathology 2021), although there is an upper limit of 75 hours. However, prior to the COVID-19 pandemic, simulation had not been widely adopted in Hong Kong. Although local speech-language pathology educators navigated telepractice in early 2020, the uptake of therapy sessions was variable amongst adult and paediatric populations. The predominantly elderly adult clients with neurogenic communication disorders at the Speech Therapy Unit of The Hong Kong Polytechnic University appeared hesitant about receiving therapy through the internet. Suboptimal internet connectivity at home, worries about technical issues, and absence of carers with adequate technological literacy were common concerns preventing adult clients from joining therapy sessions through telepractice. A similar situation has been reported in Australia, with about half of speech-language pathologists reporting that more than 80% of their clients required assistance from carers during video consultations (Filbay et al. 2021).

With difficulty recruiting sufficient adult clients with neurogenic communication disorders for telepractice to provide students with clinical placements on aphasia, the idea of simulation quickly emerged in the teaching team. Several simulation modalities have been developed for healthcare education, including the use of part-task trainers, full-body mannequins, standardised patients, virtual cases, and immersive virtual reality. A study exploring the use of simulations in communication sciences and disorders programmes across the United States demonstrated that more than half of programmes reported the use of simulation for clinical education. The most common form of simulation was standardised patients followed by computer-based simulations (Dudding and Nottingham 2018). Positive results were also noted when standardised patients portraying aphasia were used to teach interpersonal and communication skills to speech-language pathology students almost 20 years ago (Zraick et al. 2003).

A standardised patient is defined as "a person simulates an actual patient in a realistic, standardised and repeatable way" (Council of Academic Programs in Communication Sciences and Disorders 2019, p. 7), whilst a simulated patient is "a person without a history or physical signs who is trained to portray a role and/or mimic particular physical signs for the purposes of teaching or assessment" (Hill et al. 2018, p. 6). After evaluating the time constraints associated with the preparation of students' clinical placements, our teaching team was aware of the impracticality of standardising the aphasia portrayal across multiple scenario presentations. It was, therefore, decided that simulation with simulated patients would be used in our aphasia clinical placement. The use of simulated patients was also justified by the nature of clinical teaching during that period. Speech-language pathology educators were providing ongoing feedback to students, and students' performance in simulation learning was not evaluated by summative assessment (Zraick 2020).

Quality simulation learning experiences should include three components, namely, pre-briefing, the simulation scenario, and debriefing (Council of Academic Programs in Communication Sciences and Disorders 2019). Details of the three components of our simulation learning programme are summarised in Table 12.2. One unique characteristic of our simulation learning programme was that we engaged speech-language pathology students, instead of actors or patients, to serve as simulated patients. The teaching team took this approach because previous studies using medical students as simulated patients had shown that the students' professional education meant that they could be more easily trained. Also, students could benefit from developing a better appreciation of the patient's perspective and could learn from the mistakes of their peers (Mavis et al. 2002; Burgess et al. 2013).

### 12.5.3 Modified pedagogy and service delivery

Speech-language pathology students of the 2.5-year Master of Speech Therapy programme at The Hong Kong Polytechnic University normally have two clinical placements on adult clients with neurogenic communication disorders during their second year of study. Clinical educators provide a moderate degree of supervisory support to students in the first adult placement, followed by a low degree of supervisory support to students in the second one. Normally, the 32-hour first adult placement is comprised of four hours of assessment and 28 hours of treatment, all to be delivered in-person. During the COVID-19 pandemic in 2020, telepractice became the primary mode of service delivery. In addition to mode of service delivery, our teaching team also adopted new pedagogies, such as simulation and active observation, to substitute part of the conventional clinical practicum. Table 12.3 illustrates the revised composition of clinical placement hours after incorporating various pedagogies.

**TABLE 12.2** Summary of components of a simulation learning programme for speech-language pathology students

| Component | Objective | Method |
|---|---|---|
| Pre-briefing | • To introduce the simulation programme together with the intended learning outcomes and the modus operandi. | • Clinical educators briefed students on the scenario and roles of students.<br>• Students were informed of the dual role (i.e., student clinician and simulated patient) to be played by each of them and the competency expectations.<br>• Students reviewed recorded therapy sessions with guidance and rehearsed scenario presentations with their peers; clinical educators provided feedback on the desired behaviours of the simulated patient.<br>• Students were encouraged to further practice and discuss with peers before the commencement of simulation. |
| Simulation | • To provide the context for the development of professional and occupational competencies. | • Students, when playing the role of student clinician, implemented therapy according to planned objectives and methods; clinical decision-making opportunities were available during simulation.<br>• Students, when playing the role of simulated patient, presented the scenario according to instructions communicated in pre-briefing. |
| Debriefing | • To evaluate and reflect on simulation from holistic viewpoints to foster more effective clinical practice in the future. | • Students evaluated the simulation session in terms of the characteristics of the simulated clients and therapy delivered, as well as the interaction style of student clinicians.<br>• Students received timely and specific feedback from clinical educators and peers on their performance as student clinicians and simulated patients.<br>• Students were encouraged to reflect on practice, identify knowledge gaps, and plan evidence-based practice. |

Active observation was incorporated into our clinical education, as purposeful observation is believed to stimulate deep learning in clinical education. Speech-language pathology students were given an observation guide, specifying the target (who/where); focus (what); nature (how); and purpose (why) of observation. Each of them was required to submit a structured reflective journal after active observation of telepractice therapy sessions. Students were instructed to reflect on the application of treatment approach, the respective role of student clinician

**TABLE 12.3** Composition of clinical placement hours after pedagogical change

| Type of speech-language pathology service | Range of practice area | Mode of clinical placement | Clinical placement hours |
|---|---|---|---|
| Assessment | • Language<br>• Speech | In-person | 4 |
| Treatment | • Language | In-person | 4 |
| | • Speech | Telepractice | 5 |
| | • Multi-modal communication | Telepractice (active observation) | 9 |
| | | Telepractice (simulation) | 6 |
| | | In-person (simulation) | 4 |
| **Total clinical placement hours** | | | **32** |

and active observer, the learning outcomes from telepractice, and gaps in learning areas for future observation. The web-based text mining tool, Voyant Tools (Sinclair and Rockwell 2016), was used to conduct textual analysis of reflective journals submitted by 36 speech-language pathology students. The reflective journals contained a total of 44,077 words, of which 3,671 are unique word forms. Figure 12.1 shows the word cloud created from the reflective journals with words sized and positioned. The ten most frequent words in the reflective journals were "client, " "treatment," "clinician," "cue," "session," "level," "semantic," "telepractice," "word," and "different," with frequencies ranging from 147 to 1,139. A collocates graph depicting a network of higher-frequency terms that appear in proximity is visualised in Figure 12.2. A strong connection existed not only between the keywords "client" and "clinician" but also amongst "clinician," "active," "observer," and "use."

## 12.6 Unprecedented challenges in clinical education

From ideology to practice, the COVID-19 pandemic has challenged the norm of clinical education in speech-language pathology. For instance, speech-language pathology educators in Hong Kong had never found the quest to acquire PPE such a daunting task prior to the pandemic. Whilst disposable face shields were procured for hospital placements, reusable face shields were also distributed to speech-language pathology students for clinical placements in non-medical settings when there was a critical supply issue of PPE. Students have been taught not only measures to optimise the use of face shields but also how to perform proper cleaning and disinfection of reusable face shields to minimise infection risk.

The COVID outbreak affected not only speech-language pathology education through changes in hospital placements and adjustments in PPE use. Practising speech-language pathologists in the community also faced considerable struggles.

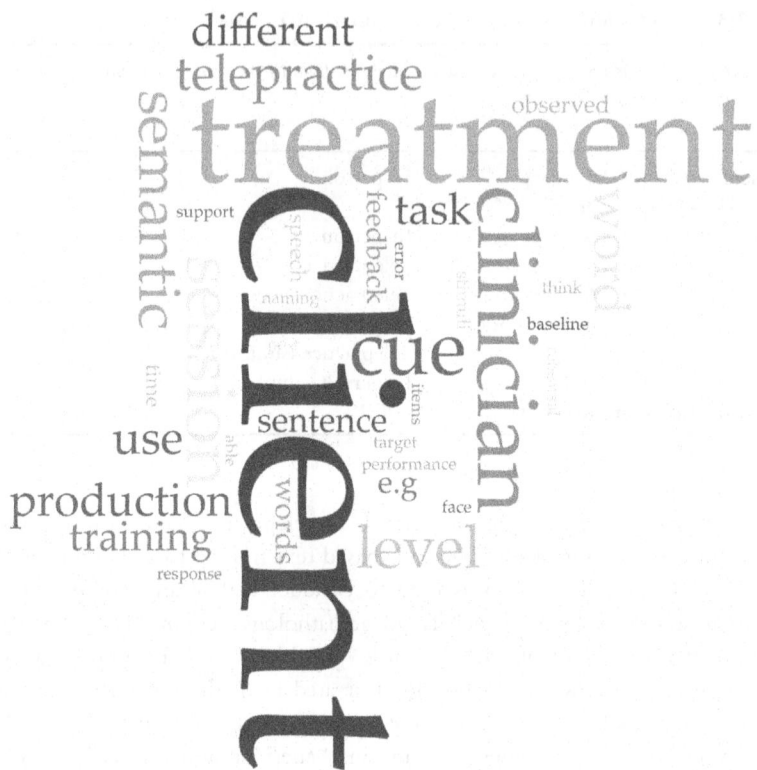

**FIGURE 12.1**  Word cloud showing the 35 most frequent words

In a study exploring the impact of COVID-19 on allied health professionals across practice settings, respondents from the audiology and speech therapy professions reported feeling more stressed than those working in social support services (Coto et al. 2020). The study did not identify explanatory factors for higher levels of perceived stress amongst audiology and speech therapy providers but mentioned that it might be related to inadequate guidance available for healthcare professionals who were not involved in the care of COVID-19 positive patients during the initial emergence of the pandemic.

Data from 302 American institutions offering communication sciences and disorders programmes in the 2019–2020 academic year showed that availability of placements, telepractice shift, and obtaining clinical hours were the top three challenges brought about by COVID-19 (Council of Academic Programs in Communication Sciences and Disorders and American Speech-Language-Hearing Association 2021a). In Hong Kong, a large proportion of speech-language pathologists work for social service organisations funded by the government. The government administers an output-based subvention system which demands

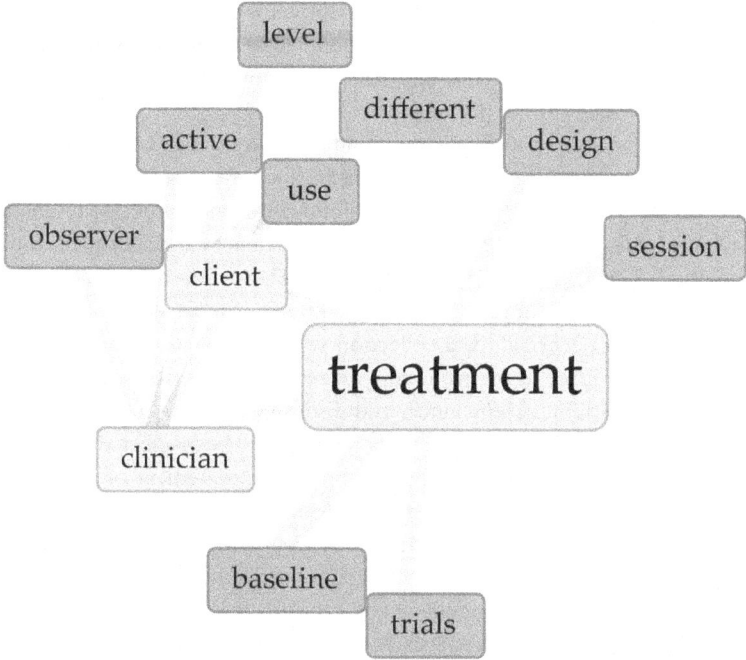

**FIGURE 12.2** Collocates graph with keywords shown in light grey and collocates shown in dark grey

regular reporting of Essential Service Requirements, Service Quality Standards, Output Standards and Outcome Standards, as well as an action plan on non-compliant areas to monitor service performance. The government has the power to withhold or terminate the subvention to social service organisations that fail to achieve a reasonable standard of performance.

When service suspension or restrictions were implemented in early 2020 by all early education and rehabilitative facilities in response to the government's infection control measures, provision of speech-language pathology services was reduced, and it became unavoidable that performance indicators of organisations would be adversely affected. Throughout 2020 to 2021, the government adopted a risk-based approach when it came to decisions about service suspension and resumption for subsidised social services. During periods when service provision was possible, speech-language pathologists at social service organisations prioritised delivering clinical services to clients over offering clinical placements to students. The same situation obtained in schools, with school-based speech-language pathologists maximising the time they offered therapy to children because of limited school hours. Whilst the shift of focus of practitioners might be understandable and legitimate, it was a severe blow to speech-language pathology education. The Hong Kong Polytechnic University, for example, was only able to secure 46% of off-campus clinical placements for a cohort of 37 speech-language pathology students in September 2020. With a severe shortage of off-campus clinical placements, university educators had no choice but to arrange more on-campus clinical placements.

Whilst clinical education challenges were commonly experienced, communication sciences and disorders departments across institutions also reported challenges in course delivery, research, student support, administration, and work-life balance (Council of Academic Programs in Communication Sciences and Disorders and American Speech-Language-Hearing Association 2021a). For course delivery, university educators had to move to online teaching in a short period of time. As far as research was concerned, data collection was reported as the most common challenge. The impact of the pandemic on research activities undoubtedly extended beyond communication sciences and disorders. In fact, 80% of higher education institutions worldwide reported that research had been affected in terms of cancellation of international travel, cancellation or postponement of scientific conferences, and delayed completion of projects (Marinoni et al. 2020).

It should be emphasised that the COVID-19 pandemic has also had an adverse impact on speech-language pathology students. Some students experienced social isolation, and extra support for students' mental health was also identified as a challenge in communication sciences and disorders departments. Non-local students, such as those from Mainland China and Macao, were particularly affected. For instance, students from Guangzhou and Macao normally spend their weekends in their home cities as those cities are located within the "one-hour living circle." The COVID-19 pandemic removed opportunities for weekly family visits since individuals in Hong Kong had to comply with the quarantine requirements of respective cities.

Some communication sciences and disorders departments in the United States also reported budgetary issues and decreased enrolment. Some 42% of programmes experienced insufficient clinical placements to achieve adequate enrolment on entry-level master's programmes for the 2019–2020 academic year (Council of Academic Programs in Communication Sciences and Disorders and American Speech-Language-Hearing Association 2021b). The entry-level master's programme at The Hong Kong Polytechnic University, by contrast, received an increased number of applications during the admissions exercise in 2020.

An American survey also found that speech-language pathology educators experienced challenges in caring for self or dependents, managing heightened workloads, and adapting to disrupted work routines (Council of Academic Programs in Communication Sciences and Disorders and American Speech-Language-Hearing Association 2021b). With speech-language pathology a predominantly female profession and women in Hong Kong primarily responsible for family caregiving and children's education, the productivity of female university educators appeared to be disproportionately affected by the work-from-home policy during the pandemic. Many local female academics had to struggle with maintaining boundaries between workplace and home. The constraints faced by female parents got worse during school closures in Hong Kong. A local academic described her routine as "teaching assistant at a primary school in the morning and academic at a university in the afternoon and evening" (Jung et al. 2021, p. 114).

## 12.7 Implications for capacity building in clinical education

The profound effects of COVID-19 may change how future speech-language pathology students are educated. COVID-19 appeared to be a catalyst for technological advancement in university teaching and learning, as well as telepractice and simulation in clinical education. The transition of clinical teaching and learning accelerated by COVID-19, though seemingly intimidating, gave the global community of speech-language pathology educators an opportunity to go through a steep learning curve by trial and error. This has had benefits and drawbacks. Telepractice may improve access to and cost-effectiveness of healthcare. Yet technological infrastructure issues and personal data protection concerns should be adequately addressed for sustainable development of this service delivery mode.

For instance, the Health Insurance Portability and Accountability Act (HIPAA) was enacted in 1996 in the United States, and national standards for protecting health information have subsequently been established. The HIPAA specifically protects individually identifiable health information in electronic form. Practitioners are responsible for compliance with regulations on privacy and security, including information storage and transmission, even as this applies to telepractice. To date, many jurisdictions including Hong Kong do not have specific legislation regulating telepractice in healthcare. Whilst the Medical Council of Hong Kong published ethical guidelines on telemedicine for physicians (The Medical Council of Hong Kong 2019), specific standards and practice details are lacking. If telepractice is to be developed as a routine service delivery mode beyond the pandemic, a unified legislation framework governing telepractice in all healthcare services would be necessary. With the advent of 5G and high penetration of smart phones in Hong Kong, older adults who have relocated to Mainland China for retirement might be able to take the advantage of telepractice for cross-border healthcare in the future (Huang et al. 2021). In fact, a survey conducted during the COVID-19 pandemic revealed that more than 60% of adults aged 55 years or above expressed willingness to try online medical consultations provided that relevant technology is well developed (Lingnan University 2020). Transforming clinical education to cater for the evolving demands of the community will be the responsibility of speech-language pathology educators going forward.

The rapid transition of clinical teaching and learning that has occurred during the COVID-19 pandemic brings renewed focus on educational scholarship. In professional practice, speech-language pathology clinicians are committed to evidence-based practice. But do speech–language pathology educators conduct evidence-based teaching? To ensure quality education and training for future speech–language pathologists, the pedagogical characteristics of simulation and active observation, as well as quality assurance of adopting alternative assessments in lieu of proctored examinations should be fully explored. Proposed changes to course delivery should be scrutinised in terms of intended learning outcomes, syllabuses, teaching and learning methodologies, assessment methods in alignment with learning outcomes, and student study effort expected. Globally, most higher education institutions are largely supported by government funding and graduates from speech–language pathology education programmes are expected to deliver high-quality clinical services to the public. Speech–language pathology educators should therefore be prudent in delivering pedagogically sound teaching instead of following popularised or customary practices. In addition to encouraging more scholarly research in speech–language pathology education, universities should devote more resources to fostering collaborative educational scholarship amongst speech–language pathology clinicians who offer off-campus clinical placements to students.

The provision of speech–language pathology education is uniquely challenging as there is a need for authentic client experiences in different clinical settings. However, the shortage of clinical placements for nursing and allied health students was a global problem even before the COVID-19 pandemic (Taylor et al. 2017). The Royal College of Speech and Language Therapists in the United Kingdom has published new guidance on practice-based learning to address the shortage of placements for speech–language pathology students and to project a culture of ownership to clinical education (Royal College of Speech and Language Therapists 2021). The professional body explicitly recommends all practising speech–language pathologists across the country, irrespective of setting or banding, share the responsibility of supporting clinical education by offering a minimum of 25 days of practice-based learning per year. It is further suggested that peer placements should be arranged where possible, and off-campus educators should attend educator training regularly. Indeed, it is only with dedicated speech–language pathology educators within and beyond universities that the global profession of speech–language pathology can thrive.

## 12.8 Summary

At the time of writing, Hong Kong is facing a substantial risk of another major outbreak in the pandemic with the emergence of the Omicron variant of SARS-CoV-2. The Hong Kong government has once again announced enhanced social distancing measures to curtail the spread of this variant. COVID-19 is neither the first nor the last infectious disease outbreak to disrupt clinical education. The shift in clinical teaching and learning that the pandemic has brought about has been radical, but the forward-thinking spirit of global educators shall prevail.

This chapter has highlighted the consequences of COVID-19 for speech-language pathology education, from the adoption of new pedagogies such as telepractice and simulation to issues of capacity building in clinical education and a much-needed increased focus on educational scholarship. The lessons that have been learnt from the pandemic can motivate the global community of educators to reflect on the future training needs of speech-language pathologists. This will undoubtedly better prepare speech-language pathologists for the pandemics that they will inevitably face.

## References

Burgess, A., Clark, T., Chapman, R., & Mellis, C. (2013). Medical student experience as simulated patients in the OSCE. *The Clinical Teacher*, 10(4), 246–250.

Canadian Alliance of Audiologists and Speech-Language Pathologists Regulators (2021). Academic equivalency framework. https://caaspr.ca/sites/default/files/2021-07/slp_aef_final_oct_18_2019copyright.pdf. Accessed 7 January 2022.

Chandrasiri, N. R., & Weerakoon, B. S. (2021). Online learning during the COVID-19 pandemic: Perceptions of allied health sciences undergraduates. *Radiography*. https://doi.org/10.1016/j.radi.2021.11.008.

Coto, J., Restrepo, A., Cejas, I., & Prentiss, S. (2020). The impact of COVID-19 on allied health professions. *PloS One*, 15(10), e0241328. doi:10.1371/journal.pone.0241328.

Council of Academic Programs in Communication Sciences and Disorders and American Speech-Language-Hearing Association (2021a). Communication sciences and disorders (CSD) education survey. Ad hoc report: COVID-19 impact on academic programs. www.asha.org/siteassets/uploadedfiles/academic/ad-hoc-report-covid-19-ay-2019-2020.pdf. Accessed 7 January 2022.

Council of Academic Programs in Communication Sciences and Disorders and American Speech-Language-Hearing Association (2021b). Communication sciences and disorders (CSD) education survey. National aggregate data report. 2019–2020 academic year. www.asha.org/siteassets/uploadedfiles/csd-education-survey-national-aggregate-data-report.pdf. Accessed 7 January 2022.

Council on Academic Accreditation in Audiology and Speech-Language Pathology (2020). Standards for accreditation. https://caa.asha.org/reporting/standards/. Accessed 7 January 2022.

Council on Academic Accreditation in Audiology and Speech-Language Pathology (2021). Coronavirus/COVID-19. https://caa.asha.org/about/coronavirus-covid-19/. Accessed 7 January 2022.

Council of Academic Programs in Communication Sciences and Disorders (2019). Best practices in healthcare simulations: Communication sciences and disorders. https://growthzonesitesprod.azureedge.net/wp-content/uploads/sites/1023/2020/03/Best-Practices-in-CSD.pdf. Accessed 7 January 2022.

Dost, S., Hossain, A., Shehab, M., Abdelwahed, A., & Al-Nusair, L. (2020). Perceptions of medical students towards online teaching during the COVID-19 pandemic: A national cross-sectional survey of 2721 UK medical students. *BMJ Open*, 10, e042378. doi:10.1136/bmjopen-2020-042378.

Dudding, C. C., & Nottingham, E. E. (2018). A national survey of simulation use in university programs in communication sciences and disorders. *American Journal of Speech-Language Pathology*, 27(1), 71–81.

Filbay, S., Hinman, R., Lawford, B., Fry, R., & Bennell, K. (2021). Telehealth by allied health practitioners during the COVID-19 pandemic: An Australian wide survey of clinicians and clients. The University of Melbourne, Australia. https://ahpa.com.au/wp-content/uploads/2021/04/Telehealth-by-allied-health-practitioners-during-the-COVID-19-pandemic.pdf. Accessed 7 January 2022.

Flanagan, B., Nestel, D., & Joseph, M. (2004). Making patient safety the focus: Crisis resource management in the undergraduate curriculum. *Medical Education*, 38(1), 56–66.

Fong, R., Tsai, C. F., & Yiu, O. Y. (2021). The implementation of telepractice in speech language pathology in Hong Kong during the COVID-19 pandemic. *Telemedicine and e-Health*, 27(1), 30–38.

Food and Health Bureau (2020). Preparedness and response plan for novel infectious disease of public health significance. www.chp.gov.hk/files/pdf/govt_preparedness_and_response_plan_for_novel_infectious_disease_of_public_health_significance_eng.pdf. Accessed 7 January 2022.

Gill, D., Whitehead, C., & Wondimagegn, D. (2020). Challenges to medical education at a time of physical distancing. *The Lancet*, 396(10244), 77–79.

Han, A. (2020). PolyU lab prints 3D face shields for medical staff. *South China Morning Post*, 25 February 2020, p. A3.

Health & Care Professions Council (2017). Standards of education and training. www.hcpc-uk.org/globalassets/resources/standards/standards-of-education-and-training.pdf?v=637660865080000000. Accessed 7 January 2022.

Hill, A. E., Ward, E., Davidson, B., McCabe, P., Purcell, A., Heard, R., McAllister, S., Hewat, S., Walters, J., Cardell, E., Howells, S., Davenport, R., Baldac, S., Penman, A., Caird, E., & Aldridge, D. (2018). *Embedding simulation in clinical training in speech pathology*. Melbourne: Speech Pathology Australia. www.speechpathologyaustralia.org.au/SPAweb/Resources_For_Speech_Pathologists/Clinical_Education/Simulation-based_Learning_Program/SPAweb/Resources_for_Speech_Pathologists/Simulation-based_Learning_Program/Simulation-based_Learning_Program.aspx?hkey=c76641bc-4318-431a-9f5e-a870af826a5a. Accessed 7 January 2022.

Hong Kong Institute of Speech Therapists (2017). Supplementary document of Competency-Based Occupational Standards (CBOS) for speech therapists in Hong Kong. www.hkist.org.hk/static/13_HKIST-A-COS-v1.pdf. Accessed 7 January 2022.

Hong Kong Institute of Speech Therapists (2019). Institutional-based assessment for speech therapy education programmes in Hong Kong. https://hkist.org.hk/static/17_HKIST-A-IBA-v1.pdf. Accessed 7 January 2022.

Hospital Authority (2021). Quality and safety annual report 2020. www.ha.org.hk/haho/ho/psrm/E_AnnualReport2020.pdf. Accessed 7 January 2022.

Huang, G., Ma, Y., & Peng, Z. (2021). Cross-border medical services for Hong Kong's older adults in Mainland China: The implications of COVID-19 for the future of telemedicine. *Journal of Aging & Social Policy*, 33(4–5), 509–521.

Jung, J., Horta, H., & Postiglione, G. A. (2021). Living in uncertainty: The COVID-19 pandemic and higher education in Hong Kong. *Studies in Higher Education*, 46(1), 107–120.

Lam, J. H. Y., Lam, T. S., Wong, C. H., Lam, W. H., Leung, C. M. E., Au, K. W. A., Lam, C. K. Y., Lau, T. W. W., Chan, Y. W. D., Wong, K. H., & Chuang, S. K. (2020). The epidemiology of COVID-19 cases and the successful containment strategy in Hong Kong-January to May 2020. *International Journal of Infectious Diseases*, 98, 51–58.

Lam, J. H. Y., Lee, S. M. K., & Tong, X. (2021). Parents' and students' perceptions of telepractice services for speech-language therapy during the COVID-19 pandemic: Survey study. *JMIR Pediatrics and Parenting*, 4(1).

Lau, J. T. F., Fung, K. S., Wong, T. W., Kim, J. H., Wong, E., Chung, S., Ho, D., Chan, L. Y., Lui, S. F., & Cheng, A. (2004). SARS transmission among hospital workers in Hong Kong. *Emerging Infectious Diseases*, 10(2), 280–286.

Lee, S. H. (2003). The SARS epidemic in Hong Kong: What lessons have we learned? *Journal of the Royal Society of Medicine*, 96, 374–378.

Lingnan University (2020). Survey finds over 60% senior citizens are willing to try online medical consultations. www.ln.edu.hk/news/20200629/survey-finds-over-60-senior-citizens-are-willing-to-try-online-medical-consultations/. Accessed 7 January 2022.

Liu, Y., Gu, Z., & Liu, J. (2021). Uncovering transmission patterns of COVID-19 outbreaks: A region-wide comprehensive retrospective study in Hong Kong. *EClinicalMedicine*, 36, 100929. https://doi.org/10.1016/j.eclinm.2021.100929.

Marinoni, G., Van't Land, H., & Jensen, T. (2020). The impact of COVID-19 on higher education around the world: IAU global survey report. www.iau-aiu.net/IMG/pdf/iau_covid19_and_he_survey_report_final_may_2020.pdf. Accessed 7 January 2022.

Mavis, B. E., Ogle, K. S., Lovell, K. L., & Madden, L. M. (2002). Medical students as standardized patients to assess interviewing skills for pain evaluation. *Medical Education*, 36(2), 135–140.

The Medical Council of Hong Kong (2019). Ethical guidelines on practice of telemedicine. www.mchk.org.hk/files/PDF_File_Ethical_Guidelines_on_Telemedicine.pdf. Accessed 7 January 2022.

National Health Service (2020). Allied health professions student support guidance during COVID-19 outbreak. www.hee.nhs.uk/sites/default/files/documents/AHP%20student%20support%20guide%20Covid-19.pdf. Accessed 7 January 2022.

Ng, J. H.-Y., Wong, C. C.-Y., Ng, C. W.-Y., & Lau, D. K,-Y. (2021). *Training the next generation speech therapists during the COVID-19 time [video file]*. Excellent Teachers on Teaching Excellence Symposium 2021. Hong Kong: The Hong Kong Polytechnic University. www.youtube.com/watch?v=8MF3FZmBQYs. Accessed 7 January 2022.

Patil, N. G., & Yan, Y. C. H. (2003). SARS and its effect on medical education in Hong Kong. *Medical Education*, 37(12), 1127–1128.

Petersen, E., Koopmans, M., Go, U., Hamer, D. H., Petrosillo, N., Castelli, F., Storgaard, M., Al Khalili, S., & Simonsen, L. (2020). Comparing SARS-CoV-2 with SARS-CoV and influenza pandemics. *The Lancet Infectious Diseases*, 20(9), e238–e244. https://doi.org/10.1016/S1473-3099(20)30484-9.

Rieder, M. J., Salvadori, M., Bannister, S., & Kenyon, C. (2004). Collateral damage: The effect of SARS on medical education. *The Clinical Teacher*, 1(2), 85–89.

Royal College of Speech and Language Therapists (2021). Practice-based learning guidance. www.rcslt.org/members/lifelong-learning/practice-based-learning/. Accessed 7 January 2022.

Seto, W., Tsang, D., Yung, R., Ching, T., Ng, T., Ho, M., Ho, L., & Peiris, J. (2003). Effectiveness of precautions against droplets and contact in prevention of nosocomial transmission of severe acute respiratory syndrome (SARS). *The Lancet*, 361(9368), 1519–1520. doi:10.1016/s0140-6736(03)13168-6.

Sinclair, S., & Rockwell, G. (2016). Voyant tools. http://voyant-tools.org/. Accessed 4 January 2022.

Speech Pathology Australia (2017). Competency-based occupational standards for speech pathologists: Entry level. www.speechpathologyaustralia.org.au/SPAweb/SPAweb/Resources_for_Speech_Pathologists/CBOS/CBOS.aspx. Accessed 7 January 2022.

Speech Pathology Australia (2019). Accreditation of speech pathology degree programs. www.speechpathologyaustralia.org.au/SPAweb/Resources_for_the_Public/University_Programs/Accreditation_Process/SPAweb/Resources_for_the_Public/University_Programs/Process.aspx?hkey=0917ee72-6b04-4479-9f51-7c7b89926539. Accessed 7 January 2022.

Taylor, C., Angel, L., Nyanga, L., & Dickson, C. (2017). The process and challenges of obtaining and sustaining clinical placements for nursing and allied health students. *Journal of Clinical Nursing*, 26(19–20), 3099–3110.

Tsang, T., & Lam, T. (2003). SARS: Public health measures in Hong Kong. *Respirology*, 8, S46–S48.

United Nations Educational Scientific and Cultural Organization (2021). One year into COVID-19 education disruption: Where do we stand? https://en.unesco.org/news/one-year-covid-19-education-disruption-where-do-we-stand. Accessed 7 January 2022.

Wong, T.-W., & Tam, W. W.-S. (2005). Handwashing practice and the use of personal protective equipment among medical students after the SARS epidemic in Hong Kong. *American Journal of Infection Control*, 33(10), 580–586.

World Health Organization (2006). *SARS: How a global epidemic was stopped*. Western Pacific Region, World Health Organization. https://apps.who.int/iris/bitstream/handle/10665/207501/9290612134_eng.pdf?sequence=1&isAllowed=y. Accessed 7 January 2022.

World Health Organization (2020a). Rational use of personal protective equipment for coronavirus disease 2019 (COVID-19): Interim guidance, 27 February 2020. https://apps.who.int/iris/handle/10665/331215. Accessed 7 January 2022.

World Health Organization (2020b). WHO Director-General's statement on IHR Emergency Committee on novel coronavirus (2019-nCoV). www.who.int/director-general/speeches/detail/who-director-general-s-statement-on-ihr-emergency-committee-on-novel-coronavirus. Accessed 7 January 2022.

World Health Organization (2021). Listings of WHO's response to COVID-19 (updated 29 January 2021). www.who.int/news/item/29-06-2020-covidtimeline. Accessed 7 January 2022.

Zraick, R. I. (2020). Standardized patients in communication sciences and disorders: Past, present and future directions. *Teaching and Learning in Communication Sciences & Disorders*, 4(3), Article 4. https://doi.org/10.30707/TLCSD4.3/KHSI3441.

Zraick, R. I., Allen, R. M., & Johnson, S. B. (2003). The use of standardized patients to teach and test interpersonal and communication skills with students in speech-language pathology. *Advances in Health Sciences Education*, 8(3), 237–248.

# 13

# CASE STUDIES OF ADULTS WITH COVID-19 INFECTION

*Louise Cummings*

Against the backdrop of large infection rates and deaths during the COVID-19 pandemic, it is easy to lose sight of the fact that it is individuals who have been most impacted by the SARS-CoV-2 virus. This chapter focuses on four such individuals. They are all women who developed COVID-19 during the first wave of the pandemic in the UK. Each has gone on to develop Long COVID. However, this is where the similarity between them ends. Three speak English as a first language. The fourth woman is a native speaker of Romanian and has a good level of English proficiency. All but one woman enjoyed good health prior to her COVID illness. Although all four women have Long COVID, only three of them report cognitive-linguistic difficulties as part of their illness. The variation between these cases is a salient reminder that COVID-19 affects people from all linguistic, social, and health backgrounds. The language profiles of these women are examined alongside the onset and development of their COVID illnesses.

---

### Case Study 1    48-year-old voice artist

#### Background

Amy (not her real name) is 48;5 years old. She is married and has two children, a son aged 15 years and a daughter aged 17 years. Amy is university educated. In 1995, she obtained a BA degree in journalism and media communications. Amy has had a portfolio career in media, wellness, and business since 2013. She is currently a professional voice artist and a skincare and beauty trainer for a company in the UK and

---

DOI: 10.4324/9781003257318-13

Ireland. She is also a part-time business coordinator for a structural engineering company. Amy has previously worked as a commercial model, a stage and TV presenter, and an actor. Prior to 2013, she worked as a radio news announcer (1993–1995) and a PR communications coordinator (1996–1999). Between 1999 and 2013, Amy volunteered as a women's pastor and provided resources to women working in prostitution. She was also a case worker with the Snowdrop Project, which helps women rescued from human trafficking. In terms of interests and hobbies, Amy describes herself as an artist and painter and a writer and blogger (e.g., she has written audio plays). She also voices fan fiction audio drama characters.

Prior to contracting COVID-19, Amy describes her overall state of health as "okay," although she has struggled with histamine intolerance and imbalanced hormones. In 1977, she had foot surgery to remove extra cartilage. In 2012, Amy had LASIK eye surgery. She had breast implants in 2014. In October 2019, Amy had a thyroid function test and was found to have subclinical (borderline) hypothyroidism. She started to take an iodine supplement. By the end of 2019, her thyroid function was back to normal and has remained normal in several subsequent tests. Amy had an abnormal smear test followed by several biopsies 18 months prior to her participation in the author's COVID language study. She recently underwent a loop procedure to treat abnormal cervical cells. Amy has had imbalanced hormones since 2012 and is working with a specialist GP on bioidentical hormones.

Amy has a well-balanced diet despite having numerous food sensitivities. Her sensitivities to certain foods have heightened significantly since becoming infected with COVID-19 in March 2020. She is sensitive to wheat (and gluten), eggs, soy, nuts, and dairy. Amy is on a strict low-histamine and low-inflammatory diet and is working with a health coach in a trial programme through Mount Sinai Hospital in New York. She avoids caffeine. Amy takes vitamin and mineral supplements including methyl B complex, vitamin C, zinc, and multiminerals. She also takes low-histamine probiotics and 1,500 mg of cannabidiol (CBD) oil twice a day. She does not smoke or vape. Amy stopped drinking alcohol three years ago because of alcohol intolerance related to the perimenopause. Even when she did consume alcohol, she had less than one drink a fortnight. Amy is 5 feet and 7 inches in height and weighs 58 kg, giving her a BMI of 19.9 (normal weight). Since her eye surgery in 2012, she has had 20/20 vision for distance but uses reading glasses. Her hearing is normal.

Amy first developed symptoms of COVID-19 on 13 March 2020. She had a low-grade fever. Her 15-year-old son developed aches, fatigue, and slight chest pain three days earlier. Amy's husband and daughter also became unwell. Amy thinks her son contracted the virus at the orthodontist's office a week before he developed symptoms. She made nine attempts to get her family tested for the virus but was unsuccessful as there was no access to these tests at the start of the pandemic in the UK. Amy remained at home during her illness. She had one visit from paramedics and made telephone calls to the non-emergency 111 service and her GP. Amy had one medical examination during her first eight weeks of illness. She took several medications to treat the symptoms of COVID-19 (see *Medication*).

Amy describes her recovery from COVID-19 as "slow and non-linear." She had a productive cough for 8–10 weeks. She reports that her lungs have continued to feel as if she is breathing through a straw. Amy has had several medical investigations following her illness. In July 2020, she had a chest X-ray, but nothing abnormal was detected. Amy was examined by an ENT specialist on 13 July 2020. Fibreoptic laryngoscopy revealed some evidence of mild reflux. Vocal cord movements were symmetrical and there was no evidence of malignancy. Amy was referred to Speech and Language Therapy. On 22 September 2020, she had CT pulmonary angiography. On 24 September, Amy had a pulmonary function test. She had an abnormal ECG at the end of September. These pulmonary and cardiac investigations revealed some heart inflammation but no lung damage due to COVID-19. However, a 24-hour ECG conducted on 14 October and an ECG conducted on 25 November were both normal. Amy had a range of blood tests (e.g., thyroid function, inflammation markers) in July, September, and October 2020, all of which produced normal results.

## Clinical symptoms

Amy experienced a wide range of symptoms during acute COVID illness. Several symptoms have persisted to the present day. She had moderate to severe breathing difficulties. They started on day 9 of her illness and caused asthma-like issues even though she has never had asthma. Amy is still having breathing difficulties. Her mild to moderate symptoms included fever, coughing, fatigue, aches and pains, headache, chest pain, and laryngitis. Amy had a low-grade fever on days 9 to 14 of her illness. On day 21, she developed a chest infection for which she took antibiotics. Her fever increased at this stage and remained high between days 21 to 25. Amy developed mild to moderate coughing in the second week of her illness. She experienced aches for the first two weeks of her illness. Some 12 weeks later, she then had aches in her muscles, hands, and feet. She took electrolytes for several weeks which helped her. Amy has had headaches, sometimes migraines, on an almost daily basis. She has experienced fluctuating mild to moderate chest pain. Recent investigations are linking this to heart inflammation rather than to lung damage. Amy had mild to moderate laryngitis for 11 weeks. She has a "raspy" voice, especially with exertion.

Amy has also had several mild symptoms during her COVID-19 illness. At around 12 weeks, she developed a rash on one of her feet after using hair dye. She had never had a reaction like this in the past. She had a sore throat which she attributes to coughing. She also had a 2-week period of cramps and diarrhea. Amy reports mostly mild fatigue that has extended beyond the acute phase of her illness. She needs to take naps every afternoon to function and must go to bed by 9:30 p.m.

Amy believes that COVID-19 has had an impact on her mental health. She reports that this "chronic, mystery illness has been a challenge for me and my family." Amy's son has had four relapses in his recovery, all seemingly triggered by strenuous physical education or athletics, and missed 16 days of school. This has been a source of stress to her. She has had to give up most of her voice over work and describes this as a huge loss to her. In July 2020, Amy started to receive counselling twice a month. This has been "incredibly helpful" to her as she comes to terms with the impact of COVID-19 on her and her family's health and livelihood.

### Daily activities

Amy's daily activities have been affected by COVID-19. Prior to her illness, she worked 35–40 hours a week. She was also a speaker at wellness conferences which required her to travel about once a month. For the first three months of her illness, Amy could not work at all as she was experiencing coughing, fatigue, and problems with breathing. Until the fifth month of her illness, she was only able to work about 10 hours a week. She can now work for about 15 hours a week but must take a nap every afternoon. Amy is spending a lot more time at home with her husband and two teenage children since contracting COVID-19. Before March 2020, she engaged in regular exercise. Amy did kickboxing once a week for fitness and high-intensity interval training once or twice a week. She also did some yoga. Currently, she is not able to undertake exercise.

It is also difficult for Amy to undertake household chores. She describes how her heart and lungs "flare up" when she unloads a full dishwasher or takes laundry in a basket downstairs. She can walk for no more than 5 minutes or climb two flights of stairs without the exertion affecting her lungs, creating chest pain, and leaving her severely out of breath. Amy tries to pace herself and schedules rest into her day. She plans her activities carefully, doing one thing a day like work or health appointments. Although Amy's social activities have changed since March 2020, she is still very connected to her friends. She used to meet female friends for coffee or brunch and male friends for coffee. Since March, she has had a few socially distanced meetings with a small group of women in her garden. Amy has a large social network of friends in the US – she is a dual British American national – and is very active on Instagram, Twitter, and LinkedIn. She has also blogged about her experience of COVID-19 and has talked about her recovery from the virus to the media.

### Medication

Amy took prescribed medications before her COVID-19 infection. They included bioidentical hormone replacement therapy: biestrogen 0.5 mg, testosterone 1.25 mg and DHEA 2.5 mg in 0.5 ml (1 pump daily in the morning with Sundays off), and progesterone 50 mg in 0.5 ml (one pump twice daily). Amy was prescribed several medications for the treatment of her COVID-19 symptoms. Around day 23 of her illness, she started taking the corticosteroid Prednisone when she developed a chest infection. Amy has taken 1 puff of Fostair (100/6 micrograms per actuation) morning and night since September 2020. Between April and July 2020, she used an Albuterol inhaler (as needed and once in morning and afternoon) and a steroid inhaler, Clenil Modulite 100 micrograms per actuation (once morning and evening). For migraines, Amy takes Sumatriptin 50 mg as needed (also taken pre-COVID).

## Communication

Amy has not noticed any significant change in cognition or language following COVID-19. She reports sometimes forgetting what she had gone into another room to pick up or the names of characters from movies, but she believes she was experiencing these problems a bit before her illness due to the perimenopause. She does not report any difficulty remembering what others have just said to her in conversation or the topic of a conversation. She can follow what others are saying in conversation and has no difficulty following the plot in a story or a film. Her ability to read and write has been unaffected by COVID-19. Amy had laryngitis for 11 weeks and still has a fluctuating "raspy" voice. As a professional voice artist, she has been trying to protect her voice as much as possible. She still displays a strong desire to communicate with others and does so multiple times every day.

For her voice problems, Amy has so far received two one-hour sessions of speech and language therapy. During the first session, Amy completed a detailed questionnaire with the therapist. Her responses were used to exclude acid reflux, identified through fiberoptic laryngoscopy, as a cause of her vocal problems. Amy had coughed persistently between March and July 2020 to clear debris from her lungs, and it was felt that this was a more significant cause of her vocal difficulties. Amy practiced voice techniques with the therapist, several of which caused chest pain and were not further pursued. The yawn-sigh technique, however, was helpful and is used by Amy before events where she must talk for long periods of time (e.g., Zoom meetings). Amy has observed a pattern in her vocal problems. Her voice will be normal for a few days, with her problems emerging again after physical exertion.

The author spoke to Amy online on 21 October 2020. It was 11:00 a.m. in the UK. The 12 language tasks described in chapter 5 were conducted during a 50-minute interaction. Amy's scores on these tasks are shown in Table 13.1. Also shown are the means and standard deviations (SD) for healthy participants and COVID (experimental) participants with cognitive-linguistic issues in the study. The reader is referred to Table 13.2 in the Appendix for age, gender, and educational profiles of participants in all comparison groups.

Amy was assessed 7 months and 8 days after the onset of her COVID illness. Despite not reporting cognitive-linguistic difficulties, she fell below the mean performance of healthy participants in eight of 12 tasks. This may simply reflect her pre-morbid cognitive-linguistic performance and is not necessarily indicative

**TABLE 13.1** Amy's raw scores on tasks in the study

| Task | Amy's scores[§] | Healthy participants Mean (SD) | COVID participants Mean (SD) |
|---|---|---|---|
| Sam and Fred (immediate recall) | 8.5/14 | 9.7 (±1.9) | 7.7 (±2.0) |
| Sam and Fred (delayed recall) | 6.5/14 | 9.3 (±2.0) | 6.5 (±2.2) |
| Cookie Theft picture description | 9.5/12 | 7.7 (±1.2) | 6.9 (±1.4) |
| Sentence generation | 5/6 | 5.2 (±0.8) | 5.0 (±1.0) |
| Letter fluency (F-A-S) | 60 | 48.0 (±10.8) | 37.0 (±11.5) |
| Category fluency (animals) | 19 | 25.8 (±4.7) | 21.7 (±6.6) |
| Category fluency (vegetables) | 23 | 15.3 (±3.7) | 15.1 (±4.4) |
| Flowerpot Incident narration | 8.5/20 | 13.8 (±2.9) | 12.3 (±2.7) |
| Cinderella narration | 29/50 | 32.0 (±5.7) | 26.9 (±7.0) |
| Procedural discourse (sandwich) | 5/8 | 6.6 (±0.9) | 6.4 (±0.9) |
| Procedural discourse (letter) | 7/8 | 6.5 (±1.4) | 6.2 (±1.3) |
| Confrontation naming | 17/20 | 17.6 (±2.0) | 17.7 (±1.8) |

[§] Figures are raw scores

of any impairment. Amy's performances on delayed recall, category fluency for animals, Flowerpot Incident narration, and sandwich-making discourse were greater than 1 standard deviation below the mean of healthy participants. In the four tasks where Amy performed above the mean of healthy participants, her Cookie Theft picture description and letter fluency performances were greater than 1 standard deviation above the mean and her category fluency for vegetables was greater than 2 standard deviations above the mean.

What is interesting is that whilst Amy's scores fell for the most part below the mean scores of healthy participants, she displayed better performance relative to people who reported cognitive-linguistic difficulties (so-called "brain fog") since their COVID illness. On six of 12 tasks, Amy exceeded the mean performance of these COVID participants. Amy registered particularly strong performances relative to COVID participants in letter fluency (2 standard deviations above COVID mean), Cookie Theft picture description, and category fluency for vegetables (both between 1 and 2 standard deviations above the COVID mean). On a further three tasks, her performance was the same as the mean scores of COVID participants. In only three tasks – category fluency for animals, Flowerpot narration, and sandwich-making procedural discourse – did Amy's scores fall below the mean scores of COVID participants. Her score for animal fluency fell within 1 standard deviation of the mean score of COVID participants, whilst her scores for Flowerpot narration and sandwich-making discourse were between 1 and 2 standard deviations below the mean. This level of performance relative to COVID participants in the study is consistent with Amy's self-report that her cognitive-linguistic functioning had not been negatively impacted by her COVID infection.

## Case Study 2   52-year-old occupational health physician

### Background

Pauline (not her real name) is 52;11 years old. She is divorced and has no children. Pauline has 18 years of formal education. She has pursued a career in medicine, obtaining her medical degree (MBChB Medicine) in 1990. In 1994, Pauline became a member of the Royal College of General Practitioners in the UK. She became a member of the Faculty of Occupational Medicine in 2002. Currently, Pauline is a trainer of communication skills to medical students, doctors, scientists, and allied health professionals. She was a Consultant in Occupational Medicine in one of her earlier roles.

Prior to contracting COVID-19, Pauline had several health difficulties. She has hypermobile Ehlers-Danlos syndrome (EDS). This is a genetic condition that causes joint problems, colitis, and other gastrointestinal disorders, bladder, autonomic nervous system, skin, and immune problems. EDS has made Pauline prone to serious bacterial infections (she is described as having "immune dysfunction"). She has had many episodes of bacterial sinusitis and multiple chest infections since she was 13 years of age. Between 1998 and 2009, Pauline received immunoglobulin treatment to prevent infections. On six occasions between 1990 and 2013, Pauline required surgery for infections in her nasal sinuses. Between December 2019 and March 2020, she received intravenous antibiotics to treat a heart and spine infection. Pauline has experienced recurrent sepsis. In 2012, she developed a spinal infection that resulted in sepsis and encephalopathy. She had to stop working at this point. In 2012, Pauline was diagnosed with dyspraxia. This is developmental in nature. Her neck is also unstable due to infection and EDS.

Pauline has a normal body weight for her age, height, and gender. She does not smoke or vape and has one glass of white wine (125ml) every two weeks. Before her spinal cord/spine problems, Pauline used to be very active. She did three hours of pilates every week. She describes her diet as "pretty well balanced," although she thinks she could probably eat less chocolate. Because of malabsorption related to EDS, Pauline is prescribed a range of vitamin and mineral supplements. She takes vitamin D (60,000 units/week); vitamin C (1 g twice a day); vitamin B complex (1 g once a day); magnesium (magnaspartate) (243 mg twice a day); and omega 3 (twice a day). She also takes probiotics. Pauline is allergic to the iodine contrast that is used in certain X-rays but has no food allergies. Her vision is near-normal in one eye while the other eye is very long-sighted. She has high-frequency hearing loss in both ears. Also, her left eardrum does not work well because of damage sustained in a past infection.

Pauline has a wide range of friends whom she met on a regular basis before the national lockdown in the UK. Many of her social activities were through church activities and exercise classes. Since formally retiring in 2012 on grounds of ill health, Pauline believes she has been able to achieve a healthy work-life balance. She has undertaken small amounts of work and pursued hobbies while managing her health limitations. Pauline is active on Facebook and has recently started campaigning for people with Long COVID along with other illness groups. She has several interests, including painting and drawing, playing the piano, music, and going to art galleries and the theatre.

Pauline first experienced symptoms of COVID-19 on 18 March 2020. Her nose was congested, and she had a "strange" dry, parched throat which was not sore. She was tested late for the virus on 5 May, 22 May, and 5 June 2020, all of which returned negative results. Pauline thinks she may have been exposed to the virus either at work – "*loads of people were ignoring guidance and coming to work with fevers, cough and sore throat*" – or through nurses who were administering intravenous antibiotics to her daily for the treatment of a spinal infection. However, she cannot be sure how she contracted the virus because although many of her nurses had coughs, they treated her before 5 March 2020, which was too early for the onset of her symptoms on 18 March 2020.

Pauline received some medical support during her acute COVID illness. On day 10 of her illness, she was admitted to Accident & Emergency with severe diarrhoea, vomiting and a high fever. From day 11 onwards, she was under the supervision of her usual bowel disease specialist team and GP. During her acute illness, Pauline took paracetamol and antibiotics. She developed bacterial sinusitis in the first 10 days of her illness and took Co-amoxiclav 625 mg three times daily for a week. Since her acute phase of illness, Pauline has had several medical investigations. She had two chest X-rays on 29 March 2020 and in early September. Nothing abnormal was detected on both occasions. In September 2020, she had a cardiac MRI, which added no new findings beyond the aneurysm of the left coronary artery detected in 2018 and the sinus of Valsalva aneurysm detected in 2015. On 9 August 2020, Pauline had an echocardiogram, which revealed a new tricuspid valve regurgitation. She continues to experience low oxygen saturation on exertion. Between March and May 2020, Pauline had appointments with her inflammatory bowel disease team for COVID colitis. In July 2020, she had a further routine review. Pauline's colitis is a severe systemic inflammatory response to infection, according to her Consultant Gastroenterologist.

### Clinical symptoms

Pauline experienced a wide range of symptoms during acute COVID illness. Five symptoms were severe: loss of taste and smell; gastrointestinal problems; aches and pains; headache; chest pain or pressure. Before contracting COVID, Pauline had an inflammatory bowel condition related to EDS. She developed severe colitis during COVID-19 infection. Between days 10–20 of her illness, she experienced severe aches and pains, leading her to beat her legs to get rid of it. Pauline had migraine-like headaches. These were worst on day 10 but also occurred in episodes later in her illness. Pauline had retrosternal chest pain briefly on day 10 and then severely from 4–6 months on exertion. She had moderate fever and moderate breathing difficulties. Pauline's breathing difficulties were most noticeable around 4 months onwards when she had more exertion, as she was too ill earlier in her illness to move much.

Pauline also had five mild symptoms: coughing, fatigue, sore throat, conjunctivitis, and skin rash. Her coughing was very mild and intermittent. Pauline experienced fatigue. In the first eight weeks of her illness, she described this as sleepiness rather than fatigue. Pauline still has a sore throat. She had conjunctivitis which became intermittent later in her illness. Pauline experienced a skin rash of varied appearance several months into her illness. She also had a hoarse voice.

Pre-COVID, Pauline had cognitive problems related to an episode of sepsis in 2012. She had short-term memory difficulties and struggled with organisation and planning. Remembering conversations, faces and names was difficult for her. Pauline could not manage a diary or write an invoice correctly. Her sense of direction was poor, a problem related to her dyspraxia. Pauline's cognitive difficulties have changed, and some have worsened since contracting COVID-19. Before her illness, Pauline struggled to remember the content of conversation but could at least remember that a conversation had taken place. Since her

COVID illness, she has no recollection of conversations even having taken place. She has noticed that her friends are commenting on this lapse of memory more often now. With flare-ups of her COVID symptoms, she can feel quite "woolly" as she weighs up what she should be doing. She feels "inanimate" and can sit rooted to the spot for hours even though she is not drowsy. Pauline finds it immensely difficult to start doing anything. This is not related to low mood and is out of character for her as she is usually good at prioritising and initiating things. It is noteworthy that since completing intravenous antibiotics for a bacterial infection in March 2020, two of Pauline's close friends had independently remarked that the cognitive difficulties she experienced pre-COVID had lessened. She was better able to complete sentences, was less confused, and was more alert than she had normally been.

Pauline believes her acute COVID illness and the restrictions used to control the virus have had a detrimental impact on her mental health. She describes being "very confused" in the first three weeks of her illness and states that she was "not fully with it" for eight weeks. She was able to cope with the 3-month national lockdown because she was so unwell. She also did painting, which kept her "sane and happy" despite being ill. However, in the last 3–4 months, she has felt angry and irritable which is out of character for her. This is because she feels lonely, cooped up, and does not agree with the COVID restrictions that have been put in place.

Pauline describes her recovery from COVID-19 as a pattern of episodic recovery and relapse following a 3-month period in which she was very ill. She is generally slightly better after each relapse. In her last major relapse in June 2020, she was very unwell again, with low blood pressure, "weird behaviour," and confusion for days. She then felt much better but thinks her white cell count must have dropped as she developed an infection of the chest and sinuses with Pseudomonas, a bacterium that affects people with immune suppression. Since October 2020, Pauline has experienced normal energy and most of her symptoms have gone. However, she still has severe chest pain, breathlessness, and low oxygen saturation, all on exertion. She reports that "something is definitely not right."

### Daily activities

Pauline's COVID illness and its consequences have compromised her daily activities. Because of lockdown, she has not been able to work.

But if circumstances had been normal, she would not have been able to do any work for 4 months on account of her illness. There has been a significant impact of her illness on her ability to engage in social and leisure activities. Pauline has been unable to see her family. She was initially housebound with a spinal infection and was then infectious with COVID and too unwell to visit relatives. Pauline cannot undertake household chores. Until recently, she needed carers four times a day as she has been too ill to cook and care for herself.

### Medication

Because of her pre-existing health problems, Pauline takes a wide range of prescribed medications. For the treatment of hypotension, she has been prescribed fludrocortisone (200 mg). For her colitis, she takes Asacol MR (1.6g three times daily) and Salofalk enema (2 g at night). Pauline takes several medications to maintain chest health. For the treatment of bronchiectasis, she uses nebulised hypertonic saline 6% once in the morning. Pauline takes Mucodyne (375 mg twice a day) to manage mucus in her respiratory tract. Occasionally, she uses a Ventolin inhaler. To manage bladder and gut problems (mast cell activation disorder/histamine intolerance), Pauline takes loratidine (10 mg twice a day), famotidine (20 mg at night), ketotifen (2 mg at night), and sodium chromoglycate (200 mg three times daily). She also uses rotating antibiotics. Pauline has been prescribed the anti-depressant sertraline (100 mg at night). For pain relief, she takes pre-gabalin (75 mg reducing to 50 mg twice a day); amitriptyline (25 mg at night); and paracetamol (1 g twice a day). Skin problems on her hands and feet are treated with Diprobase cream, Cetraben ointment and Tracolimus ointment. Pauline uses Dermol lotion to wash her skin.

### Communication

Pauline reports that COVID-19 has exacerbated some cognitive dif-ficulties that she developed following an episode of sepsis in 2012 and created some additional cognitive problems. She struggles to find words that she wants during conversation. She reports that she can-not remember the names of things and people such as the names of her friends' husbands. She also cannot remember what others have just said in conversation and the topic of conversation although both skills were already somewhat affected pre-COVID. Pauline can also have difficulty following what others are saying in conversation, especially if the interaction is formal and new information is being conveyed. However, she can manage to follow informal conversation. Pauline's ability to read and write was already affected by sepsis. However, her reading is now "even worse," and she cannot concentrate on either reading or writing. She cannot follow a plot in a story or film, although this was also an area of some difficulty pre-COVID.

Pauline has retained a strong desire to communicate with others. She is "always happy to talk." Pauline's illness and lockdown have reduced the frequency of her communication with others. She reported that after the first 3–4 months, she had almost forgotten how to speak. It was not until she started speaking with others again that she realised just how poor her language skills had become. She would stop speaking and swap syllables and words around. She could not pronounce certain words at all.

The author spoke to Pauline online on 26 October 2020. The session took place at 10:00 a.m. UK time and lasted 50 minutes. Pauline spoke at length about her COVID illness. She completed the 12 language tasks in the study. Her scores on these tasks are shown in Table 13.3, alongside means and standard deviations (SD) for healthy participants and COVID control participants in the study.

Pauline was assessed 7 months and 8 days after the onset of her COVID illness. She reported a deterioration of pre-existing cognitive difficulties following her COVID infection. This was reflected in her test performance. Pauline fell below the mean of healthy participants in 9 of 12 tasks. She was greater than 2 standard deviations below the mean on immediate recall, letter fluency, and category fluency for animals, and greater than 1 standard deviation below the mean on delayed recall and Cinderella narration. Pauline's category fluency for vegetables, Flowerpot Incident narration, and sandwich-making and letter writing discourses were all within 1 standard deviation below the mean. In the three tasks with best performance – Cookie Theft picture description, sentence generation, and confrontation naming – she returned performances that were just above the mean of healthy participants.

A similar pattern of performance was also recorded relative to COVID controls who did not report cognitive-linguistic difficulties following their COVID illness. Pauline performed below the mean of COVID controls on 8 of 12 tasks. An area of considerable difficulty was immediate recall, which fell between 3 and 4 standard deviations below the mean of these controls. Pauline's letter and category fluency for animals fell between 1 and 2 standard deviations below the mean

**TABLE 13.3** Pauline's raw scores on tasks in the study

| Task | Pauline's scores[§] | Healthy participants Mean (SD) | COVID controls Mean (SD) |
|---|---|---|---|
| Sam and Fred (immediate recall) | 5.5/14 | 9.7 (±1.9) | 10.4 (±1.5) |
| Sam and Fred (delayed recall) | 6/14 | 9.3 (±2.0) | 9.7 (±1.9) |
| Cookie Theft picture description | 8/12 | 7.7 (±1.2) | 7.7 (±0.9) |
| Sentence generation | 6/6 | 5.2 (±0.8) | 5.4 (±0.8) |
| Letter fluency (F-A-S) | 25 | 48.0 (±10.8) | 53.2 (±14.4) |
| Category fluency (animals) | 14 | 25.8 (±4.7) | 23.4 (±6.6) |
| Category fluency (vegetables) | 13 | 15.3 (±3.7) | 17.1 (±3.4) |
| Flowerpot Incident narration | 13/20 | 13.8 (±2.9) | 12.8 (±2.9) |
| Cinderella narration | 25/50 | 32.0 (±5.7) | 31.8 (±5.1) |
| Procedural discourse (sandwich) | 6/8 | 6.6 (±0.9) | 6.8 (±0.9) |
| Procedural discourse (letter) | 6/8 | 6.5 (±1.4) | 7.2 (±1.4) |
| Confrontation naming | 19/20 | 17.6 (±2.0) | 18.2 (±1.3) |

[§] Figures are raw scores

of COVID controls, a better performance than that observed relative to healthy participants. This pattern of cognitive performance below the mean of both healthy participants and COVID controls – with marked difficulties in immediate recall, letter fluency, and category fluency for animals – is consistent with Pauline's reports of a further deterioration in her cognitive functioning post-COVID.

A question of some interest is whether Pauline's COVID illness had caused new cognitive difficulties or had exacerbated her pre-existing cognitive problems. Pauline's immediate recall, letter fluency, and category fluency for animals were particularly weak areas of performance. The performance of COVID participants in the study was significantly weaker than healthy participants on all three of these tests, amongst others (see chapter 5). But whilst these difficulties had a COVID-related onset for the other COVID participants in the study, for Pauline they appeared to involve a worsening of her pre-existing difficulties. On 13 February 2015, Pauline underwent a neuropsychological assessment. This assessment, which took place after her earlier health problems, revealed significant impairments in areas of attention and memory. Although Pauline's immediate recall of story material was better than some other aspects of memory, her score was in the low average range. However, Pauline's performance on immediate recall of story material following COVID infection was lower still, with her score between 2 and 3 standard deviations below the mean of healthy participants. This suggested that, rather than giving rise to new cognitive difficulties, her COVID illness had caused some further deterioration of her cognitive abilities.

## Case Study 3   48-year-old medical practice manager

### Background

Angela (not her real name) is 48;7 years old. She is married and has two daughters aged 18 and 19 years. Both daughters are currently at university. Angela has been the manager of her husband's private medical practice since 2007. She has 18 years of formal education. In 1994, Angela graduated with a Master of General Arts. In 1998, she obtained a Montessori Diploma. Between 1998 and 2004, Angela worked as an Early Years teacher. Angela enjoys walking, reading, cooking, and travelling. She also likes going to the theatre and visiting art galleries. She describes herself as very sociable. When asked about her work-life balance, she reported having "more life than work." Angela is active on social media, using Facebook and Instagram to keep in touch with others.

Before contracting COVID-19, Angela enjoyed "very good" health. She is 5 feet and 10 inches in height and weighs 10 stone and 11 lbs, giving her a BMI of 21.7 (normal weight). She attended the gym three to four times per week where she lifted free weights and did cardiovascular exercise. Angela also walked for an hour every day with her dog. She described herself as being the fittest she has ever been. Angela has never smoked or vaped. She has one to two drinks (gin and wine) most evenings. Angela has had two surgeries to date, one in 2003 to remove a varicose vein and a tonsillectomy in 2007. She has asthma and was diagnosed with trigeminal neuralgia in 2016. Angela takes daily vitamin B12 (5,000 mg) and prescribed medications (see *Medication*). She has no allergies to food or medication and eats a well-balanced, mainly vegetarian diet, consisting of large amounts of fruit and vegetables. Angela does not eat junk food or takeaways but thinks that she could reduce her sugar intake as she "loves a chocolate biscuit." She has normal hearing, but her vision is myopic.

Angela remained at home throughout her COVID illness. Her first symptom was a slightly raised temperature of 37.8 degrees on 13 March 2020. This was followed by a cough on 15 March. After nine days of illness, Angela had a "major crash" and became bedbound. She developed breathing complications and silent hypoxia. Her $O_2$ saturation level was 93%, and her peak flow measurement was 300 litres per minute. An ambulance was sent to deliver oxygen to her at home. She opted to remain at home as her husband is a doctor and the local hospital was full. She was so unwell that she has no memory of a full week during this time. Because Angela contracted the virus prior to widespread testing in the UK, she did not receive a PCR swab for COVID-19. She believes she contracted the virus through her work as a medical practice manager. Her husband runs an acute gynaecology unit at a major teaching hospital and was treating emergency patients with no COVID screening and very little personal protective equipment. Most of his unit was infected with the virus. Some of his colleagues tested positive on PCR swabs that were performed at the hospital.

Angela had three phone calls with her GP during her acute COVID illness. On 27 August 2020, she had a chest X-ray and nothing abnormal was detected. Blood tests for rheumatoid factors, c-reactive protein, urea and electrolytes, clotting factors, white cell counts, and D-dimers were conducted on 7 September and produced negative results. Thirteen days after she first became unwell, Angela took two three-day courses of azithromycin (500 mg per day for 3 days) for secondary pleurisy. Her regular asthma medication (see *Medication*) had to be increased. Angela received five sessions of physiotherapy for tendonitis and sore joints that she developed during her acute illness.

When asked to reflect on her recovery from COVID-19 to date, Angela reported that she is about 90% recovered on a good day. However, sometimes she is "back to square one" and is so poorly that she must go to bed.

### Clinical symptoms

Angela has had a wide range of COVID symptoms. During her acute illness, she had severe breathing difficulties. Her oxygen saturation level dropped to 93% and her peak flow measurement was low. She experienced severe chest pain: "It felt like I had hit a steering wheel in a car crash." Angela has had severe fatigue which continues unabated. She describes herself as exhausted. Several of Angela's symptoms were moderate in nature, including coughing, loss of taste and smell, aches and pains, and headache. Angela's cough started lightly and then deteriorated. It lasted for 16 weeks in total. After 3 weeks of illness, Angela experienced a loss of taste and smell. She had rheumatic pains in her wrists and ankles and Achilles tendonitis. She also had a "crushing" headache behind her eyes. Angela's mild symptoms included a slight fever, with her temperature recorded at 37.8 degrees. She also had mild gastrointestinal problems, an upset stomach, for a few days. Angela experienced restless legs as she was beginning to recover.

Angela reports cognitive difficulties following her illness. She is very forgetful. She forgets to undertake day-to-day tasks. Errands are only half completed, and things that she has told others she would do are left undone. Angela has difficulty planning and organising her day. Because of limited energy, a lack of motivation and forgetfulness, she is never quite sure that she will be able to complete all her tasks in a day. In terms of the impact of COVID-19 on her mental health, Angela reports that she was "quite traumatised" by not being able to breathe.

## Daily activities

Angela reports a significant impact of COVID-19 on her daily activities. Her ability to undertake work duties has been compromised by "brain fog." She reports that this feels as if there are "blank spots" in her brain and that she must search for memories and information that she knows she has. She is forgetful and is easily distracted. Angela was physically very active before her illness and undertook some form of exercise every day. Since her illness, she has been unable to exercise. Although Angela can undertake household chores, she must do so more slowly than before her illness. She now finds large social gatherings intimidating because she does not have the energy and motivation to interact with others.

## Medication

Angela uses Nabiximols (trade name Sativex), an oromucosal spray, three times daily for pain management. For the treatment of asthma, Angela takes one puff twice daily of Symbicort Turboinhaler 200/6 inhalation powder.

## Communication

Angela has noticed some changes in her language and communication skills following her COVID illness. She reports that she "definitely needs to reach for names in her memory and trips up with words." She does not think that she processes things well. She finds that her mind is inclined to wander during conversations. This affects her ability to remember the topic of a conversation and to follow what others are saying in conversation. She can still follow the plot in a story or film. Angela's writing has been unaffected by her illness but her reading concentration is much shorter. Her desire to participate in conversation depends on how fatigued she is feeling. She reports a reduction in the frequency with which she communicates with others: "I am definitely less social than I was."

The author spoke to Angela online on 3 December 2020. It was 11:00 a.m. in the UK. The meeting lasted one hour. Angela spoke at length about the impact of COVID on her health and on her family. Her scores on the 12 language tasks in the study are shown in Table 13.4, alongside means and standard deviations (SD) for healthy participants and COVID control participants in the study.

Angela was assessed 8 months and 21 days after the onset of her COVID illness. Although she reported cognitive-linguistic difficulties following her COVID infection, her performance relative to healthy participants was above average in 9 of 12 tasks. Her category fluency performance was particularly exceptional, with the generation of animal names between 1 and 2 standard deviations above the mean and the generation of vegetable names over 3 standard deviations above the mean. But against this strong category fluency performance, there was very poor verbal recall. Angela's immediate and delayed recall were between 2 and 3 standard deviations below the mean. Her performance on Cookie Theft picture description was equally poor, with Angela's score again between 2 and 3 standard deviations below the mean of healthy participants.

Relative to COVID controls with no self-reported cognitive difficulties, Angela's performance on immediate recall and Cookie Theft picture description was poorer still. She performed between 3 and 4 standard deviations below the mean on immediate recall and her picture description was 3 standard deviations below the mean. Her category fluency performance remained equally exceptional relative to COVID controls.

Angela's self-reported cognitive-linguistic difficulties following COVID infection appear to be confirmed by her poor immediate and delayed recall of verbal material and reduced ability to be informative during picture description. She displayed above average performance relative to healthy participants and COVID controls with no self-reported cognitive-linguistic deficits in other areas. However, it is worth remarking that even this above average performance may be reduced relative to her pre-morbid cognitive-linguistic performance.

**TABLE 13.4**  Angela's raw scores on tasks in the study

| Task | Angela's scores[§] | Healthy participants Mean (SD) | COVID controls Mean (SD) |
|---|---|---|---|
| Sam and Fred (immediate recall) | 5/14 | 9.7 (±1.9) | 10.4 (±1.5) |
| Sam and Fred (delayed recall) | 5/14 | 9.3 (±2.0) | 9.7 (±1.9) |
| Cookie Theft picture description | 5/12 | 7.7 (±1.2) | 7.7 (±0.9) |
| Sentence generation | 6/6 | 5.2 (±0.8) | 5.4 (±0.8) |
| Letter fluency (F-A-S) | 58 | 48.0 (±10.8) | 53.2 (±14.4) |
| Category fluency (animals) | 33 | 25.8 (±4.7) | 23.4 (±6.6) |
| Category fluency (vegetables) | 28 | 15.3 (±3.7) | 17.1 (±3.4) |
| Flowerpot Incident narration | 16/20 | 13.8 (±2.9) | 12.8 (±2.9) |
| Cinderella narration | 33.5/50 | 32.0 (±5.7) | 31.8 (±5.1) |
| Procedural discourse (sandwich) | 7/8 | 6.6 (±0.9) | 6.8 (±0.9) |
| Procedural discourse (letter) | 7/8 | 6.5 (±1.4) | 7.2 (±1.4) |
| Confrontation naming | 18/20 | 17.6 (±2.0) | 18.2 (±1.3) |

[§] Figures are raw scores

## Case Study 4    31-year-old former college employee

### Background

Susie (not her real name) is 31;11 years old. She is single and has no children. Susie has 16 years of formal education. In 2008, she graduated from the Facultatea de Stiinte Economice Juridice si Administrative at the University of Pitesti in Romania. She studied hair art design at Blondi Hair Design Academy Wella in Bucharest between July and December 2010 and worked In several hair salons in Romania between 2008 and 2014. Susie moved from Romania to Sweden in March 2014 and lived there until June 2018. While in Sweden, she worked as a runner, bartender, and staff manager in different clubs in Stockholm. She also did freelance work with fashion TV and other companies, was a chef's assistant, and worked as a game master at Quest Room in Stockholm. Susie had an internship at Baggpipe Creative Collective in Sweden between 2015 and 2017. She was a marketing assistant between April 2017 and June 2018, a role in which she promoted artists and worked as a talent scout.

Susie moved to the UK in June 2018. She was a general assistant at University College London between August 2018 and February 2019. She then worked for nearly two years as an assistant manager/barista at Baxterstorey at Central Saint Martins, University of the Arts London. Susie attended the Oakley Academy in London in June 2019 to undertake training in hair extensions. She has not worked since February 2020 when University of the Arts London closed due to the pandemic. Susie then lost her job in October 2020 as part of COVID-related redundancies. Susie is a native Romanian speaker. She also speaks English and Spanish fluently as second languages. Susie started to learn English at school in Romania when she was seven years old.

Susie enjoyed "very good" health prior to September 2019, when she developed a severe ear infection. She was off work for 2 months and had to take four courses of antibiotics, none of which treated her infection. During this time, she experienced fatigue, anxiety, and vertigo. In February 2020, she was prescribed two further antibiotics and a steroid spray for her ears. She was admitted to hospital in the same month with pneumonia. Susie was prescribed another course of antibiotics, which successfully treated her chest infection. A short time later, her COVID symptoms started.

Susie reported no chronic health problems prior to contracting COVID-19. She is 168 cm in height and weighs 69 kg, giving her a BMI of 24.4 (normal weight). Susie stopped smoking three years ago and does not drink alcohol. In 2016, she had an appendectomy. In the same year, she also had a miscarriage. Susie is taking prescribed medication for anxiety and irritable bowel syndrome (see *Medication*). She has no food allergies but is allergic to Stemetil, which she was prescribed by an emergency room doctor for sickness and dizziness. On 26 September 2020, Susie was admitted to hospital following an oculogyric crisis related to the taking of two 5 mg Stemetil tablets. On the way to hospital in the ambulance, she began to choke due to inflammation of her throat and severe jaw clenching. Susie does not currently take vitamins and minerals, although she has taken zinc, folic acid, and oregano oil in the recent past. She reports impaired hearing and vision. Susie experiences tinnitus and has days when her hearing is poor. She has not had an audiological assessment. She describes her vision as "blurry" and reports oculomotor problems.

Susie first developed symptoms of COVID-19 in the middle of February 2020. She was talking to a friend on the telephone one evening when she suddenly became dizzy and had "a weird feeling in [her] body different from anxiety." She became pale, could no longer talk, and thought she would pass out. She recovered after two hours. The following morning, Susie woke up, went into the kitchen, and started talking to her housemates. She suddenly experienced a sharp pain in her chest and could not breathe. She described how the pain was like a sharp knife moving very quickly all over her chest. She could no longer talk and retired to her room to lie down. Susie reported then feeling as if something was moving close to her. She took it in her hands and looked at it, but it was simply her phone. When she returned to normal again, she looked at her phone and it was midnight. Susie describes herself as having lost consciousness during this time. She called the hospital and was given advice. Susie did not want to go to hospital as she was afraid of being intubated. She was continuously short of breath over the following days. She was also powerless, had muscle pains and spasms, nausea, and diarrhea, and experienced a loss of taste and smell, headaches, dizziness, and hearing loss.

During her acute COVID illness, Susie received no medical supervision. Her only medical monitoring during her recovery has been through her participation in the COVERSCAN study, a joint research initiative of Perspectum, Oxford University Hospitals NHS Trust and the Mayo Clinic. This study is mapping how COVID-19 is affecting the health of multiple organs (lungs, heart, kidney, liver, pancreas, and spleen). On 10 September 2020, Susie had a scan of her liver and heart. Her liver was healthy with a fat content of 4.3% (normal). Her cardiac scan showed normal left ventricular pumping function and no evidence of inflammation. Her blood pressure, body mass index, oxygen saturation, and blood investigations were also normal. Susie was not tested for the virus at the start of the pandemic in the UK as tests were in scarce supply but was given a clinical diagnosis of COVID-19 infection. After her acute illness, Susie received seven swab tests for the virus and an antibody test, all of which produced negative results. She cannot be certain how she contracted the virus. Her symptoms emerged one week after she was sent home from work on account of pneumonia, so her workplace is a possible setting in which exposure occurred. However, she also lives with eleven other people. After her first week of symptoms, she discovered that one of her housemates had been in bed unwell for a week. Susie does not know anyone who had a positive COVID-19 test result. When asked to describe her recovery from COVID-19 to date, she replied that she has "not recovered."

### Clinical symptoms

Susie has had a wide range of COVID symptoms. Her most severe symptoms included a loss of taste and smell (anosmia), breathing difficulties, gastrointestinal problems, fatigue, aches and pains, and chest pain/pressure. Apart from anosmia, Susie is still experiencing each of these symptoms. She had chest pain and pressure every day for the first four months of her illness. She has a relapse of this symptom every couple of weeks. Susie also had moderate fever, sore throat, and headache. Other moderate symptoms included ear pain, muscle spasms, and unusual sensations. These sensations were dizziness, strange perception of colours, and popping sounds from her nose. The dizziness Susie experienced was quite unlike the dizziness that you might experience if you get out of bed quickly. Despite drinking three litres of water every day, Susie was constantly thirsty, and her lips and skin were unusually dry. Susie also had mild coughing and skin rashes on her hands as part of her COVID illness. Other symptoms included kidney pain, heartburn, hair loss, and fluctuating low and high temperatures. Susie is also experiencing sleeplessness. She reported that on two occasions, she slept for 22 hours and 27 hours continuously, presumably due to extreme fatigue related to insomnia.

Susie reports cognitive problems following her COVID illness. She thinks that 80% of her ability to remember things has been affected by her illness. She must write things down or she will forget them. Susie describes how she cannot remember words in English and the other languages that she knows. Some of her memory lapses are potentially dangerous (e.g., leaving the door of the gas cooker open). She reports that her ability to plan and organise her day has also been compromised by as much as 80%. She postpones a lot of plans, sometimes even taking a bath to avoid doing them. Every time she plans to do something, she feels weak and powerless. Susie's anxiety has not increased during her illness apart from three or four "anxiety crises" when she was in great pain.

### Daily activities

COVID-19 has had a significant negative impact on Susie's daily activities. Before her illness, Susie occasionally went to the gym and did swimming. She also walked 2–4 km every day. She has been unable to undertake any exercise since her illness. Every time she tries to exercise, she experiences a relapse in her COVID symptoms. Susie had a well-balanced diet before her illness. Her diet has been adversely affected as her reduced energy has left her unable to cook meals for herself. She often does not have an appetite for food as well. Her reduced energy has left her unable to meet friends socially. Before her COVID illness, Susie enjoyed crafting and painting, but she has also been unable to pursue these hobbies in recent months. Susie participates in online COVID groups where she shares her symptoms with others. But beyond this, she makes limited use of social media as she is trying to relax.

When asked about the impact of her illness on her ability to perform tasks and undertake duties, Susie chose to quantify her difficulties. Her COVID illness has adversely affected 90% of her ability to perform work duties, 90% of her ability to pursue social and leisure activities, and 90% of her ability to undertake household chores.

## Medication

During her COVID illness, Susie used a Salbutamol 20 ug inhaler. She has been prescribed Citalopram 10 mg once daily for anxiety and takes Buscopan for the treatment of irritable bowel syndrome. Susie takes paracetamol 500 mg four times daily for relief of her COVID symptoms.

## Communication

Susie reports some cognitive and language disturbances following COVID-19. She forgets the names of people she has known for a long time as well as new names. Susie cannot remember what others have just said in conversation. By way of example, she recounted how a doctor gave her an address to remember, then asked her for her name, and finally asked her to recall the address. She could only recall one part of the address. When she starts to talk about something, she tends to lose what she wanted to say. She does not always understand what others are saying in conversation. This did not happen to her pre-COVID. Although she can still read and write, she struggles to remember what she has read after a few seconds. She cannot follow a plot in a film or story. Her desire to participate in conversation with others is reduced because of limited energy. She is communicating with other people with reduced frequency.

The author spoke to Susie online on 9 November 2020. It was 11:00 a.m. in the UK. The conversation lasted 1 hour and 10 minutes, during which time Susie described the significant impact of Long COVID on her daily life. Susie's performance on the language tasks described in chapter 5 is shown in Table 13.5, alongside means and standard deviations (SD) for the healthy L2 English speakers in the study.

Susie was assessed approximately 9 months after the onset of her COVID illness. Her self-reported cognitive-linguistic difficulties following her COVID illness are consistent with a pattern of poor performance in all areas. Susie performed below the mean of healthy L2 English speakers on all 12 tasks used in the study. Her strongest performances were in procedural discourse and confrontation naming, where her scores fell within 1 standard deviation below the mean scores of healthy L2 English speakers. Susie's category fluency for animals and vegetables and her immediate recall of the Sam and Fred story were between 1 and 2 standard deviations below the mean for healthy participants. Susie was not able to attempt delayed recall of the story. Sentence generation and letter fluency were between 2 and 3 standard deviations below the mean scores of healthy participants.

It is interesting that Susie's worst performances were recorded in the discourse production tasks in the study. Her scores for informativeness on these tasks ranged from between 3 and 4 standard deviations below the mean (Flowerpot Incident and Cinderella) to between 4 and 5 standard deviations below the mean (Cookie Theft). Reduced discourse informativeness was a consistent feature of the COVID participants in the study who spoke English as a first language but not COVID participants who spoke English as a second language (see chapter 5). Susie's profile

**TABLE 13.5** Susie's scores on the tasks in the study

| Task | Susie's scores[§] | Healthy L2 English speakers Mean (SD) |
|---|---|---|
| Sam and Fred (immediate recall) | 5.5/14 | 8.6 (±1.9) |
| Sam and Fred (delayed recall) | 0/14 | 8.4 (±1.8) |
| Cookie Theft picture description | 2/12 | 6.6 (±1.1) |
| Sentence generation | 2/6 | 4.6 (±1.1) |
| Letter fluency (F-A-S) | 14 | 37.0 (±10.3) |
| Category fluency (animals) | 10 | 18.6 (±4.6) |
| Category fluency (vegetables) | 5 | 10.4 (±3.2) |
| Flowerpot Incident narration | 6/20 | 12.4 (±1.7) |
| Cinderella narration | 14/50 | 34.2 (±5.9) |
| Procedural discourse (sandwich) | 4/8 | 4.6 (±0.9) |
| Procedural discourse (letter) | 5/8 | 6.1 (±1.4) |
| Confrontation naming | 12/20 | 13.1 (±4.0) |

[§] Figures are raw scores

of reduced informativeness across discourse production tasks sets her apart from other L2 English speakers with COVID. One possible explanation of this difference is that other L2 speakers of English with COVID were further into their recovery at the point of testing than Susie was – Susie was tested at 268 days (or 9 months) after the onset of her symptoms whilst the average time between symptom onset and testing for L2 English speakers with COVID was 385 days (or 13 months). Whatever ultimately explains Susie's worse discourse performance relative to other L2 English speakers with COVID, her marked difficulties in this area are indicative of the extent of her cognitive debilitation some 9 months after the onset of her COVID illness.

# APPENDIX

**TABLE 13.2** Characteristics of study participants

| Study group | N | Age (mean) | Age (range) | Gender (M/F) | Education (years) |
|---|---|---|---|---|---|
| **COVID experimental participants** | 69 | 49.1 years | 24.0–64.3 years | 5 M/64 F | 29 under 17 years<br>40 over 17 years |
| **COVID control participants** | 11 | 46.5 years | 30.9–60.6 years | 3 M/8 F | 4 under 17 years<br>7 over 17 years |
| **Healthy participants** | 26 | 48.2 years | 18.1–64.6 years | 10 M/16 F | 7 under 17 years<br>19 over 17 years |
| **L2 English control participants**[1] | 13 | 38.3 years | 18.3–60.8 years | 3 M/10 F | 1 under 17 years<br>12 over 17 years |

[1] First languages of participants: Mandarin Chinese; Cantonese Chinese; French; Spanish; Dutch

# INDEX